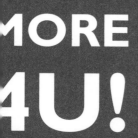

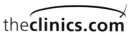

the**clinics**.com

BURTON P. DRAYER, MD, Consulting Editor

NEUROIMAGING CLINICS of North America

Stroke I: Overview and Current Clinical Practice

MICHAEL H. LEV, MD
Guest Editor

May 2005 • Volume 15 • Number 2

SAUNDERS

An Imprint of Elsevier, Inc.
PHILADELPHIA   LONDON   TORONTO   MONTREAL   SYDNEY   TOKYO

W.B. SAUNDERS COMPANY

A Division of Elsevier Inc.

1600 John F. Kennedy Boulevard • Suite 1800 • Philadelphia, Pennsylvania 19103-2899

http://www.theclinics.com

NEUROIMAGING CLINICS OF NORTH AMERICA	**Volume 15, Number 2**
May 2005	**ISSN 1052-5149**
Editor: Barton Dudlick	**ISBN 1-4160-2733-5**

Neuroimaging Clinics of North America (ISSN 1052-5149) is published quarterly by Elsevier Inc. Corporate and editorial offices: 1600 John F. Kennedy Boulevard, Suite 1800, Pennsylvania, PA 19103-2899. Accounting and circulation offices: 6277 Sea Harbor Drive, Orlando, FL 32887-4800. Periodicals postage paid at Orlando, FL 32862, and additional mailing offices. Subscription prices are USD 190 per year for US individuals, USD 290 per year for US institutions, USD 95 per year for US students and residents, USD 214 per year for Canadian individuals, USD 352 per year for Canadian institutions, USD 255 per year for international individuals, USD 352 per year for international institutions and USD 128 per year for Canadian and foreign students/residents. To receive student/resident rate, orders must be accompanied by name of affiliated institution, date of term and the *signature* of program/residency coordinator on institution letterhead. Orders will be billed at individual rate until proof of status is received. Foreign air speed delivery is included in all *Clinics* subscription prices. All prices are subject to change without notice. POSTMASTER: Send address changes to *Neuroimaging Clinics of North America*, W.B. Saunders Company, Periodicals Fulfillment, Orlando, FL 32887-4800. **Customer Service: 800-654-2452 (US). From outside of the US, call (+1) 407-345-4000. E-mail: hhspcs@harcourt.com.**

Reprints. For copies of 100 or more, of articles in this publication, please contact the Commercial Reprints Department, Elsevier Inc., 360 Park Avenue South, New York, New York 10010-1710. Tel.: (+1) 212-633-3813; Fax: (+1) 212-462-1935; E-mail: reprints@elsevier.com.

Neuroimaging Clinics of North America is covered by *Excerpta Medica/EMBASE*, the RSNA Index of Imaging Literature, Index Medicus, MEDLINE/MEDLARS, SciSearch, Research Alert, and Neuroscience Citation Index.

Printed in the United States of America.

GOAL STATEMENT

The goal of *Neuroimaging Clinics of North America* is to keep practicing radiologists and radiology residents up to date with current clinical practice in radiology by providing timely articles reviewing the state of the art in patient care.

ACCREDITATION

The *Neuroimaging Clinics of North America* is planned and implemented in accordance with the Essential Areas and Policies of the Accreditation Council for Continuing Medical Education (ACCME) through the joint sponsorship of the University of Virginia School of Medicine and Elsevier. The University of Virginia School of Medicine is accredited by the ACCME to provide continuing medical education for physicians.

The University of Virginia School of Medicine designates this educational activity for a maximum of 60 category 1 credits per year, 15 category 1 credits per issue, toward the AMA Physician's Recognition Award. Each physician should claim only those credits that he/she actually spent in the activity.

The American Medical Association has determined that physicians not licensed in the US who participate in this CME activity are eligible for AMA PRA category 1 credit.

Category 1 credit can be earned by reading the text material, taking the CME examination online at *http://www.theclinics.com/home/cme,* and completing the evaluation. After taking the test, you will be required to review any and all incorrect answers. Following completion of the test and evaluation, your credit will be awarded and you may print your certificate.

FACULTY DISCLOSURE

As a provider accredited by the Accreditation Council for Continuing Medical Education (ACCME), the Office of Continuing Medical Education of the University of Virginia School of Medicine must ensure balance, independence, objectivity, and scientific rigor in all its individually sponsored or jointly sponsored educational activities. All authors/editors participating in a sponsored activity are expected to disclose to the readers any significant financial interest or other relationship (1) with the manufacturer(s) of any commercial product(s) and/or provider(s) of commercial services discussed in an educational presentation and (2) with any commercial supporters of the activity (significant financial interest or other relationship can include such things as grants or research support, employee, consultant, stock holder, member of speakers bureau, etc.) The intent of this disclosure is not to prevent authors/editors with a significant financial or other relationship from writing an article, but rather to provide readers with information on which they can make their own judgments. It remains for the readers to determine whether the author's/editor's interest or relationships may influence the article with regard to exposition or conclusion.

The authors/editors listed below have identified no professional or financial affiliations related to their publication:
Robert H. Ackerman, MD, MPH; Luiz A. Bacheschi, MD, PhD; Joti J. Bhattacharya, MBBS, MSc, FRCR; Kathleen M. Burger, DO; Erica C.S. Camargo, MD, PhD; Verne S. Caviness, MD, DPhil; Shelagh B. Coutts, MD; Sean P. Cullen, MD; Nayeli A. Dault, SB; Andrew M. Demchuk, MD; Colin P. Derdeyn, MD; Barton Dudlick, Acquisitions Editor; Clifford J. Eskey, MD, PhD; Jeffrey Farkas, MD; Steven M. Greenberg, MD, PhD; Randall T. Higashida, MD; David N. Kennedy, PhD; Thomas Kucinski, MD; David S. Liebeskind, MD; Nikos Makris, MD, PhD; Ayrton R. Massaro, MD, PhD; Thomas P. Naidich, MD, FACR; Javier M. Romero, MD; Jonathan Rosand, MD, MS; Pina C. Sanelli, MD; John Sims, MD; Eric E. Smith, MD, FRCPC; Valarmathi Subramanian, MBBS, M Med, FRCR; Jureerat Thammaroj, MD, MSc; Stanley Tuhrim, MD; and, Andrew R. Xavier, MD.

The authors listed below have identified the following professional or financial affiliations related to their publication:
Chelsea S. Kidwell, MD is Principle Investigator for MR RESCUE Trial and Concentric Medical, the manufacturer of the Merci Retriever is providing devices for that research.
Michael H. Lev, MD has received educational grants and is on the speaker list for GE Medical Systems and Bracco Diagnostics.
Peter D. Schellinger, MD, PhD has received consulting honorariums from Boehringer Ingelheim, Ingelheim Germany and Paion, Aachen, Germany.
Lee H. Schwamm, MD, FAHA has received research support by PolyCom, Inc in the form of reduced cost telemedicine equipment. He is a member of the Act for Stroke and the INSPIRE Speakers Bureau in which IV tPA may be discussed.

Disclosure of discussion of non-FDA approved uses for pharmaceutical products and/or medical devices.
The University of Virginia School of Medicine, as an ACCME provider, requires that all authors/editors identify and disclose any "off label" uses for pharmaceutical products and/or for medical devices. The University of Virginia School of Medicine recommends that each reader fully review all the available data on new products or procedures prior to instituting them with patients.

The authors who provided disclosures will not be discussing off-label uses except:
Andrew M. Demchuk, MD will discuss tPA use beyond 3 hours from symptom onset.
Clifford J. Eskey, MD, PhD and **Pina C. Sanelli, MD** discuss acetazolamide used for challenge testing of cerebrovascular reserve ; this represents on "off-label" use of the pharmaceutical.
Chelsea S. Kidwell, MD will discuss the off-label use of tissue plasminogen activator and urokinase for intra-arterial thrombolysis.
Michael H. Lev, MD will discuss gadolinium-based contrast for MR perfusion imaging.
Lee H. Schwamm, MD, FAHA indicates that telemedicine for acute stroke treatment can be construed as an off-label use of telemedicine.
Peter D. Schellinger, MD, PhD indicates that recommendations for rt-PA in this manuscript are not consistent with regulatory approval for rt-PA in acute Stroke but represent an expert opinion/off-label rt-PA for acute ischemic stroke in extended time windows > 3 h based on modern stroke MRI diagnosis.

TO ENROLL

To enroll in the Neuroimaging Clinics of North America Continuing Medical Education program, call customer service at 1-800-654-2452 or sign up online at *http://www.theclinics.com/home/cme*. The CME program is available to subscribers for an additional annual fee of USD 156.

FORTHCOMING ISSUES

August 2005
Stroke II
Michael H. Lev, MD, *Guest Editor*

November 2005
Alzheimer's Disease
Jeffrey Petrella, MD, *Guest Editor*

RECENT ISSUES

February 2005
Ophthalmologic Neuroimaging
Mahmood F. Mafee, MD, *Guest Editor*

November 2004
Head and Neck MR Imaging
Suresh K. Mukherji, MD, *Guest Editor*

THE CLINICS ARE NOW AVAILABLE ONLINE!

Access your subscription at:
http://www.theclinics.com

CONSULTING EDITOR

BURTON P. DRAYER, MD, Dr. Charles M. and Marilyn Professor and Chairman, Department of Radiology, Mount Sinai Medical Center, New York, New York

GUEST EDITOR

MICHAEL H. LEV, MD, Associate Professor (Radiology), Department of Radiology; Director, Emergency Neuroradiology; and Director, Neurovascular Laboratory, Massachusetts General Hospital, Harvard Medical School, Boston, Massachusetts

CONTRIBUTORS

ROBERT H. ACKERMAN, MD, MPH, Senior Radiologist, Department of Radiology; Founder and Director Emeritus, Neurovascular Laboratory; and Senior Neurologist, Department of Neurology, Massachusetts General Hospital, Harvard Medical School, Boston, Massachusetts

LUIZ A. BACHESCHI, MD, PhD, Associate Professor (Neurology), Division of Neurology and Neurosurgery; and President, Postgraduate Committee, Faculdade de Medicina da Universidade de São Paulo, São Paulo, Brazil

JOTI J. BHATTACHARYA, MBBS, MSc, FRCR, Consultant Neuroradiologist, Department of Neuroradiology, Institute of Neurological Sciences, Southern General Hospital; and Honorary Senior Lecturer, Academic Department of Clinical Neurosciences, University of Glasgow, Glasgow, Scotland

KATHLEEN M. BURGER, DO, Associate/Stroke Fellow, Department of Neurology, Mount Sinai Medical Center, New York, New York

ERICA C.S. CAMARGO, MD, PhD, Research Fellow, Stroke Service, Massachusetts General Hospital, Harvard Medical School, Boston, Massachusetts

VERNE S. CAVINESS, MD, DPhil, Professor (Neurology), Department of Neurology, Harvard Medical School; Director, Center for Morphometric Analysis; and Chief, Pediatric Neurology, Massachusetts General Hospital, Charlestown, Massachusetts

SHELAGH B. COUTTS, MD, Stroke Fellow, Department of Clinical Neurosciences, Foothills Medical Center, University of Calgary, Calgary, Alberta, Canada

SEAN P. CULLEN, MD, Instructor (Radiology and Neurosurgery), Cerebrovascular Center, Interventional Neuroradiology, Brigham and Women's Hospital; and Neurointerventional Radiology, Children's Hospital, Boston, Massachusetts

NAYELI A. DAULT, SB, Research Assistant, Department of Radiology; and Research Assistant, Neurovascular Laboratory, Massachusetts General Hospital, Harvard Medical School, Boston, Massachusetts

ANDREW M. DEMCHUK, MD, Associate Professor, Department of Clinical Neurosciences, Foothills Medical Center, University of Calgary, Calgary, Alberta, Canada

COLIN P. DERDEYN, MD, Associate Professor, Mallinckrodt Institute of Radiology; and Departments of Neurology and Neurological Surgery, Washington University School of Medicine, St. Louis, Missouri

CLIFFORD J. ESKEY, MD, PhD, Assistant Professor (Radiology), Division of Neuroradiology, Dartmouth Hitchcock Medical Center, Lebanon, New Hampshire

JEFFREY FARKAS, MD, Director, Interventional Neuroradiology, Maimonides Medical Center, Brooklyn, New York

STEVEN M. GREENBERG, MD, PhD, Associate Professor (Neurology), Harvard Medical School; Associate Professor (Neurology), and Co-Director, Neurology Clinical Trials Unit, Massachusetts General Hospital, Boston, Massachusetts

RANDALL T. HIGASHIDA, MD, Clinical Professor (Radiology, Neurosurgery, and Anesthesia), Division of Neurointerventional Radiology, University of California at San Francisco Medical Center, San Francisco, California

DAVID N. KENNEDY, PhD, Assistant Professor (Neurology), Department of Neurology, Harvard Medical School; Director, Center for Morphometric Analysis, Massachusetts General Hospital, Charlestown; and Division of Health Sciences and Technology, Harvard–Massachusetts Institute of Technology, Cambridge, Massachusetts

CHELSEA S. KIDWELL, MD, University of California at Los Angeles Stroke Center, UCLA Medical Center, Los Angeles, California; and Medical Director, Washington Hospital Center; and Associate Professor, Georgetown University, Washington, DC

THOMAS KUCINSKI, MD, Private Lecturer and Senior Neuroradiologist, Department of Neuroradiology, University Medical Center Hamburg-Eppendorf, Hamburg, Germany

MICHAEL H. LEV, MD, Associate Professor (Radiology), Department of Radiology; Director, Emergency Neuroradiology; and Director, Neurovascular Laboratory, Massachusetts General Hospital, Harvard Medical School, Boston, Massachusetts

DAVID S. LIEBESKIND, MD, Assistant Professor (Neurology); Neurology Director, Stroke Imaging; and Associate Neurology Director, University of California at Los Angeles Stroke Center, UCLA Medical Center, Los Angeles, California

NIKOS MAKRIS, MD, PhD, Assistant Professor (Neurology), Department of Neurology, Harvard Medical School; and Co-director, Center for Morphometric Analysis, Massachusetts General Hospital, Charlestown, Massachusetts

AYRTON R. MASSARO, MD, PhD, Assistant Professor (Neurology), Department of Neurology; and Director, Stroke Service, Hospital São Paulo, Escola Paulista de Medicina da Universidade Federal de São Paulo, São Paulo, Brazil

THOMAS P. NAIDICH, MD, Professor, Departments of Radiology and Neurosurgery, Mount Sinai Medical Center, New York, New York

JAVIER M. ROMERO, MD, Instructor (Radiology), Department of Radiology; and Staff Member, Neurovascular Laboratory, Massachusetts General Hospital, Harvard Medical School, Boston, Massachusetts

JONATHAN ROSAND, MD, MS, Assistant Professor (Neurology), Vascular and Critical Care Neurology, Massachusetts General Hospital; and Assistant Professor (Neurology), Harvard Medical School, Boston, Massachusetts

PINA C. SANELLI, MD, Assistant Professor (Radiology), Division of Neuroradiology, New York Presbyterian Hospital, Weill Medical College of Cornell University, New York, New York

PETER D. SCHELLINGER, MD, PhD, Associate Professor (Neurology), Department of Neurology, University of Heidelberg, Heidelberg, Germany

LEE H. SCHWAMM, MD, FAHA, Associate Professor (Neurology), Harvard Medical School; Director, TeleStroke and Acute Stroke Services, Massachusetts General Hospital; and Director, Clinical Research Center, Massachusetts Institute of Technology, Boston, Massachusetts

JOHN SIMS, MD, Principal Investigator, Stroke and Neurovascular Regulation Laboratory, Charlestown; Instructor (Neurology), Harvard Medical School; and Assistant (Neurology), TeleStroke and Acute Stroke Services, Department of Neurology, Massachusetts General Hospital, Boston, Massachusetts

ERIC E. SMITH, MD, FRCPC, Instructor (Neurology), Vascular and Critical Care Neurology, Massachusetts General Hospital; and Instructor (Neurology), Harvard Medical School, Boston, Massachusetts

VALARMATHI SUBRAMANIAM, MBBS, M Med, FRCR, Consultant Diagnostic and Interventional Radiologist, Department of Radiology, Gleneagles Intan Medical Center, Kuala Lumpur, Malaysia

JUREERAT THAMMAROJ, MD, MSc, Assistant Professor (Radiology), Department of Radiology, Srinagarind Hospital, Khon Kaen University, Khon Kaen, Thailand

STANLEY TUHRIM, MD, Professor, Department of Neurology, Mount Sinai Medical Center, New York, New York

UNIVERSITY OF CALIFORNIA AT LOS ANGELES THROMBOLYSIS INVESTIGATORS, University of California at Los Angeles Stroke Center, UCLA Medical Center, Los Angeles, California

ANDREW R. XAVIER, MD, Clinical Fellow, Department of Neurosciences, University of Medicine and Dentistry–New Jersey Medical School, Newark, New Jersey

CONTENTS

New and more advanced diagnostic imaging techniques for acute stroke triage have the
potential to not only improve the quality of care but also reduce health care costs. Although
sufficiently large and methodologically sound studies with regard to cost effectiveness
of MR imaging are lacking, the overall impression is that MR imaging has revolutionized
not only the diagnosis but also the open and investigational management of neurologically
ill patients.

Neuroimaging by CT or MR imaging is necessary for the identification of hemorrhagic
stroke and provides information about its cause. The appearance of intracranial hematoma
(ICH) on CT and MR imaging evolves over time and must be understood to facilitate
accurate diagnosis. The cause of ICH varies by location. New evidence suggests that MR
imaging alone may be adequate to identify hemorrhagic stroke in the acute setting, and
that MR imaging is superior to CT for identification of chronic microbleeds and hemorrhagic conversion of infarction.

The epidemic of cardiovascular disease across most of Asia is at a different stage from
that in the West; the incidence and prevalence of stroke are increasing steadily, associated
with nutritional changes and aging of the population. Epidemiologic data, crucial in

combating stroke, have been relatively sparse in Asian populations, but a few international collaborative studies on stroke have been in progress for several years. Through these, we now know that ischemic stroke is actually the most frequent type of cerebrovascular accident in Asia, although hemorrhagic stroke remains more common in Asia than in the West. Also, the percentage of ischemic stroke attributable to intracranial vascular disease is much higher than in the West. In Japan and a few other countries, stroke rates are declining; however, increasing rates in most other countries make primary prevention of critical importance in minimizing the severe impact of this epidemic in Asia.

Stroke is one of the leading causes of mortality in Latin America, with variable incidence and prevalence throughout the continent reflecting regional socioeconomic differences. In Latin America, uncontrolled hypertension is one of the major causes of stroke, but other modifiable risk factors also play a role, such as heavy alcohol consumption and smoking. Intracerebral hemorrhage and lacunar stroke are more frequent in Latin America than in North America and Europe. There are multiple causes of stroke that are endemic to Latin America, including neurocysticercosis, Chagas' disease, sickle cell anemia, malaria, hemorrhagic fever, and snake bites.

Brainstem infarcts comprise approximately 10% of all first ischemic brain strokes. The extrinsic vascular supply to the stem is complex. The intrinsic vascularization of the stem may be conceptualized in terms of four relatively constant and distinct vascular territories designated anteromedial, anterolateral, lateral, and dorsal (or dorsolateral). The anatomic structures found within each intrinsic territory determine the symptomatology associated with infarction of that territory. This territorial anatomy permits the knowledgeable physician to plan an MR imaging examination tailored to the patient's history and to predict the patient's neurologic deficits from the MR imaging findings.

The anatomic description of the stroke lesion is an essential component of clinical diagnosis and treatment and has become an established tool in investigations into underlying stroke pathophysiology. Magnetic resonance (MR) imaging permits quantitative evaluation of the distributed consequences of the pathologic stroke insult. General properties of stroke effects have emerged using these tools. This article surveys the classes of morphometric data that are available from conventional MR images, the methods for extracting quantitative results, and samples of the application of these methods to stroke. These samples highlight anatomic-based considerations regarding the nature of stroke and its repercussions within the brain parenchyma.

The Stroke-Prone Patient: Imaging and Intervention

Positron emission tomography (PET) uniquely allows the in vivo regional measurement of several important physiologic parameters in living humans, including cerebral blood flow and oxygen metabolism. PET studies have advanced our understanding of normal human brain physiology and, as detailed in this article, our understanding of human cerebrovascular pathophysiology. This article focuses on knowledge gained from PET regarding acute ischemic stroke and chronic oligemia from arterial occlusive disease. Knowledge of the responses of the brain and its vasculature to ischemia and oligemia is growing more important with the increasing availability of CT and MR perfusion techniques.

been advocated as a triage tool for thrombolytic therapy. Recent studies have challenged the relevance of these EIS within 3 hours of stroke onset, with advanced MR and CT methods increasingly competing with unenhanced CT as the primary imaging modality for acute ischemia. Nonetheless, the insights regarding acute stroke physiology provided by studying the CT evolution of early ischemic signs continue to be valuable for the informed interpretation of all stroke images. It is these insights that comprise the topic of this article.

NEUROIMAGING
CLINICS OF
NORTH AMERICA

Neuroimag Clin N Am 15 (2005) xv – xvi

Preface

Stroke I: Overview and Current Clinical Practice

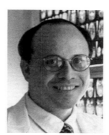

Michael H. Lev, MD
Guest Editor

...all the most acute, most powerful, and most deadly diseases, and those which are most difficult to be understood by the inexperienced, fall upon the brain.

—Hippocrates (circa 400 BC)

What am I supposed to do? No one can restore a brain!

—Dr. Leonard "Bones" McCoy
(*Star Trek* Episode #56: "Spock's Brain")

Advances in stroke neuroimaging and therapeutics since the start of the "Decade of the Brain" in 1990 have exceeded the imaginings of science fiction. Technologic developments such as diffusion/perfusion-weighted imaging, multidetector row CT angiography, and endovascular clot dissolution/retrieval strategies have occurred at a staggering pace. Improved understanding of underlying stroke pathophysiology continues to make these advances increasingly clinically relevant.

These two issues of the *Neuroimaging Clinics of North America* attempt to capture the excitement of this evolving field, making it accessible to experts and novices alike. Stroke I provides an overview of differing approaches to stroke prevention and management throughout the world, dealing primarily with

the interface between imaging and intervention. Stroke II explores the technical aspects of various neuroimaging modalities in greater detail, with special attention to their physiological underpinnings and future potential. Important differences between adult and childhood stroke are highlighted.

Certain recurrent themes emerge from the outset: diffusion imaging is the most sensitive method for the detection of infarct core (tissue likely—but not certain—to die despite early complete reperfusion of ischemic brain), although source images from the CT angiography dataset, like diffusion-weighted imaging, can also define *core*; CT angiography is more accurate than MR angiography for depicting large vessel thrombus; susceptibility MR is more sensitive than CT for detecting chronic microbleeds (the clinical relevance of which for thrombolysis exclusion, however, is unclear); and the ratio between core and salvageable penumbra (ischemic tissue that may survive with early reperfusion) might be used to extend the current limited time window for thrombolytic treatment.

The authors have done a wonderful job; they run the spectrum from "up and coming" to established leaders in their respective areas of expertise. There is some overlap—and even occasional disagreement—between authors as they review related topics from different perspectives. Such controversy befits a field undergoing such rapid evolution as stroke neuroimaging.

Acknowledgments

There are several individuals without whom these two issues would not exist. I cannot overstate the foresight of R. Gilberto Gonzalez, MD, Chief of Neuroradiology, and Walter J. Koroshetz, MD, Chief of Stroke Neurology, in both advancing novel MR and CT imaging techniques as a clinical tool for patient triage at the Massachusetts General Hospital and in supporting my career goals. Dr. Robert H. Ackerman, director emeritus of the Massachusetts General Hospital Neurovascular Laboratory, has served as a valued mentor for over 15 years. My sincere thanks go to Dr. Burton Drayer for inviting me to participate in this *Clinics* series, and I would also like to acknowledge my research assistants Jonathan Fine, Sarah Gottfried, and Erin Murphy for their editing help. Finally, my heartfelt thanks to my wife, Julie M. Goodman, PhD, not only for her detailed neuroscience editorial expertise, but also for all else that has made this work possible.

Dedication

These issues are dedicated to Marilyn Lev (1935–2003).

Michael H. Lev, MD
Department of Neurology
Massachusetts General Hospital
Harvard Medical School
55 Fruit Street
Boston, MA 02114, USA
E-mail address: mlev@partners.org

ELSEVIER
SAUNDERS

Neuroimag Clin N Am 15 (2005) 245 – 258

NEUROIMAGING
CLINICS OF
NORTH AMERICA

The Evolving Role of Advanced MR Imaging as a Management Tool for Adult Ischemic Stroke: A Western-European Perspective

Peter D. Schellinger, MD, PhD*

Department of Neurology, University of Heidelberg, Heidelberg, Germany

Stroke is the third leading cause of death after myocardial infarction and cancer, the leading cause of permanent disability in Western countries [1], and the leading cause of disability-adjusted loss of independent life-years. Aside from the tragic consequences for patients and their families, the socio-economic impact of disabled stroke survivors is clear, because patients with permanent deficits, such as hemiparesis and aphasia, typically are not able to live independently or pursue an occupation. The cost of stroke is estimated to be between $35,000 and $50,000 per survivor, per year. In the face of aging populations, the incidence and prevalence of stroke is expected to increase; therefore, an effective and widely available treatment for this devastating disease is desperately needed.

In the pre–MR-imaging era, continuing until the early 1990s, the stroke field was dominated by therapeutic nihilism. Patients were treated conservatively and sent to rehabilitation units or nursing homes. Major stroke trials performed during that time focused on secondary prevention, including two trials of carotid endarterectomy for stroke attributed to internal carotid artery stenosis [2,3]; one small negative trial for extra/intracranial bypass [4]; and trials testing the efficacy of anticoagulation (warfarin) and antiplatelet agents (acetylsalicylic acid, ticlopidine) for stroke prevention [5,6]. Heparin, low molecular weight heparins, and heparinoids, were more or less adequately tested and found to be ineffective for early or late secondary prevention of stroke [7].

Still, trials for acute stroke therapy were lacking. Anecdotal reports of acute treatment with thrombolytics were first described in the early 1960s. [8]. Small trials, however, focused only on their use for subacute stroke [9], with pilot trials for acute stroke not occurring until the early 1990s [10,11]. No diagnostic imaging modality, including angiography, was used to establish the diagnosis of stroke in these studies.

At present, the only therapy approved by the Food and Drug Administration (FDA) for improving acute ischemic stroke outcome is intravenous (IV) tissue plasminogen activator (tPA), given within 3 hours of stroke onset [12,13]. Routine tPA use, however, has been limited because of the logistical demands of such a short treatment window and the current uncertainty with regard to ischemic stroke diagnosis—leading to reluctance on the part of nonspecialists to assume the hemorrhagic risks of thrombolytic therapy. More effective treatments are needed for this potentially devastating disease because most ischemic stroke patients receive no specific acute therapy aside from aspirin (ASA), and among those treated with tPA, fewer than half recover full function. Because noncontrast CT has limited sensitivity/specificity in the initial hours after stroke, improved accuracy is needed to guide the development and application of optimal thrombolytic and other stroke therapy.

The pilot study of Haley and colleagues [14] was the first to use a cross-sectional imaging method—unenhanced CT—before thrombolytic therapy. After several negative acute stroke trials with streptokinase,

* Department of Neurology, University of Heidelberg, Im Neuenheimer Feld 400, Heidelberg 69120, Germany.
  E-mail address: Peter_Schellinger@med.uni-heidelberg.de

the National Institute of Neurological Disorders and Stroke (NINDS) group demonstrated that IV thrombolysis with recombinant tissue plasminogen activator (rt-PA) is safe and effective in patients with acute ischemic stroke but only *after* exclusion of acute intracerebral hemorrhage (ICH) by unenhanced CT and only when given within 3 hours of symptom onset. The NINDS trial was published in 1995 [12], and resulted in FDA approval of the drug in 1996. Three further trials assessed the efficacy of rt-PA beyond the 3-hour time window but yielded negative results [15–17]. Although the NINDS trial applied CT only for the purpose of ICH exclusion, later trials established criteria for the diagnosis of early *ischemic* stroke in CT [18]. Despite the poor sensitivity of noncontrast CT—31% within the therapeutic time window of 3 hours [19] and 45% to 65% at best among specialists within 6 hours [20]—and because meta-analyses suggested a therapeutic effect of rt-PA beyond the 3-hour time window (up to 4.5–6 hours in some patients [21,22]), it is surprising that modern techniques, such as CT-angiography (CTA) [23] or MR imaging, have not had a role in acute stroke imaging until recently [24].

Although Nobel prizes continue to be awarded to developers of novel imaging techniques —Hounsfield and Cormack in 1979 for CT and Lauterbur and Mansfield in 2003 for MR imaging—the most important step for a new technology is the establishment in clinical practice. The evolution from tentative reports and early research activity to the definition of possible clinical benefits to final acceptance into practice [25], is often protracted for complex technologies, such as MR imaging.

Lauterbur published his landmark paper on the derivation of position dependent information from nuclear magnetic resonance (NMR) signals using magnetic gradients in the early 1970s [26]. Despite the work that followed by Sir Peter Mansfield [27,28] and other groups, the first clinical MR imaging system was not available until 1984 and the first paramagnetic MR imaging contrast agent until 1987. The past 20 years have realized several advances in computer technology and software development, which have continuously improved the accessibility and quality of MR imaging. The earliest scans— T2-weighted, T1-weighted and PD-weighted sequence without contrast—took hours to complete. Today, multiparametric protocols can assess within 15 minutes the most complex pathophysiologic processes, facilitating a dramatic shift in the evaluation and treatment of neurologic illness. As the clinical discipline of neurology has evolved from a diagnostic to a therapeutic specialty, MR imaging has been and is being transformed into a clinical tool that impacts neurology at the bedside. With an increasing number of clinical therapeutic trials being designed, MR imaging may not only function as a diagnostic tool but also as a selection tool and surrogate endpoint for the development of new therapies [29].

Pathophysiologic concepts applied to MR imaging of acute ischemic stroke

The brain is sensitive to ischemia, with irreversible damage occurring within minutes of complete cessation of blood flow. Collateral flow sources through the Circle of Willis and leptomeningeal circulation provide some redundancy in arterial supply and can potentially help protect against death. As a result, focal arterial occlusions can produce regionally varying gradients in hypoperfusion. Electrophysiologic, biochemical and histologic data, primarily from animal models, suggest the presence of ischemic thresholds for cellular functions, such as protein synthesis, electrical excitability, and immediate or delayed cell death. Such thresholds are also influenced by ischemic duration [30] because this also contributes to tissue fate. Available information concerning ischemic thresholds in mammalian brain pertains almost exclusively to gray matter.

In the 1970s, the term "ischemic penumbra" was coined to describe the volume of brain that is dysfunctional caused by ischemic injury but is above the threshold for cell death [31,32]. This concept was first described in relation to a baboon model of middle cerebral artery occlusion [33]. In this model, a cortical region of extreme hypoperfusion around insular cortex represented the ischemic "core", with cerebral blood flow (CBF) values less than 10 mL/ 100 g/min. A surrounding "penumbral" region showed CBF values less than 20 mL/g/min, but more than 10 mL/g/min—this region may still be salvaged if blood flow is restored.

In rodent models of middle cerebral artery (MCA) occlusion, the lenticulostriate distribution represents the ischemic core that is irreversible after approximately one hour, whereas the cortical distribution has greater reversibility caused by leptomeningeal collaterals, which reduce the extent of ischemia [34]. This differential sensitivity of cortical and deep MCA distributions also helps explain the propensity for basal ganglia hemorrhage into regions of ischemic necrosis following reperfusion of MCA strokes in humans. This region is also the first and, at times, only region to be reperfused.

The target for most therapeutic interventions for focal ischemia should be ischemic tissue that can respond to treatment and is not irreversibly injured (ie, the penumbra). Until recently, only positron emission tomography (PET) and single photon emission computerized tomography (SPECT) imaging could approximately define core and penumbra thresholds. Application of these methods in the clinical setting, however, is not practical or feasible. Newer imaging techniques, such as novel MR pulse sequences, perfusion techniques, and other improvements of imaging soft- and hardware, have provided alternatives.

Noncontrast CT is the current imaging standard for acute stroke. Its status is principally because of its wide availability and its near 100% sensitivity for the detection of acute ICH—the most important differential diagnosis to ischemic stroke [35]. For infarction, several early CT signs have been described [36], and formalized CT scores have been developed [37]. The sensitivity of these findings varies widely, ranging from as low as 12% to as high as 92%, depending on the imaging features of infarction, time from clinical onset, study population, and other variables, including the availability of appropriate

clinical history at the time of image interpretation [38,39].

A post hoc analysis of the NINDS CT data yielded a 31% sensitivity for early infarct signs and a mild correlation with concurrent clinical severity assessed by the National Institutes of Health Stroke Scale (NIHSS), albeit only in the 3-hour time window [40]. Overall, the sensitivity of CT for acute ischemic stroke in the 6-hour time window can be estimated to be from approximately 40% to 60%, with substantial increase in the further hours after stroke onset [39]. CT has become the de facto diagnostic standard for acute stroke.

Two MR imaging techniques that have received much attention in the past 15 years are diffusion- and perfusion-weighted imaging (DWI and PWI) [41–44]. The phenomenon of indirectly measuring Brownian molecular motion of water with DWI was first described in 1965 [45]. The measurement of water diffusion renders pathophysiologic tissue data regarding ischemic, inflammatory, and neoplastic disease that cannot be obtained with standard MR-imaging sequences [46,47].

In addition to the qualitative DWI measurements, which have an intrinsic T2-weighted component, the

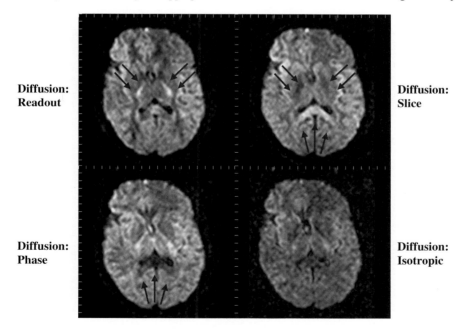

Diffusion: Readout   **Diffusion: Slice**

Diffusion: Phase   **Diffusion: Isotropic**

Fig. 1. From upper left to lower right, first three figures show diffusion in three different directions: "readout," "slice," and "phase." The arrows depict different diffusion phenomenon in the internal capsule and posterior commissure, respectively. When DWI slice is obtained perpendicular to direction of fiber tracts, there is low diffusion (hyperintense capsule on "readout" and hyperintense posterior commissure on "slice"). If obtained parallel to fiber axis, there is high diffusion (hypointense internal capsule on "slice" and hypointense posterior commissure on "phase"). On isotropic (*lower right*) DWI, effects are averaged ("trace of the diffusion tensor"), so pathologic diffusion changes are not confused with physiologic phenomenon of diffusion.

apparent diffusion coefficient (ADC) can be quantified from MR acquisitions at different b-values [48]. For structures, such as nerve fibers or tracts, that have a predominant orientation in space, the ADC is different in different directions, and the "net" ADC is determined by tensor analysis that averages the various directional components (Figs. 1 and 2). In acute stroke, whereas water diffusion is only mildly impaired along the nerve sheath axis, diffusion perpendicular to this direction is markedly decreased [49], referred to as anisotropy. In the brain, anisotropy is most pronounced in the white matter, especially in densely packed fiber structures, such as the corpus callosum and the corona radiata (Fig. 3). The effects of anisotropy can be used to obtain information regarding the regional fascicular fiber tract anatomy, which may be helpful for preneurosurgic mapping of eloquent brain regions. The expansion of these principles has led to the development of diffusion tensor imaging, which has been used to characterize myelination and demyelination [50–53].

Now that more patients have been evaluated with stroke MR imaging at early time points, partial reversal of the initial DWI lesion has been reported. These findings suggest that the early DWI lesion might be included in the therapeutic target, rather than solely be considered as the definite infarct core [54–57]. DWI lesion reversal, however, seems to be associated with ultra-early and permanent reperfusion. Therefore, in most instances—and especially in later time windows—the DWI lesion may adequately reflect permanently damaged brain tissue.

PWI uses dynamic bolus tracking to derive pixel-based concentration versus time curves, allowing the qualitative assessment of various hemodynamic parameters relative to areas of normal parenchyma [58–60]. Typical parameters are mean transit time (MTT), cerebral blood volume (CBV), CBF, and time to peak (TTP). The actual quantification of hemodynamic information has been limited by postprocessing capabilities and methods of calculating the arterial input function, detailed at length in other articles in this volume. Nonetheless, areas of relative hypoperfusion can be reliably demonstrated by current methods—of special relevance is acute ischemic stroke management [61]. Other applications, such as functional imaging with the Blood Oxygen Level Dependent (BOLD) technique, and MR spectroscopic imaging, exceed the scope of this article.

The idea that quantitative perfusion imaging is required for stroke assessment is derived from concepts of ischemic thresholds and ischemic penumbra,

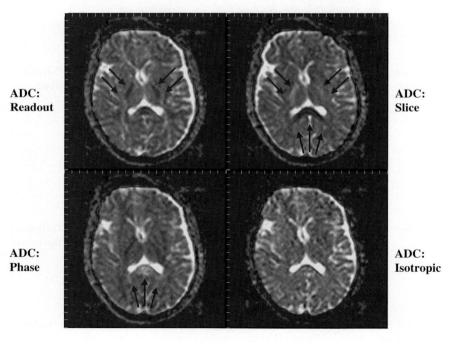

ADC: Readout

ADC: Slice

ADC: Phase

ADC: Isotropic

Fig. 2. Illustrate of anisotropy of diffusion on ADC-maps, in analogy to Fig. 1. From upper left to lower right, first three figures show ADC-maps in three different directions, "readout," "slice," and "phase." Low ADC in hypointense capsule on "readout" and in posterior commissure on "slice," with high ADC in hyperintense internal capsule on "slice" and in posterior commissure on "phase"). On isotropic (*lower right*) ADC-map effects are not present.

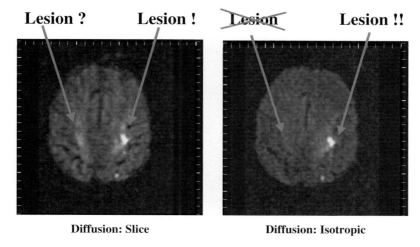

Fig. 3. Anisotropic and isotropic DWI. Definite lesion in left parietal lobe of MCA territory seen on DWI (*arrows*) maps. Lesion in right parietal lobe seen on left figure is physiologic anisotropic diffusion in corona radiata, averaged in isotropic images (*arrows*).

the premise being that if CBF could be more accurately quantified, then the tissue could be characterized as normal, reversibly ischemic, or irreversibly damaged. Unfortunately, various factors make the implementation of this concept problematic in human patients. Firstly, the duration and extent of ischemia must be known, and such information is not uniformly available, especially in the case of "wake up" strokes. Secondly, human stroke typically involves gray and white matter, whereas threshold data apply primarily to gray matter. Thirdly, whereas some human strokes, such as those caused by embolism from atrial fibrillation, typically comprise a solitary MCA occlusion, many human strokes are multifocal, or are caused by partial occlusions, and in these cases a complex topological relationship is likely to occur between "core" and "penumbra." Fourthly, mathematical approaches to account for bolus delay and dispersion are complex [62]. Finally, it is now recognized that delayed cell death occurs as a result of ischemia (apoptosis) and that recurrent sublethal ischemia can make the brain less sensitive to subsequent ischemic events (ischemic conditioning) [63].

Most authors, however, agree that even circulation time-based parameters, such as MTT or TTP, give appropriate empiric prognostic data in the clinical setting of acute ischemic stroke [64,65]. Ongoing PWI research is aimed at differentiating oligemia from critical ischemia [57], with the goal of better guiding clinical management. Time thresholding on MTT or TTP maps may increase accuracy. Neumann-Haefelin and colleagues [66] found a threshold of 4s on TTP maps to indicate moderately severe and

beyond 6s to indicate severe ischemia. Sobesky and colleagues [67] compared PWI to H_2O^{15} PET imaging and also showed that a threshold of 4s gains the best sensitivity and specificity for critical (ie, penumbral) hypoperfusion. Although hypoperfusion remains a key pathophysiologic mechanism in stroke, it is unclear whether absolute quantification of CBF at any time point is sufficient or even necessary for predicting tissue outcome.

More practically, the "ischemic penumbra" may be *operationally* defined as those brain regions that are at risk for infarction but remain salvageable based on any criteria and, hence, the target of acute stroke therapy (Fig. 4A).

The volume difference of DWI and PWI—also termed PWI/DWI mismatch—gives an approximate measure of this tissue at risk for infarction [68] (Fig. 4B). Although its nonquantitative approach suffers in part from inaccurate PWI measurements, and that DWI abnormalities may reverse [57], they serve their purpose of easy clinical application. This simple model of PWI/DWI-mismatch is sufficiently accurate in most acute stroke patients, and the stroke MR imaging findings are consistent with our understanding of the pathophysiology of acute ischemia [65,69]. According to unpublished data (Steven Warach, MD, PhD, personal communication, 2005) partial or complete DWI lesion reversal is an independent predictor of an improved outcome. However, DWI reversal is associated with early and rapid reperfusion, and this is a stronger predictor of clinical and imaging outcome [70]. Applying the mismatch concept may obviate the need for an individual time

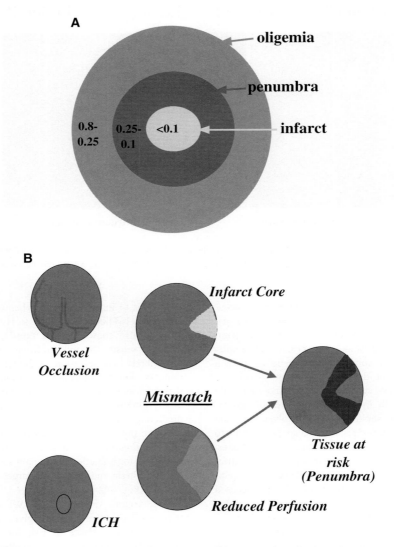

Fig. 4. (*A*) Concept of three-compartment operational model of ischemic brain tissue: infarct core is irreversibly damaged, penumbra-zone shows disturbed function but still salvageable, and oligemic-zone has preserved function and morphology. Numbers indicate CBF in mL/g/min. (*B*) Stroke MR imaging protocol: a sample comprehensive stroke imaging algorithm. Imaging triage algorithm outlined in Fig. 4 and Box 1 is based on institutional protocol, not on international guidelines. Whenever possible, informed consent should be obtained, and next of kin should be advised. International approval of IV thrombolysis is based on CT criteria within the 3-hour time window, and lysis within 3 hours of stroke onset has highest priority. Criteria based on NINDS and European Cooperative Acute Stroke Study data; one third of mild or remitting stroke patients not receiving thrombolysis have a poor outcome 103. Generating evidence by participating in randomized trials is secondary priority. Use of stroke MR imaging as triage tool for extending time window beyond 3 hours is priority 3. The 3- to 9-hour time window was chosen in parallel to DIAS trial 96. Patients with a PWI/DWI-mismatch represent an absolute indication for lysis unless exclusion criteria are met; those with PWI/DWI match might be considered for IV-thrombolysis based on the potential reversibility of DWI lesions. We included a fourth priority, if MR imagine is not available, based on analogous stroke CT criteria (CT, CT-angiography, CT-perfusion). This technique less well validated in diagnostic studies, and not at all in treatment studies. Nonetheless, preliminary data and common sense dictate that stroke CT can be used in similar fashion as stroke MR imaging, albeit with less diagnostic strength. Finally, based on combined analysis 20, if neither stroke MR imaging nor stroke CT is available, may be sufficient evidence for expanding time window for IV-lysis to 4.5 hours using unenhanced CT only as triage tool.

window for each patient, and thus allow therapeutic decision-making based on an individual's vascular and hemodynamic situation rather than the elapsed "clock" time.

Additional MR findings not captured by CT, such as early blood brain barrier disruption [71] and chronic microbleeds [72,73], may portend a poor outcome after thrombolysis and, therefore, be used to enhance patient selection, although the latter has been questioned [74]. Microbleeds are associated with a risk for hemorrhagic ischemic stroke in general [75], however, whether the one-time-risk for ICH after rt-PA treatment is increased, is, at present, unknown. Therefore, the presence of microbleeds should not influence management, but when in doubt, to increase safety, microbleeds may be used as exclusion criteria for reperfusion strategies.

Comprehensively diagnosing stroke with MR imaging

The advent of new MR imaging techniques, such as PWI and DWI in the early 1990s added another dimension to diagnostic imaging in stroke [76–79]. Several investigators found a significant correlation of DWI and PWI changes with follow-up imaging and with neurologic outcome [80–84]. Some investigators concluded that different infarct patterns can be identified by DWI and PWI in hyperacute stroke, which may allow a more rational selection of therapeutic strategies based on the presence or absence of tissue at risk [78,85–87].

The supposed lack of practicality of MR as a diagnostic tool in acutely ill patients [88–90] has been consistently disproved; however, logistical obstacles can be overcome [91,92]. Despite this, substantial doubts remain regarding the feasibility and validity of stroke MR imaging in the clinical setting [88–90]. This criticism is mainly based on a supposed lack of studies assessing sensitivity and specificity of these new imaging methods in a randomized, blinded, and controlled fashion. Also, the overuse of the term "gold standard" has added to the controversy, because there remains no such thing as an imaging gold standard for acute ischemic stroke because of the current lack of correlation of any neuroimaging method with neuropathologic findings [93]. Therefore, as a "quasi" gold standard, the diagnosis of stroke in most studies is established at follow-up, with proof of a lesion on either CT or conventional MR images together with a clinical syndrome, and a comprehensive diagnostic work-up.

Several studies have addressed the diagnostic power of stroke MR imaging for ischemic and hemorrhagic stroke. One study comparing MR imaging and CT across a broad sample of stroke patients has been published in preliminary form [79]. The authors assessed the relative accuracy of MR imaging versus CT in a representative sample of patients (n = 356) who consecutively presented to a hospital emergency department over an 18-month period and in whom the emergency physician diagnosed possible acute stroke, thus including a representative proportion of patients with not only ischemic stroke but also with non-ischemic stroke and stroke mimics. Patients with suspected acute stroke were imaged at a median of 33 minutes earlier by MR imaging than by CT. In the subset of 221 patients scanned within 12 hours from onset, four reviewers (two neuroradiologists and two stroke neurologists) interpreted all scans in a blinded and independent fashion. Acute ischemic stroke, as confirmed by final discharge diagnosis, was detected by MR imaging significantly more often than by CT (90 versus 20, $P < .0001$).

Fiebach and colleagues [94] prospectively evaluated a total of 50 patients with ischemic stroke and 4 patients with transient ischemic attacks. To avoid any bias in favor of the neuroimaging modality, patients were randomized to either MR imaging or CT first, followed by the other. Patients were excluded at the time the delay from symptom onset to one of the imaging modalities exceeded 6 hours, or the delay between the two modalities exceeded 90 minutes. The correct diagnosis of stroke was established by the clinical course and follow-up CT. Five stroke experts and four residents independently judged stroke signs and lesion size on the images. Inter-rater variability was assessed with unweighted κ-values for blinded interpretation of CT and DWI for both rating groups. The reviewers were blinded to the symptoms and signs the patients had presented with, but they knew that the cohort was an ischemic stroke population. Of the 50 patients, 55% were examined with DWI first. The mean delay from symptom onset until CT was 180 minutes; that from symptom onset until DWI was 189 minutes. The mean delay between DWI and CT was 30 minutes. Expert readers yielded, for DWI: sensitivity 91% (88%–94%), specificity 95% (75%–100%), accuracy 91% (89%–94%), positive predictive value 100% (98%–100%), and negative predictive value 47% (38%–57%). For CT, the experts reached sensitivity of 61% (52%–70%), specificity 65% (50%–100%), accuracy 61% (56%–70%), positive predictive value 96% (94%–100%), and negative predictive value 12% (9%–17%). The novices yielded, for DWI: sensitivity 81% (78%–86%), specificity 100% (100%), accuracy 82% (80%–87%), positive predictive value 100% (100%), and negative predictive value 30% (27%–36%). For CT, the novices reached sensitivity 46% (32%–64%), specificity 56% (25%–75%), accuracy 46% (35%–61%), positive predictive value 93% (90%–96%), and negative predictive value 7% (5%–11%). Inter-rater variability of lesion detection was also significantly better for DWI (CT/DWI, $\kappa = 0.51/0.84$). Assessment of lesion extent was less homogeneous on CT (CT/DWI, $\kappa = 0.38/0.62$). The differences between the two modalities were more apparent in the residents' ratings (CT/DWI: sensitivity, 46%/81%; $\kappa = 0.38/0.76$). The inter-rater variability of stroke detection on DWI decreased with the delay from symptom onset.

With regard to hemorrhage, Fiebach and colleagues [95] performed a multi-center trial of 62 prospectively acquired patients with ICH and ischemic stroke, who were assessed within 6 hours (mean 3 hours 23 minutes) with DWI, T2-MR imaging and T2*-MR imaging. The main aim of this study was to prove that stroke MR imaging can differentiate ischemic stroke from ICH within the first 6 hoursp; therefore, the spectrum of patients and controls was narrow. Baseline CT, follow-up imaging, and clinical course were used to establish the correct diagnosis of ICH and ischemic stroke, respectively. Patients were not matched for age, time since onset, or baseline stroke severity. Randomisation numbers were assigned to all scans. Three raters blindly and independently rated all scans. All three raters correctly identified all ischemic strokes and ICH; sensitivity was 100% (95% confidence interval 97.1–100%), and positive and negative predictive value and accuracy were also 100%.

Kidwell and colleagues [96] recently published a hemorrhage detection study of 200 patients imaged within 6 hours of symptom onset. They compared the accuracy of MR imaging and CT in a prospective, blinded, multicenter design. For the diagnosis of hemorrhage, MR imaging was positive in 71 patients with CT positive in 29 ($P < .001$). For the diagnosis of acute hemorrhage, MR imaging and CT were equivalent (96% concordance). Acute hemorrhage was diagnosed in 25 patients on MR imaging and CT. In 4 other patients, acute hemorrhage was present on MR imaging but not on the corresponding CT. In 49 patients, chronic hemorrhage, most often microbleeds, was visualized on MR imaging but not on CT.

Guiding therapy with stroke MR imaging: extending the time window?

Despite its benefit, as few as 1% to 2% of all stroke patients receive rt-PA [97]. Few candidates present within the time window and meet clinical criteria for thrombolysis. Educating the public to regard stroke as a treatable emergency and training emergency caregivers in the use of thrombolysis can improve use but demands a continuous effort. Health care institutions should be made aware of the potential in long-term cost savings once stroke management is optimized and thrombolytic therapy is more widely available.

Stroke physicians are frequently confronted with patients who awaken with a deficit [98] (so-called "wake up" strokes) or are unable to provide the required information because of aphasia or disorientation. At present, such patients are excluded from thrombolytic therapy, even if their CT scan is normal or has only minor ischemic change. In these patients, who might profit from rapid recanalization, thrombolysis is often withheld.

A more rational selection of therapeutic strategies based on the presence or absence of a tissue at risk, as identified by DWI and PWI patterns, can improve patient outcome. Open pilot trials have used stroke MR imaging and PWI/DWI-mismatch for treatment decisions with regard to thrombolytic therapy. MR imaging is currently used at most of the major stroke centers worldwide for management beyond the NINDS time criteria, with thrombolysis rates ranging from 10% to 25% of all patients. MR imaging has the potential to become not only the most powerful, but also the most widely and uniformly used tool to guide therapy based on individual pathophysiology, as opposed to a less accurate surrogate parameter, such as elapsed time.

With regard to extending the time window for treatment, a prospective, open-label, non-randomized multicenter trial examined the MR imaging baseline characteristics of 139 patients who presented with acute ischemic stroke within 6 hours of symptom onset, and studied the influence of IV rt-PA on MR parameters and functional outcome [99]. A significantly higher occurrence of independent outcome existed after treatment with rt-PA (76 patients versus 63 controls) despite the significantly worse baseline NIHSS score and the larger volume of tissue at risk in these patients. Another study treated patients according to the NINDS protocol within the first 3 hours (n = 115), and according to stroke MR imaging findings in the 3- to 6-hour time window (n = 48). Baseline NIHSS scores and the rate of symptomatic ICH did not differ between groups, but mortality did trend in favor of the patients receiving late rt-PA (3–6 hours) according to stroke MR imaging criteria (16.5% versus 6.3%, $P = .08$). The outcome (independent versus dependent or dead [modified Rankin scale {mRS} 0–2 versus mRS 3–6]) of the stroke

MR-imaging group was (nonsignificantly) better than in the group who received early intervention (47% versus 62.5%, odds ratio 0.54, confidence interval 0.27–1.06) based on CT and NINDS criteria. These numbers suggest that with a selection tool, such as stroke MR imaging, the time window for treating stroke using thrombolytic therapy may be substantially expanded, with improved results as compared with historical studies; however, this has not been firmly established in a randomized trial. DEFUSE (DWI Evolution For Understanding Stroke Etiology) in the United States and EPITHET (Echoplanar Imaging Thrombolysis Evaluation Trial) in Australia [100] are other MR-imaging–based open studies, which perform therapy with rt-PA in the 3- to 6-hour time window.

Two parallel phase 2 trials (DIAS: Desmoteplase in Acute Ischemic Stroke) and DEDAS: Dose Escalation study of Desmoteplase in Acute Ischemic Stroke) with a 3- to 9-hour time window for another thrombolytic drug (desmoteplase) have recently been completed; the results of DIAS trials have been presented and were published in 2005 [101]. The most important results are that high doses of desmoteplase cause excessive bleeding, whereas body-weight adapted doses lead to an increase in early reperfusion, as measured with MR imaging, and clinical improvement. Imaging parameters parallel the clinical outcome proving that the MR imaging parameters function as appropriate surrogate markers. Also, within 3 to 9 hours it does not matter at which time the therapy is given. If mismatch is present, time from symptom onset is not the relevant factor. The DEDAS study replicated these results and will be presented in 2005 (Werner Hacke, MD, PhD, personal communication, 2005).

The combination of rt-PA with glycoprotein IIb/IIIa antagonists may be a promising approach and results in increased vessel patency rates, in accordance with the cardiology literature. These trials are currently only phase 1 and 2, but will include patients in late time windows up to 24 hours after stroke onset, using MR imaging findings as inclusion criteria from the following trials:

Tirofiban plus rt-PA: SATIS or Safety of Tirofiban in Acute Ischemic Stroke (Mario Siebler, MD, PhD, personal communication, 2005)

Abciximab plus retavase: ROSIE or Reopro Retavase Reperfusion of Stroke Safety Study–Imaging Evalution (Steven Warach, MD, PhD, personal communication, 2005)

Eptifibatide plus ASA, low molecular weight heparins, rt-PA: ROSIE 2 (Steven Warach, MD, PhD, personal communication, 2005)

Box 1. Priorities of intravenous thrombolysis

Priority 1: 0–3 hours; only unenhanced CT (FDA-approved)
Level I evidence
    NINDS and meta-analyses
All patients, regardless of age, who have:
    NIHSSS > 4
    NIHSSS ≤ 4 and disabling neurologic deficit due to aphasia, paresis, complete hemianopia
CT indication
    Normal CT or only mild cortical edema with/without leucoaraiosis
CT exclusion
    ICH
    Clear-cut, "real" hypodensity
    Marked early signs: > 1/3 MCA hypodensity or ASPECTS ≤7
Priority 2: 3 to 9 hours or unknown onse. Phase I–III and randomized controlled trials
Stroke MR imaging algorithm
All patients, regardless of age, who have:
    NIHSSS >4
    NIHSSS ≤ 4 and disabling neurologic deficit
MR imaging indication for rt-PA
    PWI ≥ DWI (mismatch) including leucoaraiosis, lacune, old microbleeds:
MR imaging contraindication for rt-PA
    ICH
    DWI > 1/3 MCA vascular territory, FLAIR/T2 clear-cut hyperintensity
    PWI negative or << DWI (negative match)
Priority 3: 3–9 hours or unknown onset; stroke DWI/PWI
Priority 4: 3–9 hours or unknown onset; stroke CTA/CTP
Priority 5: 3–4.5 hours; best local practice?

The ongoing trials section in *Stroke* lists most of these new and ongoing trials [102]. Once phase 3 MR-imaging-based trials are available and yield positive results, MR imaging should become the required imaging modality, as CT has now been for nearly a decade (Box 1).

MR imaging in the design of therapeutic trials in neurology

Four major factors are hypothesized to predict tissue response and clinical efficacy in stroke trials: (1) time to treatment, (2) salvageable tissue-at-risk, (3) relevance of the patient sample to the treatment, and (4) intrinsic effectiveness of the therapeutic strategy [66]. Time is an important factor [103], but it is not the only important factor hypothesized to effect response to therapy. A clinical trial optimized on *all* features would be expected to have the most robust response.

Stroke is a special case among brain diseases because it is a single event that is not progressive beyond the initial hours and days; there is a high rate of spontaneous clinical recovery (implying that clinical improvement is less reflective of drug effect); it requires rapid diagnosis under emergency conditions (the diagnostic certainty is less); and a single discrete lesion fully captures the pathology (the clinical manifestations result from the size and location of the ischemic damage).

For stroke, the true clinical endpoint, disability, is difficult to measure and is only approximated by clinical scales. Experts do not agree on how to measure outcome using clinical scales, and the criterion of "complete recovery" used in many trials may include patients with significant disability. For these reasons, lesion volume as a biomarker is likely to be more helpful for stroke than in cancer and cardiac disorders.

Ordinarily, a drug must have a beneficial effect on a clinical endpoint or on a validated surrogate endpoint to demonstrate effectiveness and lead to registration. Current FDA regulations stipulate that for unmet medical needs for serious and life-threatening conditions, such as stroke, a drug may be approved based on a nonvalidated surrogate endpoint if it is reasonably likely to have clinical benefit. The internationally accepted regulatory standards of the International Conference on Harmonization also state that surrogate endpoints may be used as primary endpoints at the time the surrogate is likely to predict clinical outcome. Beliefs about the use of biomarkers as measures of drug activity and potential surrogates have come from fields, such as oncology or cardiology, where death or a comparably objective and reliable assessment is the relevant clinical endpoint. For these disease categories, the biomarker does not fully capture the pathology of the disease nor the clinical endpoint. However, the use of biomarkers and potential surrogates are different for brain disorders in which disability (defined by imperfect clinical rating scales) rather than death is the relevant clinical variable, and in which the biomarker (macroscopic brain lesion) more fully captures the pathology than the clinical scales.

The pharmaceutical industry has taken the initiative in investigating this final step in validation. The results of several industry-sponsored drug trials using MR imaging as a surrogate will be known over the next several years, and those studies should provide the most decisive information regarding the use of MR imaging as a measure in stroke trials. MR-imaging-based recruitment into trials with time windows of 6 hours was proved feasible, as were selection based on lesion size, location, and the PWI/DWI-mismatch. The field of stroke clinical trials continues to examine opportunities for improving trial design, such as using imaging to confirm rather than exclude pathology, and for treatment assessment. That MR imaging is increasingly used as a selection tool and an outcome measure in stroke trials reflects the growing recognition that direct pathophysiologic imaging may provide a more rational approach to stroke therapeutics. Patient selection and outcomes based exclusively on clinical assessment and nonhemorrhagic admission CT scans may no longer be appropriate for all stroke trials.

Recommendations for future research

Larger studies of DWI and PWI are needed, with clear-cut clinical details (inclusions, exclusions, and failures), blinding of analyses, valid clinical outcome measures, and comparison with routine imaging, such as CT, so that an assessment of added clinical value of the combined multiparametric stroke MR imaging protocol—including presence or absence of arterial occlusion—can be made [104]. Therefore, research should center on the use of MRA along with DWI and PWI in predicting outcome. The imaging results of randomized trials of new or existing acute stroke treatments, where suspected stroke victims receive a screening MR imaging, are a potential source of CLASS I evidence. Further improvement of imaging techniques – including CTA/CTP for use at institutions where MR imaging is not available – that can reliably differentiate irreversibly damaged ischemic infarct core from critically hypoperfused but salvageable penumbral tissue, is an important objective for ongoing and future research.

Summary

New and more advanced diagnostic imaging techniques for acute stroke triage have the potential to not only improve the quality of care, but also reduce health care costs [105–107]. Although sufficiently large and methodologically sound studies with regard to cost effectiveness of MR imaging are lacking, the overall impression is that MR imaging has revolutionized not only the diagnosis but also the open and investigational management of neurologically ill patients.

References

[1] WHO Guidelines Subcommittee. 1999 World Health Organization-International society of hypertension guidelines for the management of hypertension. J Hypertens 1999;17(2):151–83.

[2] North American Symptomatic Carotid Endarterectomy Trial (NASCET) Collaborators. Beneficial effect of carotid endarterectomy in symptomatic patients with high-grade carotid stenosis. N Engl J Med 1991; 325(7):445–53.

[3] European Carotid Surgery Trialist's (ECST) Collaborative Group. MRC European Surgery Trial. Interim results for symptomatic patients with severe (70–99%) or with mild (0–29%) carotid stenosis. Lancet 1991;337:1235–43.

[4] EC/IC Bypass Study Group. Failure of extracranial-intracranial artery bypass to reduce the risk of ischemic stroke. Results of an international randomized trial. N Engl J Med 1985;313:1191–200.

[5] Antiplatelet Trialists' Collaboration. Warfarin versus aspirin for prevention of thromboembolism in atrial fibrillation—collaborative overview of randomised trials of antiplatelet therapy–I: prevention of death, myocardial infarction, and stroke by prolonged antiplatelet therapy in various categories of patients. Stroke Prevention in Atrial Fibrillation II Study. Nouv Rev Fr Hematol 1994;36(3):213–28.

[6] Antithrombotic Trialist's Collaboration. Collaborative meta-analysis of randomised trials of antiplatelet therapy for prevention of death, myocardial infarction, and stroke in high risk patients. BMJ 2002; 324(7329):71–86.

[7] Albers GW, Amarenco P, Easton JD, et al. Antithrombotic and thrombolytic therapy for ischemic stroke. Chest 2001;119:300S–20S.

[8] Meyer JS, Gilroy J, Barnhart MI, et al. Therapeutic thrombolysis in cerebral thromboembolism. Neurology 1963;13:927–37.

[9] Schellinger PD, Fiebach JB, Mohr A, et al. Thrombolytic therapy for ischemic stroke—a review. Part I—intravenous thrombolysis. Crit Care Med 2001;29(9):1812–8.

[10] Mori E, Yoneda Y, Tabuchi M, et al. Intravenous recombinant tissue plasminogen activator in acute carotid artery territory stroke. Neurology 1992;42(5): 976–82.

[11] Yamaguchi T, Hayakawa T, Kiuchi H, Japanese Thrombolysis Study Group. Intravenous tissue plasminogen activator ameliorates the outcome of hyperacute embolic stroke. Cerebrovasc Dis 1993;3: 269–72.

[12] The National Institute of Neurological Disorders and Stroke rt-PA Stroke Study Group. Tissue plasminogen activator for acute ischemic stroke. N Engl J Med 1995;333(24):1581–7.

[13] Albers GW, Amarenco P, Easton JD, et al. Antithrombotic and thrombolytic therapy for ischemic stroke: the Seventh ACCP Conference on Antithrombotic and Thrombolytic Therapy. Chest 2004; 126(Suppl 3):483S–512S.

[14] Haley Jr EC, Brott TG, Sheppard GL, et al. The TPA Bridging Study Group. Pilot randomized trial of tissue plasminogen activator in acute ischemic stroke. Stroke 1993;24(7):1000–4.

[15] Hacke W, Kaste M, Fieschi C, et al. The European Cooperative Acute Stroke Study. Intravenous thrombolysis with recombinant tissue plasminogen activator for acute hemispheric stroke. JAMA 1995;274: 1017–25.

[16] Hacke W, Kaste M, Fieschi C, et al. Randomised double-blind placebo-controlled trial of thrombolytic therapy with intravenous alteplase in acute ischaemic stroke (ECASS II). Lancet 1998;352:1245–51.

[17] Clark WM, Wissman S, Albers GW, et al. Recombinant tissue-type plasminogen activator (Alteplase) for ischemic stroke 3 to 5 hours after symptom onset. The ATLANTIS Study: a randomized controlled trial. Alteplase Thrombolysis for Acute Noninterventional Therapy in Ischemic Stroke. JAMA 1999;282(21): 2019–26.

[18] Early CT diagnosis of hemispheric brain infarction. In: von Kummer R, Bozzao L, Manelfe C, editors. 1st edition. Berlin Heidelberg: Springer Verlag; 1995.

[19] Patel SC, Levine SR, Tilley BC, et al. Lack of clinical significance of early ischemic changes on computed tomography in acute stroke. JAMA 2001;286: 2830–8.

[20] von Kummer R, Nolte PN, Schnittger H, et al. Detectability of cerebral hemisphere ischaemic infarcts by CT within 6 h of stroke. Neuroradiology 1996; 38(1):31–3.

[21] Hacke W, Donnan G, Fieschi C, et al. Association of outcome with early stroke treatment: pooled analysis of ATLANTIS, ECASS, and NINDS rt-PA stroke trials. Lancet 2004;363(9411):768–74.

[22] Wardlaw JM, del Zoppo G, Yamaguchi T. Thrombolysis for acute ischaemic stroke. Cochrane Database Syst Rev 2002;Vol Issue 1.

[23] Knauth M, Kummer Rv, Jansen O, et al. Potential of CT angiography in acute ischemic stroke. Am J Neuroradiol 1997;18:1001–10.

[24] Mohr JP, Biller J, Hilal SK, et al. Magnetic resonance versus computed tomographic imaging in acute stroke. Stroke 1995;26(5):807–12.

[25] Jackson A. Technical progress in neuroradiology and its application. In: Demaerel P, editor. Recent advances in diagnostic neuroradiology. Berlin Heidelberg: Springer-Verlag; 2001. p. 23–46.

[26] Lauterbur P. Image formation by induced local interactions: examples employing nuclear magnetic resonance. Nature 1973;242:190–1.

[27] Mansfield P, Maudsley AA. Line scan proton spin imaging in biological structures by NMR. Phys Med Biol 1976;21(5):847–52.

[28] Mansfield P, Maudsley AA. Medical imaging by NMR. Br J Radiol 1977;50(591):188–94.

[29] Warach S. Use of diffusion and perfusion magnetic resonance imaging as a tool in acute stroke clinical trials. Curr Control Trials Cardiovasc Med 2001;2(1):38–44.

[30] Hossman KA. Viability thresholds and the penumbra of focal ischemia. Ann Neurol 1994;36(4):557–65.

[31] Astrup J, Siesjö B, Symon L. Thresholds in cerebral ischemia—the ischemic penumbra. Stroke 1981;12:723–5.

[32] Belayev L, Saul I, Curbelo K, et al. Experimental intracerebral hemorrhage in the mouse: histological, behavioral, and hemodynamic characterization of a double-injection model. Stroke 2003;34(9):2221–7.

[33] Branston NM, Strong AJ, Symon L. Extracellular potassium activity, evoked potential and tissue blood flow. Relationships during progressive ischaemia in baboon cerebral cortex. J Neurol Sci 1977;32(3):305–21.

[34] Memezawa H, Minamisawa H, Smith ML, et al. Ischemic penumbra in a model of reversible middle cerebral artery occlusion in the rat. Exp Brain Res 1992;89(1):67–78.

[35] Larrue V, von Kummer RR, Muller A, et al. Risk factors for severe hemorrhagic transformation in ischemic stroke patients treated with recombinant tissue plasminogen activator: a secondary analysis of the European-Australasian Acute Stroke Study (ECASS II). Stroke 2001;32(2):438–41.

[36] Grond M, von Kummer R, Sobesky J, et al. Early computed-tomography abnormalities in acute stroke. Lancet 1997;350(9091):1595–6.

[37] Barber PA, Demchuk AM, Zhang J, et al. Validity and reliability of a quantitative computed tomography score in predicting outcome of hyperacute stroke before thrombolytic therapy. ASPECTS study group. Alberta stroke programme early CT score. Lancet 2000;355(9216):1670–4.

[38] Baron JC, vonKummer R, del Zoppo GJ. Treatment of acute ischemic stroke. Challenging the concept of a rigid and universal time window. Stroke 1995;26:2219–21.

[39] Mullins ME, Lev MH, Schellingerhout D, et al. Influence of the availability of clinical history on the noncontrast CT detection of acute stroke. AJR 2002;179(1):223–8.

[40] Griffiths PD, Wilkinson ID, Mitchell P, et al. Multimodality MR imaging depiction of hemodynamic changes and cerebral ischemia in subarachnoid hemorrhage. Am J Neuroradiol 2001;22(9):1690–7.

[41] Warach S, Chien D, Li W, et al. Fast magnetic resonance diffusion-weighted imaging of acute human stroke. Neurology 1992;42(9):1717–23.

[42] Heiland S, Reith W, Forsting M, et al. Perfusion-weighted magnetic resonance imaging using a new gadolinium complex as contrast agent in a rat model of focal cerebral ischemia. J Magn Reson Imaging 1997;7:1109–15.

[43] Ostergaard L, Weisskoff RM, Chesler DA, et al. High resolution measurement of cerebral blood flow using intravascular tracer bolus passages, part I: mathematical approach and statistical analysis. Magn Reson Med 1996;36:715–25.

[44] Moseley ME, Wendland MF, Kucharczyk J. Magnetic resonance imaging of diffusion and perfusion. Top Magn Reson Imaging 1991;3(3):50–67.

[45] Stejskal EO, Tanner JE. Spin diffusion measurements: spin echoes in the presence of a time-dependent field gradient. J Chem Phys 1965;42:288–92.

[46] Le Bihan D, Breton E, Lallemand D, et al. MR imaging of intravoxel incoherent motions: application to diffusion and perfusion in neurologic disorders. Radiology 1986;161(2):401–7.

[47] Le Bihan D, Turner R, Douek P, et al. Diffusion MR imaging: clinical applications. Am J Roentgenol 1992;159:591–9.

[48] Tanner JE, Stejskal EO. Restricted self-diffusion of protons in colloidal systems by the pulsed-gradient, spin-echo method. J Chem Phys 1968;49:1768–77.

[49] Basser PJ, Pierpaoli C. Microstructural and physiological features of tissues elucidated by quantitative-diffusion-tensor MRI. J Magn Reson B 1996;111:209–19.

[50] Le Bihan D, Mangin JF, Poupon C, et al. Diffusion tensor imaging: concepts and applications. J Magn Reson Imaging 2001;13(4):534–46.

[51] Pierpaoli C, Jezzard P, Basser PJ, et al. Diffusion tensor MR imaging of the human brain. Radiology 1996;201:637–48.

[52] Neil JJ, Shiran SI, McKinstry RC, et al. Normal brain in human newborns: apparent diffusion coefficient and diffusion anisotropy measured by using diffusion tensor MR imaging. Radiology 1998;209:57–66.

[53] Ono J, Harada K, Takahashi M, et al. Differentiation between dysmyelination and demyelination using

magnetic resonance diffusional anisotropy. Brain Res 1995;671:141–8.

[54] Kidwell CS, Saver JL, Mattiello J, et al. Thrombolytic reversal of acute human cerebral ischemic injury shown by diffusion/perfusion magnetic resonance imaging. Ann Neurol 2000;47(4):462–9.

[55] Fiehler J, Foth M, Kucinski T, et al. Severe ADC decreases do not predict irreversible tissue damage in humans. Stroke 2002;33(1):79–86.

[56] Fiehler J, Knudsen K, Kucinski T, et al. Predictors of apparent diffusion coefficient normalization in stroke patients. Stroke 2004;35(2):514–9.

[57] Kidwell CS, Alger JR, Saver JL. Beyond mismatch: evolving paradigms in imaging the ischemic penumbra with multimodal magnetic resonance imaging. Stroke 2003;34(11):2729–35.

[58] Villringer A, Rosen BR, Belliveau JW, et al. Dynamic imaging with lanthanide chelates in normal rat brain: contrast due to magnetic susceptibility effects. Magn Reson Med 1988;6:164–74.

[59] Rosen BR, Belliveau JW, Vevea JM, et al. Perfusion imaging with NMR contrast agents. Magn Reson Med 1990;14:249–65.

[60] Rosen BR, Belliveau JW, Chien D. Perfusion imaging by nuclear magnetic resonance. Magn Reson Q 1989;5(4):263–81.

[61] Schlaug G, Benfield A, Baird AE, et al. The ischemic penumbra: operationally defined by diffusion and perfusion MRI. Neurology 1999;53(7):1528–37.

[62] Weisskoff RM, Chesler D, Boxerman JL, et al. Pitfalls in MR measurements of tissue blood flow with intravascular tracers: which mean transit time? Magn Reson Med 1993;29:553–9.

[63] Wegener S, Gottschalk B, Jovanovic V, et al. Transient ischemic attacks before ischemic stroke: preconditioning the human brain? A multicenter magnetic resonance imaging study. Stroke 2004;35(3):616–21.

[64] Baird AE, Lovblad KO, Dashe JF, et al. Clinical correlations of diffusion and perfusion lesion volumes in acute ischemic stroke. Cerebrovasc Dis 2000;10(6):441–8.

[65] Schellinger PD, Fiebach JB, Jansen O, et al. Stroke magnetic resonance imaging within 6 hours after onset of hyperacute cerebral ischemia. Ann Neurol 2001;49(4):460–9.

[66] Neumann-Haefelin T, Wittsack HJ, Wenserski F, et al. Diffusion- and perfusion weighted MRI. The DWI/PWI mismatch region in acute stroke. Stroke 1999;30:1591–7.

[67] Sobesky J, Weber OZ, Lehnhardt FG, et al. Which time-to-peak threshold best identifies penumbral flow? A comparison of perfusion-weighted magnetic resonance imaging and positron emission tomography in acute ischemic stroke. Stroke 2004;35(12):2843–7.

[68] Warach S. Tissue viability thresholds in acute stroke: the 4-factor model. Stroke 2001;32(11):2460–1.

[69] Schellinger PD, Fiebach JB, Hacke W. Imaging-based decision making in thrombolytic therapy for ischemic stroke: present status. Stroke 2003;34(2):575–83.

[70] Chalela JA, Kang DW, Luby M, et al. Early magnetic resonance imaging findings in patients receiving tissue plasminogen activator predict outcome: insights into the pathophysiology of acute stroke in the thrombolysis era. Ann Neurol 2004;55(1):105–12.

[71] Latour LL, Kang DW, Ezzeddine MA, et al. Early blood-brain barrier disruption in human focal brain ischemia. Ann Neurol 2004;56(4):468–77.

[72] Kidwell CS, Saver JL, Villablanca JP, et al. magnetic resonance imaging detection of microbleeds before thrombolysis: an emerging application. Stroke 2002;33(1):95–8.

[73] Nighoghossian N, Hermier M, Adeleine P, et al. Old microbleeds are a potential risk factor for cerebral bleeding after ischemic stroke: a gradient-echo t2*-weighted brain MRI study. Stroke 2002;33(3):735–42.

[74] Derex L, Nighoghossian N, Hermier M, et al. Thrombolysis for ischemic stroke in patients with old microbleeds on pretreatment MRI. Cerebrovasc Dis 2004;17(2–3):238–41.

[75] Tsushima Y, Aoki J, Endo K. Brain microhemorrhages detected on T2*-weighted gradient-echo MR images. Am J Neuroradiol 2003;24(1):88–96.

[76] Davalos A, Toni D, Iweins F, et al. Neurological deterioration in acute ischemic stroke: potential predictors and associated factors in the European cooperative acute stroke study (ECASS) I. Stroke 1999;30(12):2631–6.

[77] Bertram M, Bonsanto M, Hacke W, et al. Managing the therapeutic dilemma: patients with spontaneous intracerebral hemorrhage and urgent need for anticoagulation. J Neurol 2000;247(3):209–14.

[78] Chalela JA, Haymore J, Schellinger PD, et al. Acute stroke patients are being underfed—a nitrogen balance study. Neurocrit Care 2004;1(3):331–4.

[79] Chalela JA, Ezzeddine M, Latour LL, et al. Reversal of perfusion and diffusion abnormalities after intravenous thrombolysis for a lacunar infarction. J Neuroimaging 2003;13:152–4.

[80] Benfield Y, Prasad PV, Edelman RR, et al. On the optimal b value for measurement of lesion volumes in acute human stroke by diffusion weighted imaging. Paper presented at: ISMRM, Fourth Scientific Meeting. Book of abstracts. 1996.

[81] Baird AE, Benfield A, Schlaug G, et al. Enlargement of human cerebral ischemic lesion volumes measured by diffusion-weighted magnetic resonance imaging. Ann Neurol 1997;41(5):581–9.

[82] Sorensen AG, Buonanno FS, Gonzalez RG, et al. Hyperacute stroke: evaluation with combined multisection diffusion-weighted and hemodynamically weighted echo-planar MR imaging. Radiology 1996;199(2):391–401.

[83] Tong DC, Yenari MA, Albers GW, et al. Correlation of perfusion- and diffusion-weighted MRI with

NIHSS score in acute (<6.5 hour) ischemic stroke. Neurology 1998;50(4):864–70.

[84] Barber PA, Darby DG, Desmond PM, et al. Prediction of stroke outcome with echoplanar perfusion- and diffusion-weighted MRI. Neurology 1998;51:418–26.

[85] Eckstein HH, Schumacher H, Dorfler A, et al. Carotid endarterectomy and intracranial thrombolysis: simultaneous and staged procedures in ischemic stroke. J Vasc Surg 1999;29(3):459–71.

[86] Adams Jr HP, Adams RJ, Brott T, et al. Guidelines for the early management of patients with ischemic stroke: a scientific statement from the stroke council of the American Stroke Association. Stroke 2003;34(4):1056–83.

[87] Budson AE, Schlaug G, Briemberg HR. Perfusion- and diffusion-weighted magnetic resonance imaging in transient global amnesia. Neurology 1999;53(1):239–40.

[88] Powers WJ, Zivin J. Magnetic resonance imaging in acute stroke: not ready for prime time. Neurology 1998;50(4):842–3.

[89] Powers WJ. Testing a test: a report card for DWI in acute stroke. Neurology 2000;54(8):1549–51.

[90] Zivin JA, Holloway RG. Weighing the evidence on DWI: caveat emptor. Neurology 2000;54(8):1552.

[91] Schellinger PD, Jansen O, Fiebach JB, et al. Feasibility and practicality of MR imaging of stroke in the management of hyperacute cerebral ischemia. Am J Neuroradiol 2000;21(7):1184–9.

[92] Buckley BT, Wainwright A, Meagher T, et al. Audit of a policy of magnetic resonance imaging with diffusion-weighted imaging as first-line neuroimaging for in-patients with clinically suspected acute stroke. Clin Radiol 2003;58(3):234–7.

[93] Engelhorn T, von Kummer R, Reith W, et al. What is effective in malignant middle cerebral artery infarction: reperfusion, craniectomy, or both? An experimental study in rats. Stroke 2002;33(2):617–22.

[94] Fiebach JB, Jansen O, Schellinger PD, et al. Serial analysis of the apparent diffusion coefficient time course in human stroke. Neuroradiology 2002;44:294–8.

[95] Fiebach JB, Schellinger PD, Gass A, et al. stroke magnetic resonance imaging is accurate in hyperacute intracerebral hemorrhage. A multicenter study on the validity of stroke imaging. Stroke 2004;35(2):502–7.

[96] Kidwell CS, Chalela JA, Saver JL, et al. Comparison of MRI and CT for detection of acute intracerebral hemorrhage. JAMA 2004;292(15):1823–30.

[97] Kaste M. Approval of alteplase in Europe: will it change stroke management? Lancet Neurol 2003;2(4):207–8.

[98] Fink JN, Kumar S, Horkan C, et al. The stroke patient who woke up: clinical and radiological features, including diffusion and perfusion MRI. Stroke 2002;33(4):988–93.

[99] Röther J, Schellinger PD, Gass A, et al. Intravenous effect of thrombolysis on MRI parameters and functional outcome in acute stroke <6h. Stroke 2002;33(10):2438–45.

[100] Parsons MW, Barber PA, Chalk J, et al. Diffusion- and perfusion-weighted MRI response to thrombolysis in stroke. Ann Neurol 2002;51(1):28–37.

[101] Hacke W, Albers G, Al-Rawi Y, et al. The Desmoteplase in Acute Ischemic Stroke Trial (DIAS): a phase II MRI-based 9-hour window acute stroke thrombolysis trial with intravenous desmoteplase. Stroke 2005;36(1):66–73.

[102] Major ongoing stroke trials. Stroke 2003;34(6):E61–72.

[103] Marler JR, Tilley BC, Lu M, et al. Early stroke treatment associated with better outcome: the NINDS rt-PA stroke study. Neurology 2000;55(11):1649–55.

[104] Keir SL, Wardlaw JM. Systematic review of diffusion and perfusion imaging in acute ischemic stroke. Stroke 2000;31(11):2723–31.

[105] Demaerel P. Guidelines for brain MR imaging. In: Demaerel P, editor. Recent advances in diagnostic neuroradiology. Berlin Heidelberg: Springer-Verlag; 2001. p. 91–105.

[106] Gleason S, Furie KL, Lev MH, et al. Potential influence of acute CT on inpatient costs in patients with ischemic stroke. Acad Radiol 2001;8:955–64.

[107] Barber PA, Zhang J, Demchuk AM, et al. Why are stroke patients excluded from TPA therapy?: an analysis of patient eligibility. Neurology 2001;56(8):1015–20.

ELSEVIER
SAUNDERS

Neuroimag Clin N Am 15 (2005) 259 – 272

NEUROIMAGING
CLINICS OF
NORTH AMERICA

Hemorrhagic Stroke

Eric E. Smith, MD, FRCPC[a,b,*], Jonathan Rosand, MD, MS[a,b],
Steven M. Greenberg, MD, PhD[b,c]

[a]Vascular and Critical Care Neurology, Massachusetts General Hospital, Boston, MA, USA
[b]Harvard Medical School, Boston, MA, USA
[c]Neurology Clinical Trials Unit, Massachusetts General Hospital, Boston, MA, USA

Hemorrhagic stroke accounts for approximately 15% of all stroke and is classified according to anatomic compartmentalization as intracerebral hemorrhage (ICH) (approximately two thirds) or subarachnoid hemorrhage (SAH) (approximately one third) [1]. This article discusses the use of CT and MR imaging for the differential diagnosis of ICH; for a detailed review of SAH, which is typically attributed to aneurysm rupture or severe trauma, the reader is referred elsewhere [2]. Topics to be discussed include the CT and MR imaging appearance of ICH, the differential diagnosis of ICH by location, and the imaging evaluation of acute stroke with regard to hemorrhage.

CT appearance of intracerebral hemorrhage

The CT appearance of hemorrhage is determined by the degree of attenuation of the x-ray beam, which is proportional to the density of hemoglobin protein (relative to plasma concentration) within the hematoma.

Immediately following vessel rupture, the hematoma consists of a collection of red blood cells, white blood cells, platelet clumps, and protein-rich serum

This work was supported by National Institutes of Health Grant K23 NS046327.

* Corresponding author. Stroke Service, VBK 802, Massachusetts General Hospital, 55 Fruit Street, Boston, MA 02114.

E-mail address: eesmith@partners.org (E.E. Smith).

that has a heterogeneous appearance on CT with attenuation in the range of 30–60 Hounsfield units (HU), depending on the degree of plasma extrusion [3]. In this hyperacute phase, hemorrhage may be difficult to distinguish from normal cortex because of similar attenuation. Over minutes to hours, a fibrin clot forms with an increase in attenuation to 60–80 HU (Fig. 1A) [3]. Clot retraction and extrusion of serum can further increase attenuation to as high as 80–100 HU in the center of the hematoma. The degree of attenuation may be reduced in patients with severe anemia [4], impaired clot formation due to coagulopathy, or volume averaging with adjacent tissue. Vasogenic edema evolves around the hematoma within hours and may continue to increase for up to 2 weeks after hemorrhage onset [5].

Over the following days, cells and protein are broken down and scavenged by macrophages, leading to slowly decreasing attenuation, with the greatest decrease at the periphery of the hematoma and more gradual evolution toward the center (Fig. 1B and C) [6]. Within 4 to 9 days, the hematoma attenuation decreases to that of normal cortex, and within 2 to 3 weeks to that of normal white matter [3].

The CT recognition of subacute intracerebral hematoma can be challenging because the attenuation is similar to that of normal brain tissue, although mass effect may still be present. MR imaging can confirm subacute hematoma. As time goes on, attenuation continues to decrease to levels below that of the normal brain. Eventually, the hematoma resolves into a fluid-filled or slit-like cavity that may be difficult to visualize on CT (Fig. 1D). Contrast enhancement is not present in the initial days following ICH but may

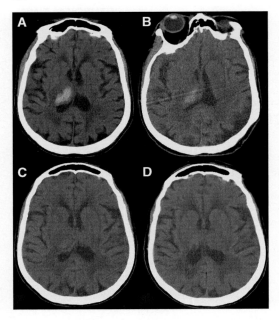

Fig. 1. CT appearance of hemorrhage. Serial CT scans of right thalamic hematoma. (*A*) Acute ICH in the right thalamus with mean attenuation 65 HU. (*B*) CT performed 8 days later than (*A*); the periphery of the hematoma is now isodense to the brain while the center of the hematoma has mean attenuation 45 HU. (*C*) CT performed 13 days later than (*A*) shows continued evolution of the hematoma with decreasing attenuation. (*D*) CT performed 5 months later than (*A*) shows a small area of encephalomalacia in the location of the previous hemorrhage.

develop at the periphery in weeks to months [7], sometimes leading to diagnostic confusion with brain tumor or abscess.

A blood-fluid level may be seen in medium to large ICH within the first hours after onset; the dependent portion displays higher attenuation (Fig. 2) due to sedimentation of cellular elements [8]. This finding may be more common in ICH caused by anticoagulation [9], but it is not specific and has also been described in ICH due to hypertension, trauma, tumor, or arterial-venous malformation. The association with shorter time interval from ICH onset, and in some cases with anticoagulation, has led to speculation that incomplete clotting is required for blood-fluid level formation.

MR appearance of intracerebral hemorrhage

The physics of MR imaging of hemorrhage is complex; multiple reviews have covered this topic in detail [10,11]. A brief explanation is warranted here, however, because an understanding of the signal characteristics of hemorrhage, as well as their evolution over time, is essential for radiologic interpretation.

The MR signal intensity of hemorrhage is dependent on both the chemical state of the iron atoms within the hemoglobin molecule and the integrity of the red blood cell membrane [12]. Iron can be either diamagnetic or paramagnetic, depending on the state of its outer electron orbitals. In the paramagnetic state, it alters the T1 and T2 relaxation times of water protons through magnetic dipole–dipole interactions and susceptibility effects. Dipole–dipole interactions shorten both the T1 and T2 relaxation times but have a greater effect on T1. Susceptibility effect is present when iron atoms are compartmentalized within the red cell membrane, causing magnetic field inhomogeneity, with resulting loss of phase coherence and selective shortening of the T2 relaxation time. After degradation of red cell membranes, the iron becomes more homogenously distributed, and this effect is nullified. Other factors that influence signal characteristics to a lesser extent include protein content, brain edema, oxygen tension, blood–brain barrier breakdown, thrombus formation, and clot retraction [11].

Both the chemical environment surrounding the hemoglobin iron atom and red cell membrane integrity undergo relatively predictable changes after ICH. The following section enumerates these changes in MR signal characteristics during the different phases of ICH evolution (Fig. 3 and Table 1).

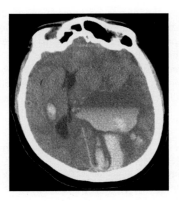

Fig. 2. CT with blood-fluid level. A 77-year-old woman was admitted with coma of 4 hours' duration. CT scan shows massive left hemispheric hematoma with blood-fluid level. No history of anticoagulation or coagulopathy.

Effect of hematoma evolution on MR imaging appearance of intracerebral hemorrhage

Hyperacute phase

The hyperacute phase of the hematoma is seen immediately following extravasation of blood into the brain parenchyma. At this stage the red cell membrane is intact, and the hemoglobin molecule is normally saturated with oxygen (oxy-hemoglobin). Specifically, the iron atoms contained within the heme portions of the hemoglobin molecule are bound to oxygen. This is the only phase of hematoma in which the iron atoms have no unpaired electrons in their outer orbitals and are therefore "diamagnetic," without exaggerated T1 relaxation or susceptibility effects. The ICH signal characteristics are thus not primarily attributable to iron but instead to the increased spin density of the hematoma relative to uninvolved brain tissue. Hyperacute hematoma appears slightly hypointense or iso-intense on T1-weighted images and slightly hyperintense on T2-weighted images (see Fig. 3); this pattern resembles that of many other pathologic conditions of the brain. Even early in the hyperacute phase, however, there is often deoxy-hemoglobin at the periphery of the hematoma, which appears as a thin rim of T2 hypointensity. This pattern can help differentiate hyperacute hematoma from other brain pathologies [13–16].

Acute phase

The acute phase, which begins within hours of ICH, is characterized by deoxy-hemoglobin. Deoxygenation occurs first at the periphery of the hematoma and progresses toward the center. This pattern appears because intrahematoma oxygen tension is lowest in the periphery, where red cells are adjacent to oxygen-starved tissue, and highest in the center, because red cells do not use oxygen for their metabolism. The iron atoms of deoxy-hemoglobin have five ligands

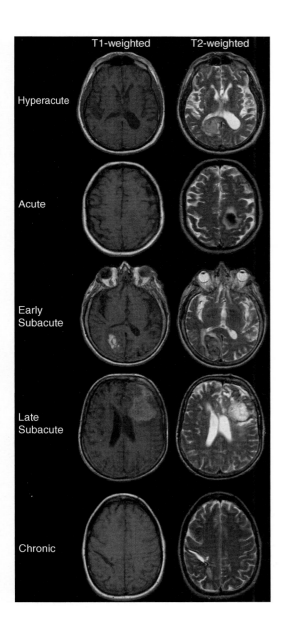

Fig. 3. MR imaging appearance of hemorrhage on T1-weighted (*left column*) and T2-weighted (*right column*) sequences for the different stages of hematoma (*rows*). Examples are selected from various patients. Hyperacute: There is relative isointensity on the T1-weighted and hyperintensity on the T2-weighted sequence of this right occipital hematoma. A small degree of vasogenic edema surrounds the hematoma. On the T2-weighted sequence there is a thin rim of hypointensity that is barely detectable in the periphery; this is caused by susceptibility effect from deoxy-hemoglobin. Acute: The marked hypointensity on the T2-weighted sequence of this left frontal hematoma is caused by susceptibility effect from deoxy-hemoglobin. Early subacute: The hyperintensity on the T1-weighted sequence of this right occipital hematoma is caused by the oxidation of deoxy-hemoglobin to met-hemoglobin. Late subacute: The hyperintensity on the T2-weighted sequence of this large left frontal hematoma results from the loss of susceptibility effect caused by degradation of the red cell membranes. The degree of vasogenic edema is lesser compared with earlier phases. Chronic: A former large right frontal hematoma has resolved into a slit-like cavity with a rim of hypointensity on the T2-weighted sequence caused by hemosiderin deposition.

Table 1
Evolution of MR imaging signal characteristics with time

Phase	Time	Iron-containing molecule	Iron oxidation state	Red cell membranes	T1	T2	T2*
Hyperacute	Hours	Oxyhemoglobin	Fe^{2+}	Intact	↓	↑	
Acute	Hours to days	Deoxyhemoglobin	Fe^{2+}	Intact	iso, ↓	↓	↓
Early subacute	Days to 1 week	Methemoglobin	Fe^{3+}	Intact	↑↑	↓	
Late subacute	1 week to months	Methemoglobin	Fe^{3+}	Degraded	↑↑	↑	
Chronic	≥ months	Hemosiderin	Fe^{3+}	Degraded	iso, ↓	↓	↓

Abbreviations: Fe, iron; iso, isointense relative to normal brain; ↑, hyperintense relative to brain, ↓, hypointense relative to brain.

and four unpaired electrons and hence are para-magnetic. Susceptibility effect is present because the iron is compartmentalized within intact red cell membranes, resulting in hypointensity on T2-weighted images that is due to increased T2* relaxation (see Fig. 3). Magnetic dipole–dipole inter-actions are prevented by the three-dimensional atomic structure of deoxy-hemoglobin, which blocks access of water protons to iron atoms. T1 relaxation times are therefore not shortened, and there is iso- or slight hypointensity on T1-weighted images (see Fig. 3). Sometimes a thin rim of T1 hyperintensity can be seen in the periphery of the hematoma, caused by early oxidation of intracellular deoxy-hemoglobin to intracellular met-hemoglobin.

Early subacute phase

After several days, the early subacute phase begins. The production of reducing substances de-clines with failure of red cell metabolism, and the iron atoms are oxidized to the ferric state, Fe^{3+}, to produce met-hemoglobin. Magnetic dipole–dipole interactions can occur because the three-dimensional structure of met-hemoglobin exposes the iron atoms to water protons. This pattern leads to decreased T1 relaxation times and marked hyperintensity on T1-weighted images. Susceptibility effect is present because the red cell membranes remain intact, and hence there is continued hypointensity on T2-weighted images (see Fig. 3).

Late subacute phase

Over several days to weeks, the red cell membranes are degraded, and the late subacute phase begins. Susceptibility effect is lost because met-hemoglobin is no longer locally sequestered within red cell membranes; it freely diffuses within the hematoma cavity, resulting in a locally homogeneous magnetic field. This pattern leads to T2* lengthening, and hence to increased hyperintensity, on T2-weighted images (see Fig. 3).

Chronic phase

Over the ensuing months, the hematoma enters the chronic phase. The degree of hyperintensity on T1- and T2-weighted images lessens as the concen-tration of met-hemoglobin decreases with protein breakdown. The center of the hematoma may evolve into a fluid-filled cavity with signal characteristics identical to cerebrospinal fluid, or the walls of the cavity may collapse, leaving only a thin slit (see Fig. 3). As proteins are degraded, the iron atoms become liberated from the heme molecules, scav-enged by macrophages, and converted into ferritin, which can be recycled. In most cases, however, the degree of iron deposition overwhelms the recycling capacity, with the excess being locally concentrated in hemosiderin molecules. The iron in hemosiderin does not have access to water protons and therefore exerts only susceptibility effect without significant dipole–dipole interactions, leading to marked hypo-intensity on T2-weighted images. This hypointensity is seen at the rim of the hematoma cavity and may persist indefinitely.

In practice, there is considerable variability in the orderly progression of hematoma signal change over time. The evolution of these signal characteristics may be influenced by a number of factors, including ICH size, oxygen tension, integrity of the blood–brain barrier, the presence of rebleeding, the effi-ciency of the patient's intrinsic repair processes, and the presence of an underlying lesion such as an arte-riovenous malformation or tumor [11]. It is common to see different stages appear simultaneously. For these reasons, "dating" of bleed onset using MR imaging data alone is intrinsically imprecise.

MR imaging pulse sequences and intracerebral hemorrhage appearance

Hematoma signal characteristics are determined by the specific MR imaging pulse sequence applied. Higher magnetic field strength increases sensitivity to susceptibility effects and therefore should allow easier identification of hemorrhage. Fast spin-echo (FSE) sequences are less sensitive to magnetic susceptibility effects, owing to multiple 180° refocusing pulses, whereas echo planar imaging (EPI) and gradient recalled echo (GRE) sequences, which lack a 180° pulse, are more sensitive. Therefore, the use of FSE with relatively low-field-strength magnets, a common situation in clinical practice, is associated with a lesser degree of T2-hypointensity than is that of EPI or GRE sequences on higher-strength magnets [10,17,18].

To overcome these limitations, GRE sequences should be used whenever the identification of hemorrhage is clinically important. The GRE sequence—also known as susceptibility-weighted or T2*-weighted sequence—employs a partial flip angle without a refocusing pulse. In contrast to the use of the 180° spin-echo refocusing pulse, this method does not compensate for signal loss due to magnetic field inhomogeneities, thus producing a stronger susceptibility effect. This pattern increases sensitivity for hematoma detection in the acute and chronic stages, because the already strong susceptibility effect causes extreme hypointensity on GRE sequences (Fig. 4) [10,19]. A relative disadvantage of the GRE sequence, however, is that artifactual signal loss is generated at the boundary of tissues that normally exhibit differences in susceptibility. This signal loss is particularly prominent at the pneumatized sinuses at the skull base and may obscure underlying lesions in those areas.

Small hemosiderin deposits due to chronic, prior asymptomatic hemorrhage, sometimes referred to as "microbleeds" [20], are often only visualized on the GRE sequence. These may provide a clue to other-wise unsuspected underlying amyloid angiopathy, cavernous malformations, or hypertensive microvascular disease [21–23]. Evidence suggests that, although most hemosiderin deposits persist indefinitely, as many as 20% may become unapparent at 2 years [24]. Because most of these deposits are long lasting, the GRE sequence can be used to determine the cumulative hemorrhagic "history" of the patient over a prolonged period of time.

Causes of intracerebral hemorrhage

Large cohort studies have identified the following risk factors for hemorrhagic stroke: age, hypertension, African-American or Hispanic ethnicity, smoking, excessive alcohol consumption, prior ischemic stroke, low serum cholesterol, and anticoagulant medications [25]. Age and hypertension account for the greatest risk to the population. It must be recognized, however, that ICH is not a single pathologic entity and may result from a number of diseases with differing pathophysiology and risk factors. It is the responsibility of the radiologist to recognize findings that may support or refute the underlying differential diagnostic causes of ICH (Box 1). Radiologic clues to the cause of ICH may come from the topographic pattern, the signal characteristics, and the presence of other related lesions.

Effect of location on cause of intracerebral hemorrhage

The causes of ICH vary by location. The frequency of primary ICH at different sites, when not

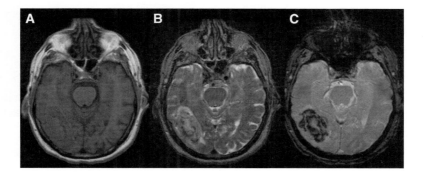

Fig. 4. GRE sequence. T1- (*A*) and T2-weighted (*B*) MR imaging sequences show acute hematoma of the right occipital lobe. Areas of hypointensity are seen on the T2-weighted sequence (*B*), caused by susceptibility effect from intracellular deoxy-hemoglobin. The susceptibility effect is far more conspicuous on the GRE sequence (*C*).

Box 1. Causes of intracerebral hemorrhage

Hypertension
Cerebral amyloid angiopathy
Vascular malformations
  Arteriovenous malformation
  Arteriovenous dural fistula
  Cavernous hemangioma
Hemorrhagic transformation of ischemic stroke
  Related to arterial infarction
  Related to venous infarction
Vasculitis
Moyamoya disease
Coagulopathy
  Related to anticoagulant use
  Related to thrombolytic use
  Thrombocytopenia
  Decreased synthesis of clotting factors (eg, hemophilia, liver disease)
  Increased consumption of clotting factors (eg, disseminated intravascular coagulation)
Brain tumor
Aneurysm
  Ruptured berry aneurysm
  Ruptured mycotic aneurysm
Related to sympathomimetic drug use
  Amphetamines
  Cocaine
  Phenylpropanolamine
  Ephedrine
Trauma

Table 2
Location of primary of intracranial hematoma

Location	No. of cases	%
Lobar	114	35
Striatum (putamen and caudate nucleus)	89	27
Thalamus	64	19
Cerebellum	34	10
Multiple	14	4
Brainstem	12	4
Intraventricular	3	1

Location of ICH in 330 consecutive patients age >18 y with primary ICH admitted to Massachusetts General Hospital between January 2001 and December 2004. Hemorrhages due to trauma, infarction, aneurysm, coagulopathy, tumor or vascular malformations were excluded. ICH in the striatum, thalamus, cerebellum and brainstem was most common (60%); these locations are typical for hypertensive hemorrhage.

risk factor for nonlobar but not lobar ICH (relative risk = 1.0) [26]. Conversely, apolipoprotein E genotype was a strong risk factor for lobar but not nonlobar ICH. The lack of association between hypertension and lobar ICH is notable and suggests

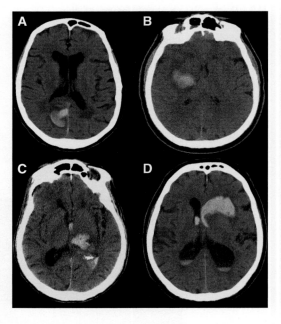

Fig. 5. Lobar and deep hemispheric ICH. (*A*) Lobar ICH in the medial right occipital lobe. (*B*) Putaminal ICH originating from the posterior right putamen. (*C*) Left thalamic ICH dissecting medially into the ventricular system, with hemorrhage in the third and ipsilateral lateral ventricle. (*D*) Left caudate hemorrhage extending laterally into the white matter and medially into the ventricular system.

due to identifiable structural lesions, is shown in Table 2.

Supratentorial hemorrhages should be stratified into lobar and nonlobar ICH (Fig. 5). "Lobar ICH" is defined as hemorrhage at the superficial part of the brain, where bleeding is centered at the cortico–subcortical boundary. "Deep ICH" is defined as hemorrhage in the deeper internal supratentorial compartment, with the hemorrhage centered principally in the putamen, head of the caudate nucleus, or thalamus. The site of origin can be difficult to determine when the hemorrhage is massive; in cases where both deep and subcortical structures are involved, the site of origin is more likely to be deep.

A population-based study comparing lobar to nonlobar ICH showed that hypertension was a strong that lobar and nonlobar hemorrhage have different causes. Most cases of deep ICH in the elderly are caused by hypertensive vasculopathy [27], whereas most lobar ICH in the elderly is caused by cerebral amyloid angiopathy (CAA). Pathologic evidence of CAA was found in 74% of lobar ICH patients over 55 years of age in a North American cohort [28]. Even among the elderly with hypertension, most lobar ICH was due to CAA [28]. In younger normotensive patients, particularly those aged less than 45 years [29], prevalence of both hypertensive vasculopathy and CAA is reduced. Therefore, other causes of deep and lobar ICH, such as vascular malformation, underlying tumor, underlying cavernous malformation, and hypertensive crisis induced by exogenous sympathomimetic drugs, should be considered in this age group.

Brain stem hemmorhage

Brain stem hemorrhage (Fig. 6) most often occurs in the pons. Common causes include hypertensive vasculopathy, arteriovenous malformation, and cavernous malformation [30]. Mortality exceeds 60% when hypertension is the causative agent but is less for vascular malformation [30].

Cerebellar hemorrhage

Cerebellar hemorrhage (Fig. 7) is a neurosurgical emergency because the limited volume capacity of the posterior fossa leads to compression of critical brain stem structures. Typical complications of cerebellar hemorrhage include brain stem compression with cranial nerve palsy, respiratory arrest, upward and downward cerebellar herniation, and ventricular compression with acute obstructive hydrocephalus [31]. Prompt neurosurgical consultation is manda-

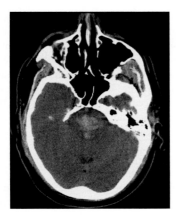

Fig. 6. Brain stem ICH. Hemorrhage is present in the central pons with extension into the aqueduct of Silvius.

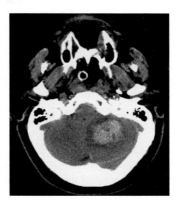

Fig. 7. Cerebellar ICH. Hemorrhage is present in the left lateral cerebellum with mild surrounding vasogenic edema.

tory; suboccipital craniectomy with hematoma resection may be life saving. Causes of cerebellar ICH include hypertension, arteriovenous malformation, and, rarely, CAA [31,32].

Intraventricular hemorrhage

Intraventricular hemorrhage is uncommon without parenchymal involvement. Before concluding an absence of parenchymal involvement, one should carefully examine the head of the caudate and thalamus, because even minute hemorrhage in these locations may quickly rupture into the ventricular system. Primary intraventricular hemorrhage has been associated with hypertension, anterior communicating artery aneurysm, anticoagulation, vascular malformation, moyamoya disease, and intraventricular neoplasm [33,34].

Multiple simultaneous intracranial hematoma

Multiple simultaneous ICH at different locations is uncommon and has been associated with coagulopathy, infarction, tumor, CAA, vasculitis, and hypertension [35,36].

Specific causes of intracerebral hemorrhage

ICH due to hypertensive vasculopathy, CAA, or an unknown cause is often referred to as "primary ICH" to distinguish it from ICH due to other defined causes, such as vascular malformation, tumor, trauma, and infarction. The following section describes the imaging features of primary ICH, as well as several important causes of secondary ICH.

Hypertensive hemorrhage

Even in this era of improving blood pressure control, hypertensive vasculopathy remains the most common cause of ICH, although the incidence is declining [37]. Chronic hypertension causes a degenerative cerebral microangiopathy, characterized by hyalinization of the walls of small arteries and arterioles, and ultimately fibrinoid necrosis. Small areas of red cell extravasation may be associated with vessel wall cracking or microaneurysmal dilatation of the arteriole (also referred to as Charcot-Brouchard aneurysms) [38].

ICH caused by hypertension most commonly results from rupture of the 50- to 200-μm–diameter lenticulostriate arteries that arise from the middle cerebral artery stem, leading to putaminal or caudate hemorrhage. It may also result from rupture of small perforating branches that arise from the basilar artery, leading to pontine or thalamic bleeds (see Figs. 5 and 6). Larger hematomas often dissect into the ventricles. Hypertensive vasculopathy is also a common cause of cerebellar ICH (see Fig. 7).

Cerebral amyloid angiopathy

CAA is caused by the deposition of β-amyloid in the arterial media/adventitia of the small arteries/arterioles in the meninges, cortex, and cerebellum. Affected vessels have eosinophilic walls that stain homogeneously with Congo red and demonstrate apple-green birefringence when viewed under polarized light [39]. The major risk factors for CAA-related hemorrhage are age and the presence of either the apolipoprotein E ε4 allele—which is associated with greater amyloid burden [40]—or the apolipoprotein E ε2 allele, which is associated with more severe vasculopathic change [41,42]. CAA-related hemorrhage is rare in persons aged less than 55 years, although the incidence increases exponentially in subsequent decades [43]. Recurrent hemorrhage is more frequent in CAA-related lobar ICH than in hypertensive ICH [44]. The risk of future recurrence is higher in patients with an apolipoprotein E ε2 or ε4 allele [45], moderate-to-severe white matter lesion burden [46], increased baseline number of MR imaging–detectable hemorrhages [47], and increased rate of new MR-detectable microbleeds [47].

CAA causes lobar hemorrhage in the cortex or subcortical white matter of the cerebrum [43] or, more rarely, the cerebellum [32]. Dissection into the subarachnoid space is common, whereas ventricular extension is uncommon. Rarely, CAA may present with solely sulcal SAH, thus mimicking aneurismal SAH [48]. CAA is frequently associated with clinically silent microbleeds remote from the symptomatic ICH (Fig. 8) [21]. Elderly patients with lobar ICH and multiple lobar microbleeds are highly likely to have CAA; the high specificity of this

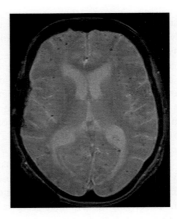

Fig. 8. Clinically silent microbleeds in amyloid angiopathy. A 72-year-old woman presented with cognitive impairment; cortical biopsy showed amyloid angiopathy. MR imaging–GRE sequence showed numerous cortical microbleeds with sparing of the deep hemispheric structures, including thalamus and basal ganglia. These lesions were not seen on the T2-weighted sequence. Sulcal vessels and calcification can also appear as small areas of hypointensity on the GRE sequence and must be distinguished from microbleeds.

radiographic syndrome has been incorporated into a rating scale for diagnostic certainty of CAA [28]. The presence of any microbleeds in deep hemispheric locations should, conversely, put the diagnosis of CAA in doubt.

Warfarin-related hemorrhage

The strongest risk factor for warfarin-related hemorrhage is intensity of anticoagulation; age and history of ischemic stroke are additional independent risk factors [49]. The superimposed presence of leukoaraiosis appears to further increase risk [50,51]. A substantial proportion of elderly patients who have warfarin-related hemorrhage have underlying CAA [52]. Most studies have found no difference in hemorrhage location between patients taking and those not taking warfarin [53], although others have found an excess of cerebellar hemorrhage [54]. Warfarin-related hematomas are more likely to expand [55] and to have fatal outcomes [56].

Vascular malformations

Vascular malformations that can bleed include arteriovenous malformations, arteriovenous dural fistulas, and cavernous malformations (also known as cavernomas). Both venous angiomas (also known as developmental venous anomalies [DVAs]) and

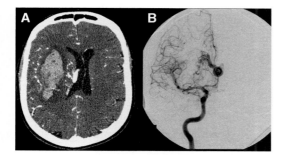

Fig. 9. ICH due to arteriovenous malformation. CT angiogram (*A*) shows a large acute hemorrhage in the right hemisphere, with multiple feeding vessels in the periventricular white matter. There is a large draining vein along the lateral wall of the right lateral ventricle. Catheter angiography (*B*, anteroposterior view of right carotid injection) confirms the presence of arteriovenous malformation.

capillary telangiectasias are generally benign lesions, which are almost never associated with hemorrhage (although as many as 25% of DVAs are associated with an underlying cavernoma). Arteriovenous malformations and arteriovenous dural fistulas can be difficult to detect without conventional catheter arteriography; suggestive but not sensitive imaging findings include dilated feeding and draining vessels on MR T2-weighted sequences, CT angiography, or MR angiography, as well as patchy enhancement (Fig. 9) [57]. Similarly, cavernous malformations are typically "silent" on all imaging modalities unless they have recently or previously bled. When recent, they may appear as "popcorn"-like lesions on T2-weighted MR images because of the presence of multiple small hemorrhages of different ages arising from the same lesion (Fig. 10). When they are

chronic, the hemosiderin from prior macro- or microhemorrhage may only be detectable on MR GRE sequences. These lesions may be multiple and familial [57].

Hemorrhagic transformation of brain infarction

Infarcted brain tissue has a propensity to bleed. A common classification scheme differentiates between hemorrhagic infarction, which does not produce mass effect and is usually asymptomatic, and parenchymal hematoma, which is more extensive and may be associated with neurologic deterioration [58]. Hemorrhage due to brain infarction may be recognized by the presence of surrounding cytotoxic edema conforming to an arterial territory, but it may be difficult to diagnose when early massive hemorrhage obscures the underlying infarct [59]. Venous infarction carries a higher risk for bleeding than arterial infarction, although anticoagulation treatment is typically *indicated*—not contraindicated—in the setting of venous thrombosis [60].

Brain tumors

Brain tumors are associated with neovascularity, incompetence of the blood–brain barrier, and an increased risk for hemorrhage [61]. Tumors with a particular propensity to hemorrhage include glioblastoma multiforme, oligodendroglioma, and certain metastases such as melanoma, renal cell carcinoma, choriocarcinoma, and thyroid carcinoma (mnemonic: MR/CT). Lung cancer is also frequently hemorrhagic [61–64]. In some cases, the tumor may be asymptomatic and unrecognized until presentation with hemorrhage.

The CT and MR imaging characteristics of tumor-associated hematoma are often atypical and complex,

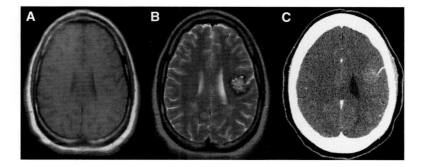

Fig. 10. Cavernous malformation. T1- (*A*) and T2-weighted (*B*) MR sequences show a large cavernous malformation in the left frontal lobe. T2-weighted sequence (*B*) shows a heterogenous central core of variable hyperintensity surrounded by a deeply hypointense rim, caused by hemorrhage of various ages surrounded by hemosiderin-stained tissue. CT angiogram (*C*) reveals this lesion to be associated with a venous angioma.

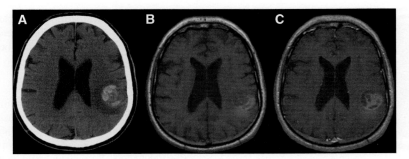

Fig. 11. ICH originating within brain tumor. CT scan (*A*) shows acute hemorrhage with marked surrounding edema. T1-weighted MR imaging (*B*) shows hyperintensity within the hematoma, consistent with met-hemoglobin (subacute hemorrhage). Following contrast administration (*C*), there is a marked increased central hyperintensity on the T1-weighted sequence. Biopsy showed an underlying glioblastoma multiforme.

because the blood may be of multiple ages and may be admixed with abnormal neoplastic tissue containing cysts and necrosis. Evolution of the MR signal changes is often delayed, possibly because of extremely low intratumoral partial pressure of oxygen, and hemosiderin formation may be absent [65,66]. The location may be atypical for hemorrhage caused by cerebrovascular disease, and there may be multiple simultaneous hemorrhages. The degree of vasogenic edema surrounding tumor-associated hemorrhage is greater than that in primary ICH and persists even into the chronic phase of hematoma [67]. Administration of contrast may reveal tumor enhancement (Fig. 11); the specificity of this enhancement for tumor is reduced in the subacute phase by enhancement of the hematoma capsule. In some cases, hemorrhage may completely obscure the underlying lesion; repeat imaging after hematoma resolution can allow tumor detection.

Ruptured saccular aneurysm

Blood from a ruptured saccular aneurysm enters the subarachnoid space under great pressure and may dissect into the brain parenchyma. Parenchymal hematoma is seen in 4% to 19% of patients with SAH due to saccular aneurysm and is highly correlated with the location of the ruptured aneurysm [68]. The most common locations are the medial frontal lobe adjacent to a ruptured anterior communicating artery or anterior cerebral artery aneurysm (Fig. 12) and the temporal lobe adjacent to a ruptured middle cerebral artery aneurysm. In some cases, the amount of associated subarachnoid blood may be minimal. When ICH is immediately adjacent to the subarachnoid space at the base of the brain or basal interhemispheric fissure, vascular imaging

should be strongly considered to exclude saccular aneurysm.

Cerebral contusion

Brain contusion deserves mention because of the potential for misclassification as hemorrhagic stroke when a history of trauma cannot be elicited—for example, in a patient found alone and confused. Contusions frequently occur in the basal anterior frontal and temporal lobes, where the brain is adjacent to the bony floor of the anterior and middle cranial fossa [69]. They may also be seen in the cortex either on the same side as the injury or as contrecoup. Contusions may be multiple and are often associated with other evidence of trauma, such as

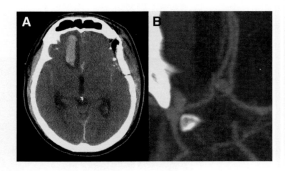

Fig. 12. ICH due to ruptured saccular aneurysm. CT scan (*A*) shows hemorrhage in the right medial basal frontal lobe. Subarachnoid hemorrhage is seen in both sylvian fissures and in the interhemispheric fissure. (A left skull defect with mild pneumocephalus is due to recent craniotomy for aneurysm clipping.) Maximum intensity projection images from the preoperative CT angiogram (*B*) reveal an anterior communicating artery aneurysm as the bleeding source.

skull fracture, subdural hematoma, and epidural or subgaleal hematoma.

Imaging evaluation for hemorrhage in the acute stroke setting

Management decisions in the acute stroke setting rely on the differentiation of hemorrhagic from ischemic stroke. Imaging is required to make this differentiation, because there are no clinical features that reliably predict hemorrhagic stroke [1]. Demonstration of hemorrhagic absence identifies ischemic stroke patients who may be eligible for thrombolysis, whereas demonstration of hemorrhagic presence may, in the future, identify acute ICH patients eligible for medical therapies to prevent continued bleeding. One such therapy currently under investigation is recombinant activated factor VII, which has shown promising results in a phase II study [70].

CT has traditionally been preferred over MR imaging for identification of ICH. CT scanning is faster, less expensive, and more widely available; it can be safely performed in patients with contraindications to MR, including claustrophobia. Moreover, the sensitivity of conventional MR imaging for hyperacute hematoma detection has been questioned, because the oxy-hemoglobin stage of hemorrhage is isointense to water (see Table 1) [10]. Ample evidence indicates, however, that even in the earliest stages of hemorrhage, deoxy-hemoglobin is present in the lesion periphery, with corresponding hypointensity on T2 and GRE sequences [13–16].

MR imaging has potential advantages over CT in the evaluation of ischemic stroke, both for delineating the extent of infarction with diffusion-weighted imaging (DWI) and detecting the presence of hemorrhagic complications with GRE sequences. MR may be superior to CT for the detection of early hemorrhagic conversion of infarction [71–73], and, in patients who undergo intra-arterial thrombolysis, it may be better at distinguishing between hemorrhage and contrast extravasations (postlysis "blush") into infarcted regions [74].

MR imaging is definitely more sensitive than CT for the detection of chronic microbleeds [71], which have been linked in at least one report to a higher risk of subsequent hemorrhagic transformation of infarction [75]. Although it has been suggested [76,77]—though not proved [78]—that the presence of baseline microbleeds could be a risk factor for major hemorrhage following thrombolysis, this hypothesis has yet to affect clinical management.

Two blinded studies have compared CT and conventional MR imaging with MR GRE sequence for the detection of acute ICH in stroke patients. One study, which used acute ICH cases and selected ischemic stroke controls, found that MR imaging detected ICH with 100% sensitivity and 100% specificity [79]. The other study, which used a multicenter prospective cohort design, found that GRE MR imaging was more sensitive than CT for both the diagnosis of hemorrhagic transformation and the detection of chronic microbleeds. As noted earlier, however, GRE MR imaging is sensitive but not specific: 3 of 29 acute ICH cases in this study were misclassified as chronic ICH. This lack of specificity may help to explain why inter-rater reliability for detection of ICH was lower for MR imaging ($\kappa = .75$ to $.82$) than for CT ($\kappa = .87$ to $.94$). Moreover, although GRE is sensitive for ICH detection, its sensitivity for SAH detection is dubious at best; the one case of SAH in the study discussed earlier was not detected by GRE [71]. The available data therefore suggest that it is feasible to use MR as the sole imaging modality for acute stroke evaluation, but that expert interpretation should be available and that caution should be exercised when excluding SAH.

The relative role of CT angiography or MR angiography in the emergent evaluation of the ICH patient has not been fully defined. Vascular imaging has the potential to identify secondary causes of ICH that might require urgent surgical treatment, such as saccular aneurysm or vascular malformation [80]. In one study, extravasation of CT angiography contrast into the hematoma, possibly representing active bleeding, was seen in 46% of patients studied at a mean of 4.5 hours and was associated with increased mortality [81].

Summary

Neuroimaging by CT or MR is necessary for the detection of hemorrhagic stroke and provides important data regarding the cause of stroke. Serial changes in the CT and MR appearance of hematoma attributable to temporal evolution must be assessed to assure accurate diagnosis. Emerging evidence suggests that the use of MR imaging alone may be adequate for identifying hemorrhage in acute stroke patients and that GRE MR imaging is superior to both CT and conventional spin-echo MR imaging sequences for the detection of chronic microbleeds and hemorrhagic conversion of infarction.

References

[1] Mohr JP, Caplan LR, Melski JW, et al. The Harvard Cooperative Stroke Registry: a prospective registry. Neurology 1978;28(8):754–62.

[2] Lasner TM, Raps EC. Clinical evaluation and management of aneurysmal subarachnoid hemorrhage. Neuroimaging Clin N Am 1997;7(4):669–78.

[3] Bergstrom M, Ericson K, Levander B, et al. Variation with time of the attenuation values of intracranial hematomas. J Comput Assist Tomogr 1977;1(1):57–63.

[4] Kasdon DL, Scott RM, Adelman LS, et al. Cerebellar hemorrhage with decreased absorption values on computed tomography: a case report. Neuroradiology 1977;13(5):265–6.

[5] Inaji M, Tomita H, Tone O, et al. Chronological changes of perihematomal edema of human intracerebral hematoma. Acta Neurochir Suppl 2003;86: 445–8.

[6] Dolinskas CA, Bilaniuk LT, Zimmerman RA, et al. Computed tomography of intracerebral hematomas. I. Transmission CT observations on hematoma resolution. AJR Am J Roentgenol 1977;129(4):681–8.

[7] Messina AV. Computed tomography: contrast enhancement in resolving intracerebral hemorrhage. AJR Am J Roentgenol 1976;127(6):1050–2.

[8] Ichikawa K, Yanagihara C. Sedimentation level in acute intracerebral hematoma in a patient receiving anticoagulation therapy: an autopsy study. Neuroradiology 1998;40(6):380–2.

[9] Pfleger MJ, Hardee EP, Contant Jr CF, et al. Sensitivity and specificity of fluid-blood levels for coagulopathy in acute intracerebral hematomas. AJNR Am J Neuroradiol 1994;15(2):217–23.

[10] Bradley Jr WG. MR appearance of hemorrhage in the brain. Radiology 1993;189(1):15–26.

[11] Atlas SW, Thulborn KR. Intracranial hemorrhage. In: Atlas SW, editor. Magnetic resonance imaging of the brain and spine. 3rd edition. Philadelphia: Lippincott Williams & Wilkins; 2002. p. 773–832.

[12] Gomori JM, Grossman RI, Goldberg HI, et al. Intracranial hematomas: imaging by high-field MR. Radiology 1985;157(1):87–93.

[13] Linfante I, Llinas RH, Caplan LR, et al. MRI features of intracerebral hemorrhage within 2 hours from symptom onset. Stroke 1999;30(11):2263–7.

[14] Patel MR, Edelman RR, Warach S. Detection of hyperacute primary intraparenchymal hemorrhage by magnetic resonance imaging. Stroke 1996;27(12): 2321–4.

[15] Wiesmann M, Mayer TE, Yousry I, et al. Detection of hyperacute parenchymal hemorrhage of the brain using echo-planar T2*-weighted and diffusion-weighted MRI. Eur Radiol 2001;11(5):849–53.

[16] Wintermark M, Maeder P, Reichhart M, et al. MR pattern of hyperacute cerebral hemorrhage. J Magn Reson Imaging 2002;15(6):705–9.

[17] Allkemper T, Tombach B, Schwindt W, et al. Acute and subacute intracerebral hemorrhages: comparison of MR imaging at 1.5 and 3.0 T—initial experience. Radiology 2004;232(3):874–81.

[18] Wolansky LJ, Holodny AI, Sheth MP, et al. Double-shot magnetic resonance imaging of cerebral lesions: fast spin-echo versus echo planar sequences. J Neuroimaging 2000;10(3):131–7.

[19] Liang L, Korogi Y, Sugahara T, et al. Detection of intracranial hemorrhage with susceptibility-weighted MR sequences. AJNR Am J Neuroradiol 1999;20(8): 1527–34.

[20] Fazekas F, Kleinert R, Roob G, et al. Histopathologic analysis of foci of signal loss on gradient-echo T2*-weighted MR images in patients with spontaneous intracerebral hemorrhage: evidence of microangiopathy-related microbleeds. AJNR Am J Neuroradiol 1999;20(4):637–42.

[21] Greenberg SM, Finklestein SP, Schaefer PW. Petechial hemorrhages accompanying lobar hemorrhage: detection by gradient-echo MRI. Neurology 1996;46(6): 1751–4.

[22] Jeong SW, Jung KH, Chu K, et al. Clinical and radiologic differences between primary intracerebral hemorrhage with and without microbleeds on gradient-echo magnetic resonance images. Arch Neurol 2004; 61(6):905–9.

[23] Kato H, Izumiyama M, Izumiyama K, et al. Silent cerebral microbleeds on T2*-weighted MRI: correlation with stroke subtype, stroke recurrence, and leukoaraiosis. Stroke 2002;33(6):1536–40.

[24] Messori A, Polonara G, Mabiglia C, et al. Is haemosiderin visible indefinitely on gradient-echo MRI following traumatic intracerebral haemorrhage? Neuroradiology 2003;45(12):881–6.

[25] Smith EE, Koroshetz WJ. Epidemiology of stroke. In: Furie KL, Kelly PJ, editors. Current clinical neurology: handbook of stroke prevention in clinical practice. Totowa (NJ): Humana Press; 2004. p. 1–17.

[26] Woo D, Sauerbeck LR, Kissela BM, et al. Genetic and environmental risk factors for intracerebral hemorrhage: preliminary results of a population-based study. Stroke 2002;33(5):1190–5.

[27] Fisher CM. Pathological observations in hypertensive cerebral hemorrhage. J Neuropathol Exp Neurol 1971; 30(3):536–50.

[28] Knudsen KA, Rosand J, Karluk D, et al. Clinical diagnosis of cerebral amyloid angiopathy: validation of the Boston criteria. Neurology 2001;56(4):537–9.

[29] Zhu XL, Chan MS, Poon WS. Spontaneous intracranial hemorrhage: which patients need diagnostic cerebral angiography? A prospective study of 206 cases and review of the literature. Stroke 1997; 28(7):1406–9.

[30] Rabinstein AA, Tisch SH, McClelland RL, et al. Cause is the main predictor of outcome in patients with pontine hemorrhage. Cerebrovascular Diseases 2004; 17(1):66–71.

[31] Ott KH, Kase CS, Ojemann RG, et al. Cerebellar hemorrhage: diagnosis and treatment. A review of 56 cases. Arch Neurol 1974;31(3):160–7.

[32] Itoh Y, Yamada M, Hayakawa M, et al. Cerebral amyloid angiopathy: a significant cause of cerebellar as well as lobar cerebral hemorrhage in the elderly. J Neurol Sci 1993;116(2):135–41.

[33] Angelopoulos M, Gupta SR, Azat Kia B. Primary intraventricular hemorrhage in adults: clinical features, risk factors, and outcome. Surg Neurol 1995;44(5): 433–6.

[34] Marti-Fabregas J, Piles S, Guardia E, et al. Spontaneous primary intraventricular hemorrhage: clinical data, etiology and outcome. J Neurol 1999;246(4): 287–91.

[35] Maurino J, Saposnik G, Lepera S, et al. Multiple simultaneous intracerebral hemorrhages: clinical features and outcome. Arch Neurol 2001;58(4):629–32.

[36] Tucker WS, Bilbao JM, Klodawsky H. Cerebral amyloid angiopathy and multiple intracerebral hematomas. Neurosurgery 1980;7(6):611–4.

[37] Furlan AJ, Whisnant JP, Elveback LR. The decreasing incidence of primary intracerebral hemorrhage: a population study. Ann Neurol 1979;5(4):367–73.

[38] Fisher CM. Cerebral miliary aneurysms in hypertension. Am J Pathol 1972;66(2):313–30.

[39] Vinters HV, Gilbert JJ. Cerebral amyloid angiopathy: incidence and complications in the aging brain. II. The distribution of amyloid vascular changes. Stroke 1983;14(6):924–8.

[40] Greenberg SM, Briggs ME, Hyman BT, et al. Apolipoprotein E epsilon 4 is associated with the presence and earlier onset of hemorrhage in cerebral amyloid angiopathy. Stroke 1996;27(8):1333–7.

[41] Greenberg SM, Vonsattel JP, Segal AZ, et al. Association of apolipoprotein E epsilon2 and vasculopathy in cerebral amyloid angiopathy. Neurology 1998;50(4): 961–5.

[42] McCarron MO, Nicoll JA, Stewart J, et al. The apolipoprotein E epsilon2 allele and the pathological features in cerebral amyloid angiopathy-related hemorrhage. J Neuropathol Exp Neurol 1999;58(7):711–8.

[43] Vinters HV. Cerebral amyloid angiopathy. A critical review. Stroke 1987;18(2):311–24.

[44] Bailey RD, Hart RG, Benavente O, et al. Recurrent brain hemorrhage is more frequent than ischemic stroke after intracranial hemorrhage. Neurology 2001; 56(6):773–7.

[45] O'Donnell HC, Rosand J, Knudsen KA, et al. Apolipoprotein E genotype and the risk of recurrent lobar intracerebral hemorrhage. N Engl J Med 2000; 342(4):240–5.

[46] Smith EE, Gurol ME, Eng JA, et al. White matter lesions, cognition, and recurrent hemorrhage in lobar intracerebral hemorrhage. Neurology 2004;63(9): 1606–12.

[47] Greenberg SM, Eng JA, Ning M, et al. Hemorrhage burden predicts recurrent intracerebral hemorrhage after lobar hemorrhage. Stroke 2004;35(6):1415–20.

[48] Ohshima T, Endo T, Nukui H, et al. Cerebral amyloid angiopathy as a cause of subarachnoid hemorrhage. Stroke 1990;21(3):480–3.

[49] Hylek EM, Singer DE. Risk factors for intracranial hemorrhage in outpatients taking warfarin. Ann Intern Med 1994;120(11):897–902.

[50] Smith EE, Rosand J, Knudsen KA, et al. Leukoaraiosis is associated with warfarin-related hemorrhage following ischemic stroke. Neurology 2002;59(2):193–7.

[51] Gorter JW. Major bleeding during anticoagulation after cerebral ischemia: patterns and risk factors. Stroke Prevention in Reversible Ischemia Trial (SPIRIT). European Atrial Fibrillation Trial (EAFT) study groups. Neurology 1999;53(6):1319–27.

[52] Rosand J, Hylek EM, O'Donnell HC, et al. Warfarin-associated hemorrhage and cerebral amyloid angiopathy: a genetic and pathologic study. Neurology 2000; 55(7):947–51.

[53] Hart RG, Boop BS, Anderson DC. Oral anticoagulants and intracranial hemorrhage. Facts and hypotheses. Stroke 1995;26(8):1471–7.

[54] Kase CS, Robinson RK, Stein RW, et al. Anticoagulant-related intracerebral hemorrhage. Neurology 1985;35(7):943–8.

[55] Flibotte JJ, Hagan N, O'Donnell J, et al. Warfarin, hematoma expansion, and outcome of intracerebral hemorrhage. Neurology 2004;63(6):1059–64.

[56] Rosand J, Eckman MH, Knudsen KA, et al. The effect of warfarin and intensity of anticoagulation on outcome of intracerebral hemorrhage. Arch Intern Med 2004;164(8):880–4.

[57] Barnes B, Cawley CM, Barrow DL. Intracerebral hemorrhage secondary to vascular lesions. Neurosurg Clin N Am 2002;13(3):289–97.

[58] Fiorelli M, Bastianello S, von Kummer R, et al. Hemorrhagic transformation within 36 hours of a cerebral infarct: relationships with early clinical deterioration and 3-month outcome in the European Cooperative Acute Stroke Study I (ECASS I) cohort. Stroke 1999;30(11):2280–4.

[59] Smith EE, Fitzsimmons AL, Nogueira RG, et al. Spontaneous hyperacute postischemic hemorrhage leading to death. J Neuroimaging 2004;14(4):361–4.

[60] de Bruijn SF, de Haan RJ, Stam J. Clinical features and prognostic factors of cerebral venous sinus thrombosis in a prospective series of 59 patients. For the Cerebral Venous Sinus Thrombosis Study Group. J Neurol Neurosurg Psychiatry 2001;70(1):105–8.

[61] Little JR, Dial B, Belanger G, et al. Brain hemorrhage from intracranial tumor. Stroke 1979;10(3):283–8.

[62] Kondziolka D, Bernstein M, Resch L, et al. Significance of hemorrhage into brain tumors: clinicopathological study. J Neurosurg 1987;67(6):852–7.

[63] Wakai S, Yamakawa K, Manaka S, et al. Spontaneous intracranial hemorrhage caused by brain tumor: its incidence and clinical significance. Neurosurgery 1982;10(4):437–44.

[64] Mandybur TI. Intracranial hemorrhage caused by metastatic tumors. Neurology 1977;27(7):650–5.

[65] Destian S, Sze G, Krol G, et al. MR imaging of hemorrhagic intracranial neoplasms. AJR Am J Roentgenol 1989;152(1):137–44.

[66] Atlas SW, Grossman RI, Gomori JM, et al. Hemorrhagic intracranial malignant neoplasms: spin-echo MR imaging. Radiology 1987;164(1):71–7.

[67] Tung GA, Julius BD, Rogg JM. MRI of intracerebral hematoma: value of vasogenic edema ratio for predicting the cause. Neuroradiology 2003;45(6): 357–62.

[68] Abbed KM, Ogilvy CS. Intracerebral hematoma from aneurysm rupture. Neurosurg Focus 2003;15(4):E4.

[69] Adams JH, Doyle D, Graham DI, et al. The contusion index: a reappraisal in human and experimental nonmissile head injury. Neuropathol Appl Neurobiol 1985;11(4):299–308.

[70] Mayer SA, Brun NC, Begtrup K, et al. Recombinant activated factor VII for acute intracerebral hemorrhage. N Engl J Med 2005;352(8):777–85.

[71] Kidwell CS, Chalela JA, Saver JL, et al. Comparison of MRI and CT for detection of acute intracerebral hemorrhage. JAMA 2004;292(15):1823–30.

[72] Nighoghossian N, Hermier M, Berthezene Y, et al. Early diagnosis of hemorrhagic transformation: diffusion/perfusion–weighted MRI versus CT scan. Cerebrovasc Dis 2001;11(3):151–6.

[73] Weingarten K, Filippi C, Zimmerman RD, et al. Detection of hemorrhage in acute cerebral infarction. Evaluation with spin-echo and gradient-echo MRI. Clin Imaging 1994;18(1):43–55.

[74] Greer DM, Koroshetz WJ, Cullen S, et al. Magnetic resonance imaging improves detection of intracerebral hemorrhage over computed tomography after intra-arterial thrombolysis. Stroke 2004;35(2):491–5.

[75] Nighoghossian N, Hermier M, Adeleine P, et al. Old microbleeds are a potential risk factor for cerebral bleeding after ischemic stroke: a gradient-echo T2*-weighted brain MRI study. Stroke 2002;33(3):735–42.

[76] Chalela JA, Kang DW, Warach S. Multiple cerebral microbleeds: MRI marker of a diffuse hemorrhage-prone state. J Neuroimaging 2004;14(1):54–7.

[77] Kidwell CS, Saver JL, Villablanca JP, et al. Magnetic resonance imaging detection of microbleeds before thrombolysis: an emerging application. Stroke 2002; 33(1):95–8.

[78] Derex L, Nighoghossian N, Hermier M, et al. Thrombolysis for ischemic stroke in patients with old microbleeds on pretreatment MRI. Cerebrovasc Dis 2004;17(2–3):238–41.

[79] Fiebach JB, Schellinger PD, Gass A, et al. Stroke magnetic resonance imaging is accurate in hyperacute intracerebral hemorrhage: a multicenter study on the validity of stroke imaging. Stroke 2004;35(2):502–6.

[80] Eshwar Chandra N, Khandelwal N, Bapuraj JR, et al. Spontaneous intracranial hematomas: role of dynamic CT and angiography. Acta Neurol Scand 1998;98(3): 176–81.

[81] Becker KJ, Baxter AB, Bybee HM, et al. Extravasation of radiographic contrast is an independent predictor of death in primary intracerebral hemorrhage. Stroke 1999;30(10):2025–32.

ELSEVIER
SAUNDERS

Neuroimag Clin N Am 15 (2005) 273 – 282

NEUROIMAGING
CLINICS OF
NORTH AMERICA

Stroke in Asia

Jureerat Thammaroj, MD, MSc[a],
Valarmathi Subramaniam, MBBS, M Med, FRCR[b],
Joti J. Bhattacharya, MBBS, FRCR, MSc[c,d,*]

[a]*Department of Radiology, Srinagarind Hospital, Khon Kaen University, Khon Kaen, Thailand*
[b]*Department of Radiology, Gleneagles Intan Medical Center, Kuala Lumpur, Malaysia*
[c]*Department of Neuroradiodiogy, Institute of Neurological Sciences, Southern General Hospital, Glasgow, UK*
[d]*Academic Department of Clinical Neurosciences, University of Glasgow, Glasgow, UK*

Stroke is the second leading global cause of death after ischemic heart disease. Although the incidence of cerebrovascular disease has decreased progressively in most Western countries in the latter part of the twentieth century, the emergence of a growing epidemic of coronary artery disease (CAD) and stroke in much of Asia is equally striking. With more than half the population of the world living in Asia, stroke would be expected to have a major impact on the continent. Indeed, the World Health Organization (WHO) has estimated that in 1990 alone, 2.1 million Asians died of stroke [1].

In contrast to CAD, stroke is a markedly heterogeneous disorder. Whereas most coronary artery syndromes are caused by atheroma of large- and medium-sized intracardiac vessels, ischemic stroke may be caused by a variety of other pathologic conditions, including intracranial small vessel disease, cardioembolism, and prothrombotic disorders. Until the last decade, data on stroke in the diverse populations of Asia were sparse by comparison with the extensive literature on cerebrovascular disease in the West, although there has been a growing recognition of differences in disease patterns.

In the following brief survey, we provide an overview of ischemic stroke in Asia, underscoring dif-

ferences in epidemiology and pathologic findings compared with stroke in the West. We focus mainly on ischemic stroke, although acknowledging that hemorrhagic stroke in the Far East also shows certain differences from the West. For example, compared with the United States, there is a lower incidence of aneurysmal subarachnoid hemorrhage in Southeast Asia and, conversely, a higher incidence in Japan. We focus on cerebrovascular disease in countries in the following three regions: South Asia (eg, India, Pakistan), Southeast Asia (eg, Indonesia, Malaysia, Philippines, Singapore, Thailand, Vietnam), and East Asia (eg, China, Japan, Korea, Taiwan).

Epidemiologic data

There are wide disparities in per capita income among Asian countries, ranging from developed Japan and the urban economies of Singapore and Hong Kong SAR, on one side, to less affluent countries, such as India, Pakistan, and Indonesia on the other. Similarly, in much of Asia, there is great variation in access to medical care, ranging from world-class medical centers in some urban areas to rudimentary primary care in others.

Clearly, the ideal way to study the burden of diseases generally, and stroke in particular, is by community-based studies using standardized diagnostic criteria with verified diagnoses. Hospital-based studies on stroke are also useful but are more prone to selection bias, influenced to varying degrees in differ-

---

* Corresponding author. Department of Neuroradiology, Institute of Neurological Sciences, Southern General Hospital, 1345 Govan Road, Glasgow G51 4TF, UK.

E-mail address: j.j.bhattacharya@clinmed.gla.ac.uk (J.J. Bhattacharya).

ent countries by factors like wealth, health insurance, stroke specialization in the receiving center, confidence in diagnosis by the referring physician, and proximity to health care facilities.

The landmark Framingham Heart Study in Massachusetts, which commenced in 1948 [2], identified the classic risk factors for vascular disease (indeed, the term *risk factor* was coined by the Framingham researchers), which include hypertension, diabetes mellitus (DM), cigarette smoking, hypercholesterolemia, and obesity. Over the last half-century, numerous studies in Western Europe and North America, such as the population-based Oxford Community Stroke Project [3] and hospital-based German Stroke Data Bank [4], have helped to clarify the frequency of stroke subtypes as well as the relative roles of risk factors for stroke and heart disease.

Broadly speaking, these studies suggest that approximately 80% of strokes are ischemic and 20% are hemorrhagic in Western populations. Of ischemic strokes, approximately 20% to 25% are cardioembolic and 20% are attributable to large vessel atheroma, 20% to small vessel occlusion, 5% to other causes (eg, dissection), and the remainder to undetermined causes. Cardiovascular mortality (from coronary and stroke disease) is declining in developed countries, with CAD outweighing stroke [5].

In Asia, only Japan has produced a similar body of epidemiologic data, although the last 2 decades have seen growing stroke research from many other countries, documenting the emergence of a cardiovascular disease epidemic [6]. Rapid economic development in many Asian countries since World War II has been accompanied by improvements in nutritional status and life expectancy. In India, for example, life expectancy was approximately 40 years in the 1950s and rose to greater than 60 years in the 1990s [7].

CAD, hypertension, DM, and cancer tend to emerge as leading sources of mortality in a population when life expectancy reaches 50 to 60 years, replacing death from infectious disease, the so-called "epidemiologic transition" [6]. In developing countries, cardiovascular diseases had become a significant cause of death by the mid-1970s, some 50 years later than in the West. Specific differences in disease patterns have been described, including a higher incidence of hemorrhagic stroke in Asian populations. Generally, however, risk factors for cardiovascular disease and early death after acute stroke are similar to those in North America and Europe; for example, diabetic and elderly patients have higher death rates regardless of stroke subtype [8]. It is striking that deaths attributable to cerebrovascular disease occur at a younger age in developing countries in the East. In developed countries, 23% of deaths attributable to cerebrovascular disease occur at an age less than 70 years, whereas in India, 53% occur at an age less than 70 years [9].

The precise genetic-environmental interactions accounting for differences between Western and Eastern populations (and between those within Asia) are far from fully understood. The last decade, however, has seen a growing number of more rigorous studies on Asian vascular disease, often involving international collaboration, such as the International Collaborative Study of Cardiovascular Disease in Asia (China and Thailand) [10], the Asia Pacific Cohort Studies Collaboration (multiple Asian countries as well as Australia and New Zealand) [11], the Eastern Stroke and Coronary Heart Disease Collaborative Research Group (Japan and China) [12], and the Sino-MONICA project (China) [13]. Problems remain in comparing data between different studies and countries, as highlighted by Sudlow and Warlow [14]. Comparisons are meaningful only if they are based on studies that use similar definitions, methods, and data presentation.

With regard to risk factors, for example, it is increasingly recognized that each reduction in systolic blood pressure (SBP) of 10 mm Hg is associated with a decrease in stroke risk of approximately 33% in subjects aged 60 to 79 years in the Asia-Pacific region and in the West [15]. The association is continuous down to levels of at least 115/75 mm Hg (many previous studies used older definitions of hypertension, SBP ≥ 160 mm Hg and diastolic pressure ≥ 95 mm Hg).

The use of CT scanning for determining stroke subtype and the presence of hemorrhage is similarly variable across studies. As CT scanning has become more widely available, the frequency of stroke of undetermined cause has fallen and more accurate subtyping has ensued. Zhang and colleagues [16] showed that over the decade since 1991, CT use increased from approximately 50% to more than 90% in the Chinese populations studied (Table 1).

Japan

Japan is unique in Asia, with the world's second largest economy and a gross domestic product per capita among the highest globally. As a fully developed country, the level of health care exceeds that of many Western nations. As in most developed countries, there has been a progressive decline in stroke mortality in recent years. Indeed, between 1965 and 1990, stroke deaths decreased by 60% [17]. Nevertheless, stroke accounts for 14.2% of deaths in

Table 1
Proportion of stroke subtypes in patients 25 years of age or greater, among 12 populations in China, between 1991 and 2000

Monitor year	Total cases (N)	SAH (%)	ICH (%)	CI (%)	Und (%)	CT (%)
1991	1007	1.3	16.8	30.2	51.7	49.4
1992	1073	0.7	13.0	33.5	52.8	48.5
1993	1205	1.4	19.3	35.0	44.3	57.3
1994	1267	0.8	20.8	39.8	38.6	61.5
1995	1265	1.7	26.6	50.8	20.9	79.4
1996	1482	1.6	23.9	55.3	19.2	81.0
1997	1577	1.8	28.9	57.1	12.2	88.5
1998	1644	1.6	25.0	53.8	19.6	80.8
1999	1615	2.3	29.0	58.8	9.9	90.8
2000	1601	1.1	28.5	61.9	8.5	91.4
Total	**13,736**	**1.5**	**23.9**	**49.3**	**25.3**	**75.3**

As the use of CT increased (see last column), the proportion of undetermined stroke declined rapidly and the percentage of CI increased most strikingly.
Abbreviations: ICH, intracranial hemorrhage; SAH, subarachnoid hemorrhage.
From Zhang LF, Yang J, Hong Z, et al for the Collaborative Group of China Multicenter Study of Cardiovascular Epidemiology. Proportion of different subtypes of stroke in China. Stroke 2003;34:2091–6; with permission.

Japan and remains the third leading cause of death after heart disease and cancer [18]. Interestingly, although it is frequently stated that cerebral hemorrhage is the most common cause of stroke in Asian populations, Morikawa and coworkers [17] showed that between 1977 and 1991, the proportion of brain hemorrhages decreased from 23.6% to 16.4%, whereas cerebral infarction (CI) increased from 64.1% to 73.6%. In spite of the overall reduction in stroke, its incidence in Japan remains higher than in most other industrialized nations.

East Asia

Death rates from stroke in East Asian countries, including China, Japan, and Taiwan, exceed 100 per 100,000 persons and are higher than in New Zealand or Australia (50–80 per 100,000 persons) [19]. China remains a country of great contrasts, including that in the degree of development of varying areas. In Hong Kong, per capita GDP is similar to that of many Western countries. Urban areas like Beijing and Shanghai show rapidly rising levels of affluence, yet many rural areas remain at a lower level of development. China is at a stage of epidemiologic transition in which diseases of industrialization (eg, cerebrovascular disease) are becoming more prevalent than diseases of underdevelopment (eg, infectious diseases).

In spite of some difficulties, the Sino-MONICA project has been successful in providing cardiovascular data from a wide range of Chinese populations. Stroke incidence and mortality have been revealed as high compared with world averages. Stroke is the most common cause of death, and the burden of stroke in the Chinese population is rising progressively, with major health and economic implications. Conversely, as in much of Asia, rates of coronary events are currently below world averages [13]. Although, as in Japan, ischemic stroke is dominant, hemorrhagic stroke accounts for up to 30% of stroke cases and remains more common than in populations in the West [16].

In Taiwan and Korea, stroke is the second most common cause of death, with ischemic stroke more common but hemorrhage also substantially higher than in the West. In Taiwan, deaths attributable to cerebrovascular disease increased rapidly after World War II but have decreased since the early 1980s. Hypertension is the most significant risk factor for all major stroke types and is most strongly associated with cerebral hemorrhage. Antihypertension campaigns in Taiwan since 1986 have contributed to a reduction in the incidence and fatality of stroke [20]. Similarly, in Korea, the epidemiologic transition associated with rapid development has resulted in a rapidly rising stroke incidence. Since the mid 1980s, however, age-adjusted mortality from stroke has decreased progressively, although the proportion attributable to ischemic stroke has increased. The prevalence of hypertension also fell during this period, although fat intake and total serum cholesterol increased [21].

South Asia

In India, the burden of stroke is growing with increasing urbanization, a pattern reflected in other South Asian countries. With its large population, difficulties in gathering and validating epidemiologic data in India are significant. Nevertheless, several community-based studies are available that suggest the prevalence of stroke to be approximately 203 per 100,000 persons. Stroke deaths are more difficult to quantify but have been estimated at 1.2% of total deaths [22]. Mortality from cardiovascular diseases is progressively increasing, likely associated with the steady rise in prevalence of hypertension as well as changing dietary habits, including increased fat intake [7]. By 2015, cerebrovascular disease is predicted to account for more than 30% of all deaths and stroke is predicted to have a major impact on already stretched medical resources [23]. It is notable that South Asian migrants to countries in the West have shown excessive susceptibility to cardiovascular diseases. This may reflect the prevalence of DM, impaired glucose tolerance, and central obesity as well as high levels of triglycerides and low levels of high-density lipoprotein (HDL) cholesterol in South Asian migrants, a pattern similar to that seen in urban areas in India [24].

Southeast Asia

Southeast Asia is a region of great contrasts, with some countries, such as Malaysia and Thailand, showing rapid industrialization and urbanization, whereas others, such as Vietnam, still have a mainly rural population. Death rates from stroke, although increasing, seem to be lower than in East Asian countries and have been estimated to be below 20 per 100,000 persons in Thailand, Malaysia, Indonesia, and the Philippines [19]. Nevertheless, stroke remains the third leading cause of death in Malaysia and Indonesia but not among the top three in Thailand or the Philippines.

Most epidemiologic data (predominantly hospital based) comes from Thailand, Malaysia, and Singapore. Interestingly, a recent study in Singapore showed higher incidences of stroke in Chinese and Indian men than in Malaysian men but with the highest incidence in Malaysian women [25]. Recent studies from Chulalongkorn University in Bangkok reveal that 78% of stroke admissions had CI and 22% had hemorrhagic infarction. Risk factors in Thailand were similar to those in the West, with hypertension showing the strongest association. Stroke incidence and prevalence were highest in urban areas, probably related to distribution of risk factors. Polpinit and colleagues [26] confirmed a lower prevalence of hypertension in rural areas of Khon Kaen than that reported for Bangkok. DM and CAD were associated with extracranial carotid stenosis more strongly than with intracranial disease.

Stroke pathologic findings in Asian populations

Cerebral hemorrhage as a stroke subtype has been noted to be more common in populations in the East than in the West and has even been deemed the major stroke subtype in Japan and China [7]. Studies into the 1980s reported high rates of hemorrhage; in a community-based survey of stroke in China, Li and coworkers [27] cited the incidence of hemorrhagic stroke at 44%. More recent studies from the mid-1980s in Japan and the 1990s in China, when CT scanning became more widely used in diagnosing stroke, clearly reveal that ischemic stroke is now the dominant subtype, however. It is unclear whether the rate of cerebral hemorrhage really declined over this period or if previous studies were not sufficiently robust. Nevertheless, it seems certain that cerebral hemorrhage is currently more frequent throughout most of Asia (20%–30% of strokes compared with 15%–20% in the West).

The pattern of atheromatous disease distribution in Asian nations is different from that in Western nations. In white populations, extracranial atheromatous disease is predominant, whereas in Asians (eg, Chinese, Indian, Japanese, Korean, Thai), intracranial stenoses seem more common (Figs. 1 and 2) [28–30].

Within Asia, rates of intracranial stenosis also vary. Chinese populations show higher rates than Japanese or Korean populations [31].

The association of coronary and extracranial carotid artery atherosclerosis is well recognized in white populations as well as in Japanese [32]. This close relation, however, does not apply to the intracranial arteries. Although it seems that the balance of risk factors predisposing to intra- or extracranial atherosclerosis may be different, there is conflicting evidence regarding which factors are most frequently associated with which locations [33]. Thus, in Korean subjects with extracranial stenosis, DM is associated with coexisting intracranial stenosis [34]. Yasaka and colleagues [35] found DM, hypercholesterolemia, and age to be associated with extracranial atherosclerosis in Japanese subjects, whereas hypertension was more strongly associated with middle cerebral artery disease. Changing lifestyles in Japan

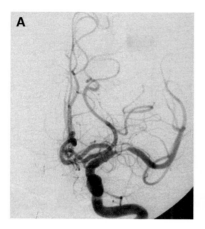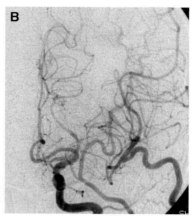

Fig. 1. A 34-year-old Japanese man with a right-sided clinical deficit. (*A*) Cerebral angiography demonstrates proximal stenosis of the left middle cerebral artery (MCA). There were no associated cardiac abnormalities and no evidence of cardioembolism. This is the typical intracranial pattern of atherothrombotic disease across much of Asia. (*B*) Treatment in this case was by extracranial-intracranial bypass rather than by MCA stenting. (Courtesy of Shushi Kominami, MD, Tokyo, Japan.)

in the last few decades, including dietary changes, have been associated with increasing levels of DM and hypercholesterolemia. Koyama and coworkers [36] conducted a comparative study on the changing pattern of intracranial atherosclerosis and coronary artery stenosis from 1974 to 2001, which showed a marked decline in intracranial disease over this period. The increasing proportion of extracranial stenosis in Japan is thus coming to resemble the pattern in the West and may foreshadow changes in other parts of Asia (Fig. 3).

The frequency of small vessel disease in Asia is less widely appreciated. Studies from Taiwan (29%)

[37], Sri Lanka (41%) [38], and Japan (38.8%) [18] suggest that levels of lacunar infarction are higher than in the West. Interestingly, in a large hospital-based registry, Kimura and colleagues [18] demonstrated a lacunar infarction rate (38.8%) lower than that previously identified in the 3-decade–long community-based Hisayama Study (56%) as well as a correspondingly higher atherothrombosis rate [39]. This may reflect improved medical management of hypertension in Japan in recent years.

Originally described in Japan and long believed to be a largely Asian form of cerebrovascular disease, moyamoya disease has now been described in all

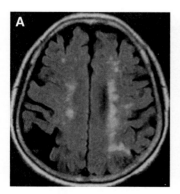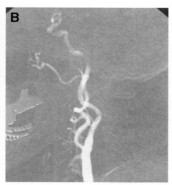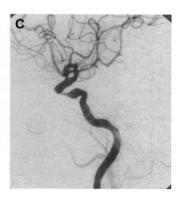

Fig. 2. A 76-year-old Korean woman with hypertension, who presented with right arm weakness and slowly improving aphasia. (*A*) Fluid-attenuated inversion recovery MR imaging shows multiple high signal lesions in the left middle cerebral artery–anterior cerebral artery border zone area. (*B*) Roadmap angiogram shows a normal carotid bulb. (*C*) Selective internal carotid arteriogram shows severe stenosis of a cavernous segment of the left internal carotid artery, a frequent site of involvement in Asian populations. (Courtesy of Dae Chul Suh, MD, Seoul, Korea.)

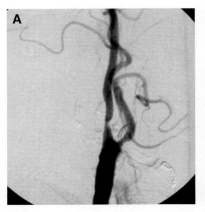
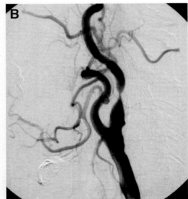

Fig. 3. Left (*A*) and right (*B*) common carotid angiograms in a 66-year-old Japanese man with a history of transient ischemic attacks. Extracranial stenosis, as in this case, has become the predominant form of atherosclerosis in Japan, as it is in the West. (Courtesy of S. Kominami, Tokyo, Japan.)

parts of the world. The term *moyamoya* ("puff of smoke") refers to the florid pattern of proliferating collateral vessels at the base of the brain seen at angiography, which is related to the progressive severe stenosis of the distal internal carotid and proximal portions of the anterior and middle cerebral arteries (Fig. 4).

Primary moyamoya disease must be distinguished from moyamoya syndrome, in which a similar pattern of collateral vessels develops in response to proximal occlusive disease of known cause. The largest number of cases has been described in Japan [40], with China and Korea also reporting significant numbers. The disease affects all age groups, but the highest incidence is in children less than 10 years of age. In children, infarction or transient ischemic attacks are typical, whereas adults may also present with hemorrhage.

Pathologic features include fibrocellular thickening of the intima, with smooth muscle cell proliferation, tortuosity, and duplication of the internal elastic lamina. There is usually no evidence of associated atheroma [41]. The cause of the disease is unknown, but the clustering mainly in East Asian populations and Japan, and a 10% familial incidence, suggest genetic inheritance. Indeed, recent reports have suggested linkage to chromosomes 3, 6, and 17 [42].

In contrast, familial small vessel occlusive syndrome (cerebral autosomal dominant arteriopathy with subcortical infarcts and leukoencephalopathy [CADASIL]) was initially described in whites. CADISIL is characterized by autosomal dominant

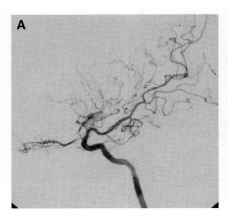
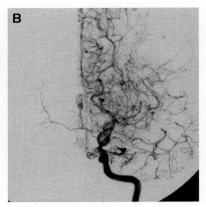

Fig. 4. Lateral (*A*) and frontal (*B*) internal carotid artery angiograms. A 34-year-old Japanese woman presented with progressive neurologic deficit. Cerebral angiography demonstrated occlusion of the proximal anterior and middle cerebral arteries and a network of small basal collateral vessels typical of moyamoya disease. (Courtesy of S. Kominami, Tokyo, Japan.)

inheritance, vascular dementia at 30 to 60 years of age without known risk factors for cerebrovascular disorders, and recurrent transient ischemic attacks with migrainous headache. In 90% of white patients, mutations are found in the Notch3 gene on chromosome 19. Now identified in Asia populations [43,44] as well, it is notable that the Notch3 mutation is less common in Japan, being present in only 25% of patients [45]. Unlike in the West, where Alzheimer's disease is the dominant form of dementia, vascular dementia seems to be more common in Asia. This raises the possibility that CADASIL may actually also be more common in Asia. An unusual variant, cerebral autosomal recessive arteriopathy with subcortical infarcts and leukoencephalopathy (CARASIL), has been described mainly in Japanese patients with autosomal recessive inheritance and several unique features, including frequent consanguinity, associated spinal deformity, and alopecia [46]. The causative gene has not been identified.

Stroke resources and treatment

In 1997, the WHO convened the Asia Pacific Consensus Forum on Stroke Management, which resulted in the Melbourne Declaration on Stroke Management [47]. It has been widely recognized that the global burden of stroke is increasing in concert with aging of the world population. This is particularly striking in Asia, where an increase in risk factors, such as smoking and the adoption of Western diets, is also occurring. The conference stressed the importance of primary prevention, secondary prevention, acute stroke management, organization of stroke services, and economic issues. It also highlighted rehabilitation, evaluation of quality of care, public education, and particular problems of remote and rural areas. It was accepted that the level of adoption of management recommendations would vary between countries, reflecting particular health priorities and national economies.

The availability and quality of medical services varies widely in as vast and populous a continent as Asia, but some generalizations can be made. Typically, rural populations, (most populations in many countries) have limited access to advanced medical care; hence, the pressing need for public health education and primary prevention strategies. Conversely, urban populations in many Asian areas have ready access to medical facilities that rival any in the world. It is difficult to give definitive figures for the availability of stroke management resources in Asia. In 2000, Poungvarin and coworkers [48] published a survey of epidemiologic data from nine Asian countries, notably excluding China and Japan. The wide range of availability of neurologic services, stroke units, and imaging equipment in these countries is apparent (Table 2). Over the last 5 years there

Table 2
National health resources of nine Asian countries published in 2000

National health resource	Singapore	Malaysia	India	Thailand	Indonesia	China (Hong Kong)	Philippines	Taiwan	Korea
Neurologists	21	15	405	150	303	30	99	414	674
Neurosurgeons	15	16	483	150	43	41	40	172	923
Hospitals	25	—	13,700	—	—	—	1111	596	21,121[a]
Public	NA	102	—	788	—	41	—	—	—
Private	NA	200	—	255	—	—	—	—	—
General	—	—	—	—	830	—	—	—	—
Specialist	—	—	—	—	96	—	—	—	—
Teaching	5	5	146	12	30	2	7	26	252
Hospital beds	10,446	42,500	810,000	90,740	110,460	29,342	35,571	112,380	N/A
Public	8346	35,000	—	80,259	58,912	24,940	—	39,3923	—
Private	2100	7500	—	10,481	54,548	4402	—	72,457	—
Stroke units	2	0	5	1	1	3	1	7	4
CT scanners	13	22	510	150	35	0	25	264	700
MR imaging scanners	5	10	203	20	10	9	6	38	160

Abbreviations: NA, not applicable; N/A, not available.
  [a] Including clinics.
Data from Asian Acute Stroke Advisory Panel (AASAP). Stroke epidemiological data for nine Asian countries. J Med Assoc Thai 2000;83:3.

has been further expansion of resources in many countries; in India, for example, there were 8–10 stroke units by 2002 [49].

Of note, in comparison to Table 2, Japan had by far the highest number of CT and MR imaging scanners per capita of any Organisation for Economic Co-operation and Development (OECD) country in 2000, with 84 CT scanners per million persons and 23 MR imaging units. In contrast, the average numbers of CT and MR imaging scanners per million persons in OECD countries were 17.7 and 6.5, respectively [50]. Aggressive management policies directed at "brain attacks," with rapid imaging and thrombolytic therapy, are widely available only in countries like Japan, Singapore, Taiwan, and Korea. In other countries, these clinical and neuroradiologic services as well as interventions like carotid stenting and endarterectomy are available primarily to specific groups living near urban centers, once again underscoring the importance of primary prevention.

Caution must be exercised, however, regarding the applicability of guidelines between different populations, an issue that has generally received little attention. Evidence-based guidelines in the United States are derived from research performed in North America and Europe but are often applied in clinical care throughout the world.

For example, in the United States, aspirin is recommended to reduce the risk of cardiovascular events in patients with a 3% or more 5-year risk of coronary heart disease [51] and would prevent at least twice as many events as the number of potential hemorrhagic complications. As we have seen, however, the incidence of coronary heart disease in Asia is lower, whereas the frequency of stroke, hemorrhagic stroke in particular, is much higher. Indeed, the 5-year CAD risk of asymptomatic middle-aged Japanese men has been estimated to be only 0.8%; hence, this group may actually be harmed by widespread use of aspirin prophylaxis. Thus, different thresholds may apply, and uncritical adoption of guidelines may not always be of benefit to differing populations [52]. Once again, this emphasizes the need for further robust data applicable to Asia.

Nonetheless, the association of hypertension with stroke, for example, is so strong that the decline in average diastolic blood pressure of approximately 4 mm Hg seen in Japan in recent decades could explain much of the marked decrease in stroke during this period [12]. This suggests that population-wide lowering of blood pressure by lower salt intake, higher potassium intake, more exercise, reduced obesity, and availability of pharmacologic agents has the potential for enormous reduction of stroke in Asia.

Summary

The epidemic of cardiovascular disease across most of Asia is at a different stage from that in the West; the incidence and prevalence of stroke are increasing steadily, associated with nutritional changes and aging of the population. Epidemiologic data, crucial in combating stroke, have been relatively sparse in Asian populations, but a few international collaborative studies on stroke have been in progress for several years. Through these, we now know that ischemic stroke is actually the most frequent type of cerebrovascular accident in Asia, although hemorrhagic stroke remains more common in Asia than in the West. Also, the percentage of ischemic stroke attributable to intracranial vascular disease is much higher than in the West. In Japan and a few other countries, stroke rates are declining; however, increasing rates in most other countries make primary prevention of critical importance in minimizing the severe impact of this epidemic in Asia.

References

[1] Murray CJL, Lopez AD, editors. The global burden of disease, vol. 1. Boston: Harvard University Press; 1996. p. 118–201.

[2] Kannel WB. The Framingham Study: its 50-year legacy and future promise. J Atheroscler Thromb 2000;6: 60–6.

[3] Bamford J, Sandercock P, Dennis M, et al. A prospective study of acute cerebrovascular disease in the community: the Oxfordshire Community Stroke Project 1981–86, I: methodology, demography and incident cases of first-ever stroke. J Neurol Neurosurg Psychiatry 1988;51:1373–80.

[4] Grau AJ, Weimar C, Buggle F, et al for the German Stroke Data Bank Collaborators. Risk factors, outcome, and treatment in subtypes of ischemic stroke: the German Stroke Data Bank. Stroke 2001; 32:2559–66.

[5] Thom TJ, Epstein FH, Feldman JJ, et al. Total mortality and mortality from heart disease, cancer, and stroke from 1950 to 1987 in 27 countries: highlights of trends and their interrelationships among causes of death. NIH publication no. 92–3088. Washington, DC: US DHHS PHS, National Institutes of Health; 1992.

[6] Reddy KS, Yusuf S. Emerging epidemic of cardiovascular disease in developing countries. Circulation 1998;97:596–601.

[7] Singh RB, et al. Hypertension and stroke in Asia: prevalence, control and strategies in developing countries for prevention. J Hum Hypertens 2000;14:749–63.

[8] Wong KS. Asian Acute Stroke Advisory Panel. Risk factors for early death in acute ischemic stroke and

intracerebral hemorrhage. A prospective hospital based study in Asia. Stroke 1999;30:2326–30.

[9] Murray CJL, Lopez AD. Global comparative assessments in the health sector. Geneva, Switzerland: World Health Organization; 1994.

[10] He J, Neal B, Gu D, et al for the InterASIA Collaborative Group. International collaborative study of cardiovascular disease in Asia: design, rationale, and preliminary results. Ethn Dis 2004;14:260–8.

[11] Zhang X, Patel A, Horibe H, et al for the Asia Pacific Cohort Studies Collaboration. Cholesterol, coronary heart disease, and stroke in the Asia Pacific region. Int J Epidemiol 2003;32:563–72.

[12] Rodgers A, MacMahon S, Yee T, et al for the Eastern Stroke and Coronary Heart Disease Collaborative Research Group. Blood pressure, cholesterol, and stroke in eastern Asia. Lancet 1998;352:1801–7.

[13] Wu Z, Yao C, Zhao D, et al. Sino-MONICA Project, a collaborative study on trends and determinants in cardiovascular diseases in China, part I: morbidity and mortality monitoring. Circulation 2001;103:462–8.

[14] Sudlow CL, Warlow CP. Comparing stroke incidence worldwide: what makes studies comparable. Stroke 1996;27:550–8.

[15] Lawes CMM, Bennett DA, Feigin VI, et al. Blood pressure and stroke, an overview of published reviews. Stroke 2004;35:1024–33.

[16] Zhang LF, Yang J, Hong Z, et al for the Collaborative Group of China Multicenter Study of Cardiovascular Epidemiology. Proportion of different subtypes of stroke in China. Stroke 2003;34:2091–6.

[17] Morikawa Y, Nakagawa H, Naruse Y, et al. Trends in stroke incidence and acute case fatality in a Japanese rural area: the Oyabe study. Stroke 2000;31:1583–7.

[18] Kimura K, Kazui S, Minematsu K, et al for the Japan Multicenter Stroke Investigators' Collaboration. Analysis of 16,922 patients with acute ischemic stroke and transient ischemic attack in Japan. A hospital-based prospective registration study. Cerebrovasc Dis 2004; 18:47–56.

[19] Khor GL. Cardiovascular epidemiology in the Asia-Pacific region. Asia Pac J Clin Nutr 2001;10:76–80.

[20] Hung TP. Changes in mortality from cerebrovascular disease and clinical pattern of stroke in Taiwan. J Formos Med Assoc 1993;92:687–96.

[21] Suh I. Cardiovascular mortality in Korea: a country experiencing epidemiologic transition. Acta Cardiol 2001;56:75–81.

[22] Anand K, Chowdhury D, Singh KB, et al. Estimation of mortality and morbidity due to strokes in India. Neuroepidemiology 2001;20:208–11.

[23] Bulatao RA, Stephens PW. Global estimates and projections of mortality by cause. Preworking paper 1007. Washington, DC: Population, Health, and Nutrition Department, World Bank; 1992.

[24] Reddy KS. Cardiovascular disease and diabetes in migrants: interaction between nutritional changes and genetic background. In: Shetty PS, McPherson K, editors. Diet, nutrition and chronic disease: lessons

from contrasting worlds. Chichester, UK: Wiley; 1997. p. 71–5.

[25] Heng DM, Lee J, Chew SK, et al. Incidence of ischaemic heart disease and stroke in Chinese, Malays and Indians in Singapore: Singapore Cardiovascular Cohort Study. Ann Acad Med Singapore 2000;29: 231–6.

[26] Polpinit A, Ungsununtawiwat M, Bhuripanyo K, et al. The prevalence and risk factors of hypertension in population aged 30–65 years in rural area, Amphoe Phon, Khon Kaen. J Med Assoc Thai 1992; 75:259–66.

[27] Li SC, Schoenberg BS, Wang CC, et al. Cerebrovascular disease in the People's Republic of China: epidemiologic and clinical features. Neurology 1985;35: 1708–13.

[28] Caplan LR, Gorelick PB, Hier DB. Race, sex and occlusive cerebrovascular disease: a review. Stroke 1986;17:648–55.

[29] Padma MV, Gaikwad S, Jain S, et al. Distribution of vascular lesions in ischaemic stroke: a magnetic resonance angiographic study. Natl Med J India 1997;10: 217–20.

[30] Suh DC, Lee SH, Kim KR, et al. Pattern of atherosclerotic carotid stenosis in Korean patients with stroke: different involvement of intracranial versus extracranial vessels. AJNR Am J Neuroradiol 2003;24: 239–44.

[31] Leung SY, Ng TH, Yuen ST, et al. Pattern of cerebral atherosclerosis in Hong Kong Chinese. Severity in intracranial and extracranial vessels. Stroke 1993;24: 779–86.

[32] Uehara T, Tabuchi M, Hayashi T, et al. Relationship between atherosclerosis in the cerebral and coronary arteries: cerebral and coronary angiographic findings in 17 patients. Jpn J Stroke 1994;16:109–16.

[33] Uehara T, Tabuchi M, Hayashi T, et al. Asymptomatic occlusive lesions of carotid and intracranial arteries in Japanese patients with ischemic heart disease: evaluation by brain magnetic resonance angiography. Stroke 1996;27:393–7.

[34] Lee SJ, Cho SJ, Moon HS, et al. Combined extracranial and intracranial atherosclerosis in Korean patients. Arch Neurol 2003;60:1561–4.

[35] Yasaka M, Yamaguchi T, Shichiri M. Distribution of atherosclerosis and risk factors in atherothrombotic occlusion. Stroke 1993;24:206–11.

[36] Koyama S, Saito Y, Yamanouchi H, et al. Marked decrease of intracranial atherosclerosis in contrast with unchanged coronary artery stenosis in Japan. Nippon Ronen Igakkai Zasshi 2003;40:267–73 [in Japanese].

[37] Yip PK, Jeng JS, Lee TK, et al. Subtypes of ischemic stroke. A hospital-based stroke registry in Taiwan (SCAN-IV). Stroke 1997;28:2507–12.

[38] Gunatilake SB, Jayasekera BA, Premawardene AP. Stroke subtypes in Sri Lanka: a hospital based study. Ceylon Med J 2001;46:19–20.

[39] Tanizaki Y, Kiyohara Y, Kato I, et al. Incidence and risk factors for subtypes of cerebral infarction in a

general population: the Hisayama study. Stroke 2000;
31:2616–22.

[40] Fukui M. Current state of study on moyamoya disease in Japan. Surg Neurol 1997;47:138–43.

[41] Fukui M, Kono S, Sueishi K, et al. Moyamoya disease. Neuropathology 2000;20(Suppl):S61–4.

[42] Inou TK, Ikezaki K, Sasazuki T, et al. Linkage analysis of moyamoya disease on chromosome 6. J Child Neurol 2000;15:179–82.

[43] Suwanwela N, Srikiatkhachorn A, Tangwongchai S, et al. Mutation of the Notch 3 gene in a Thai cerebral autosomal dominant arteriopathy with subcortical infarcts and leukoencephalopathy family. J Med Assoc Thai 2003;86(2):178–82.

[44] Moon SY, Kim HY, Seok JI, et al. A novel mutation (C67Y) in the NOTCH3 gene in a Korean CADASIL patient. J Korean Med Sci 2003;18:141–4.

[45] Santa Y, Uyama E, Chui de H, et al. Genetic, clinical and pathological studies of CADASIL in Japan: a partial contribution of Notch3 mutations and implications of smooth muscle cell degeneration for the pathogenesis. J Neurol Sci 2003;212:79–84.

[46] Yanagawa S, Ito N, Arima K, et al. Cerebral autosomal

recessive arteriopathy with subcortical infarcts and leukoencephalopathy. Neurology 2002;58:817–20.

[47] Donnan G, Davis S, Chambers B, et al. Asia Pacific Consensus Forum on Stroke Management. Stroke 1998;29(8):1730–6.

[48] Asian Acute Stroke Advisory Panel (AASAP). Stroke epidemiological data for nine Asian countries. J Med Assoc Thai 2000;83:1–7.

[49] Hastak SM. Relevance of stroke units to stroke care: from nihilism to cautious optimism. Neurol India 2002; 50(Suppl 1):S64–5.

[50] Lafortune G, Morgan D. Health at a Glance—OECD Indicators 2003: briefing note (Japan). Available at: http://www.oecd.org/dataoecd/20/5/16502622.pdf. Accessed August 15, 2005.

[51] Hayden M, Pignone M, Phillips C, et al. Aspirin for the primary prevention of cardiovascular events: a summary of the evidence for the US Preventive Services Task Force. Ann Intern Med 2002;136:161–72.

[52] Morimoto T, Fukui T, Lee TH, et al. Application of US guidelines in other countries: aspirin for the primary prevention of cardiovascular events in Japan. Am J Med 2004;117:459–68.

ELSEVIER
SAUNDERS

Neuroimag Clin N Am 15 (2005) 283 – 296

NEUROIMAGING
CLINICS OF
NORTH AMERICA

Stroke in Latin America

Erica C.S. Camargo, MD, PhD[a],*, Luiz A. Bacheschi, MD, PhD[b],
Ayrton R. Massaro, MD, PhD[c],[d]

[a]Stroke Service, Department of Neurology, Massachusetts General Hospital, Harvard Medical School, Boston, MA, USA
[b]Division of Neurology and Neurosurgery, Faculdade de Medicina, Universidade de São Paulo, São Paulo, Brazil
[c]Department of Neurology, Escola Paulista de Medicina, Universidade Federal de São Paulo, São Paulo, Brazil
[d]Stroke Service, Hospital São Paulo, Escola Paulista de Medicina, Universidade Federal de São Paulo, São Paulo, Brazil

Stroke is one of the leading causes of mortality in Latin America, with variable incidence and prevalence throughout the continent reflecting regional socioeconomic differences. In Latin America, uncontrolled hypertension is one of the major causes of stroke, but other modifiable risk factors also play a role, such as heavy alcohol consumption and smoking. Intracerebral hemorrhage and lacunar stroke are more frequent in Latin America than in North America and Europe. There are multiple causes of stroke that are endemic to Latin America, including neurocysticercosis, Chagas' disease, sickle cell anemia, malaria, hemorrhagic fever, and snake bites.

Burden of stroke in Latin America

Cerebrovascular disease is among the major causes of mortality and neurologic dependency in industrialized countries. According to recent statistics, approximately 730,000 North Americans have a new or recurrent stroke each year [1]. Despite evidence that stroke is one of the largest worldwide public health problems, research funds dedicated to this disease remain small relative to those of cardiac disease and cancer [2].

Although mortality related to stroke has significantly decreased since 1950, in large part, attributable to better control of risk factors, such as arterial hypertension, recent statistics from Rochester, Minnesota have revealed an alarming increase in stroke incidence [3–5]. Among possible factors that could account for this are the more precise noninvasive diagnosis of less severe stroke cases, the presence of previously unidentified risk factors, and an increase in the number of survivors of myocardial infarction who suffer subsequent strokes [5].

There are great regional variations in stroke mortality worldwide. This can be appreciated by comparing the high mortality rates related to stroke in Eastern Europe with the smaller rates of Western nations. This is largely attributable to better control of risk factors in the typically higher socioeconomic status (SES) Western countries [6].

The same is true within Latin America, where there are marked geographic, ethnic, cultural, and socioeconomic differences, despite otherwise "homogeneous" groups of predominantly Portuguese- and Spanish-speaking populations. Among the most important of these disparities is the differential access of rural versus urban populations to medical services. This difference influences the estimates of disease prevalence in the few epidemiologic studies of stroke

Dr. Camargo is supported by a scholarship from Coordenação de Aperfeiçoamento de Pessoal de Nível Superior, Brazil.

* Corresponding author. Stroke Service, Department of Neurology, Massachusetts General Hospital, Harvard Medical School, VBK 802, 55 Fruit Street, Boston, MA 02114–2622.

E-mail address: ecamargo@partners.org (E.C.S. Camargo).

neuroimaging.theclinics.com

from Latin America, and thus biases assessment of the real dimension of this health problem [7].

Stroke epidemiology in Latin America

Coronary heart disease (CHD) and stroke remain leading causes of mortality in Latin America, despite trends toward reduced mortality from all cardiovascular diseases [8–10]. In Brazil, a nationwide study demonstrated that stroke has been the leading cause of death over the past 20 years; indeed, stroke has recently been declared an "epidemic" in Latin America by the Pan American Health Organization [9,11].

Studies from various Latin American countries have revealed annual incidence rates ranging from 0.89 to 1.83 per 1000 and prevalence rates of 1.74 to 5.6 per 1000 in the general population [12–15]. The wide variations in these rates could be attributable to environmental factors, different lifestyles (eg, rural versus urban), regional educational campaigns, and other socioeconomic inequalities in Latin America [7,12].

Stroke risk factors in Latin America

In multiethnic Latin American populations, ischemic and hemorrhagic stroke are strongly linked to vascular risk factors, most notably hypertension [10,16,17]. The relation between modifiable and nonmodifiable risk factors influences the frequency of ischemic stroke subtypes, as evidenced by the relatively high rates of atherosclerotic intracranial disease seen in some regions of Latin America [18]. Additionally, ethnic disparities and genetic predispositions might play a role in the pathophysiology of different stroke subtypes, again, especially with regard to the occurrence of more intracranial than extracranial atherosclerotic disease as a cause of stroke in younger patients [18–22].

Hypertension is a major risk factor for stroke in Latin America, with a prevalence ranging from 20% to 23% in the general population and from 60% to 80% in stroke victims, both of which are higher than the fraction of strokes attributable to hypertension in other continents [13,14,19,23–25]. Inadequate medical treatment (in up to 80% of patients) and poor compliance are factors that increase the risk for ischemic and hemorrhagic stroke [10,25,26]. Hypertensive arteriopathy in Latin America has been shown to be the most significant risk factor for up to 43% of ischemic strokes and 64% of hemorrhagic strokes [14,27,28].

Other "classic" cardiovascular risk factors are highly prevalent in Latin American stroke sufferers: smoking has been reported in 23% to 50%, cardiac disease in 16% to 35%, diabetes in 17% to 25%, dyslipidemia in 4% to 38%, antecedent stroke in 13% to 25%, and heavy alcohol consumption in 9% to 40% [13,14,19,25,29]. Some of these risk factors are more frequent among Latin Americans than among North Americans. This has been demonstrated for moderate to high alcohol consumption and smoking in a hospital-based study from Buenos Aires, Argentina and Boston, Massachusetts [24]. The association between smoking and death attributable to stroke, however, was not observed in a large epidemiologic study conducted in Brazilian metropolitan areas [30]. This underscores how local factors can differentially affect stroke risk profiles in various Latin American countries. In this regard, regional dietary habits, such as the high intake of saturated fats attributable to meat, which is common in Argentina and Brazil, have also been hypothesized to influence the elevated rates of CHD and stroke in some regions, although this has yet to be confirmed in epidemiologic studies [10].

Stroke in Latin America: socioeconomic implications

SES may contribute to the regional differences observed in epidemiologic studies of stroke [8]. Low SES can impede access to adequate medical care; associated lower educational levels are correlated with diminished adherence to medical preventive strategies [26,31,32]. In Latin America, SES divides the population roughly into two broad groups: (1) patients with access to appropriate medical care, who have risk factors similar to those of industrialized western countries, and (2) patients with lower SES, who are burdened by factors related to their condition, of which Chagas' disease (CD) is one of the most representative examples [33,34].

Stroke subtypes

Relative frequencies of ischemic and hemorrhagic strokes vary widely in the many Latin American populations, as demonstrated in Table 1 [13,14, 25,29]. The prevalence of cerebral hemorrhage is consistently higher in all these Latin American series than in analogous studies of white cohorts, however,

Table 1
Relative frequencies of ischemic and hemorrhagic stroke, and hemorrhagic stroke subtypes, in Latin American registries

First author, year [Ref.]	Location	Study design registry	Strokes (n)	Ischemic stroke, n (%)	Hemorrhagic stroke		
					Total N (%)	ICH n (%)[a]	SAH n (%)[a]
Del Brutto, 1993 [14]	Guayaquil, Ecuador	Hospital	500	313 (62.6)	187 (37.4)	177 (35.4)	—
Cabral, 1993 [13]	Joinville, Brazil	Metropolitan	320[b]	235 (73.4)	85 (26.6)	59 (18.5)	26 (8.10)
Nogales-Gaete, 2000 [25]	Santiago, Chile	Hospital	450[c]	229 (51.0)	207 (46.0)	153 (34.0)	54 (12.0)
Saposnik, 2001 [29]	Buenos Aires, Argentina	Hospital	361	250 (69.0)	111 (31.0)	84 (23.4)	27 (7.60)

[a] Indicates the percentage relative to all strokes.
[b] 320 cases of first stroke, from a total of 429 incident strokes in the year 1995.
[c] Included 14 cases of patients with transient ischemic attacks.

with rates of hemorrhage among Latin Americans similar to those among Asians [14].

Hemorrhagic stroke

Intracerebral hemorrhage (ICH) is the most common type of hemorrhagic stroke in Hispanics, and its frequency differs more from that reported in temperate climate countries than does the frequency of subarachnoid hemorrhage (SAH) (see Table 1) [14,28,29]. Of the locations for ICH, lobar (26%–42%) and putaminal (26%–39%) hemorrhages are the most common, followed by posterior fossa (13.5%–17%) and thalamus hemorrhages.

The reasons for these elevated rates of ICH remain unclear. Although it is known that the high prevalence of hypertensive arteriopathy plays a role in this phenomenon, some studies have alluded to interactions of multiple risk factors. In a hospital-based study, Saposnik and colleagues [24] have shown that white stroke patients in Buenos Aires had significantly higher frequencies of hemorrhagic stroke than did white stroke patients in Boston, which could be attributable not only to differences in risk factors and patients' age but to dietary habits and regional factors. When comparing nonwhites and whites from both regions, however, nonwhites had a higher frequency of hemorrhagic stroke, which could be explained by genetic predisposition.

In another hospital-based series of 151 ICH cases, Del Brutto and coworkers [28] determined that hypertensive arteriopathy was the cause of stroke in 42% of the diagnosable cases, followed by rupture of a saccular aneurysm or vascular malformation in 22%. In an elegant case-control study of 140 patients with

ICH in Santiago, Chile, Diaz and colleagues [35] found that 25.7% of patients had significantly heavier alcohol intake (>402.5 g/wk) than did controls and that this habit carried an adjusted odds ratio (OR) of 4.5 for ICH. Of note, this risk factor was only significant for the subset of patients less than 65 years of age. Mortality attributable to ICH has been shown to range from 30% in a Brazilian multiethnic series of 100 ICH cases to 80% in patients with hemorrhage expansion (Ayrton Massaro, MD, PhD, personal communication, 2005) [36].

Other causes of hemorrhagic stroke specific to Latin America, because of their occurrence in tropical and underdeveloped areas, have been described in case reports and small series. These include neurocysticercosis (NCC, which can cause SAH); malaria; and hemorrhagic fevers, such as Dengue, yellow fever, and Hantavirus [11,37]. Snake bites are an additional health problem in rural tropical areas and account for a large proportion of deaths in the Indian tribes of the Amazon [11]. Cerebral hemorrhage, ICH or SAH, has been reported in 2.6% to 5% of snake bite victims [38,39]. More rarely, snake bites have been reported to cause ischemic infarction [40,41].

Ischemic stroke

There are many causes of ischemic stroke that are unique to tropical and underdeveloped nations and have epidemiologic importance in Latin America. With the increasing number of Latin American immigrants to North America, it is imperative that endemic diseases of the tropics be considered in the differential diagnosis of ischemic stroke in immigrants

Table 2
Ischemic stroke subtypes in Latin American registries

First author, year [Ref.]	Location	Ischemic strokes n	Large artery n (%)			Cardioembolic n (%)	Small artery n (%)	Other n (%)	Uknown n (%)
			Total	Intracranial	Extracranial				
Del Brutto, 1993 [14]	Guayaquil, Ecuador	313	23 (7.3)	11 (3.5)	12 (3.8)	44 (14.1)	135 (43.1)	19 (6.1)	92 (29.4)
Cabral, 1993 [13]	Joinville, Brazil	235	48 (20.4)	—	—	29 (12.3)	49 (20.9)	11 (4.7)	98 (41.7)
Diaz, 2001 [19]	Santiago, Chile	110	46 (41.8)	—	—	30 (27.3)	27 (24.5)	7 (6.4)	0
Saposnik, 2001 [29]	Buenos Aires, Argentina	250	31 (12.4)	—	—	53 (21.2)	105 (42)	16 (6.4)	45 (18)

[42]. In what follows, we discuss some of these prevalent Latin American diseases in detail.

Ischemic stroke subtypes

Various studies have shown that the frequencies of ischemic stroke subtypes in Latin American populations are different than those in white populations (Table 2) [13,14,19,29]. One of the most striking findings is the elevated frequency of small vessel or lacunar infarcts in the Latin American registries, most probably attributable, again, to uncontrolled hypertension. Intracranial atherosclerosis has consistently been shown to be a more frequent cause of ischemic stroke in Latin America than extracranial carotid disease, similar to that which occurs in Africans and Asians, and can account for as much as 60% of cases of large artery strokes (Figs. 1 and 2) [18,19].

Cardioembolic stroke in Latin America is most commonly associated with the classic risk factors seen worldwide, and atrial fibrillation plays a major role in this stroke subtype. Additionally, CD and

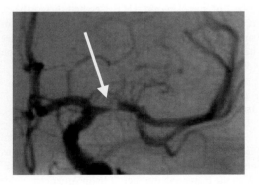

Fig. 1. Digital subtraction angiography demonstrates severe intracranial stenosis of the proximal M1 segment of the left MCA (*arrow*).

rheumatic heart disease are important causes of cardioembolic stroke in Latin Americans [43].

Chagas' disease: a public health challenge

CD is endemic in almost all Latin America, where there are an estimated 16 to 18 million people chronically infected by the protozoan parasite *Trypanosoma cruzi*, a substantial proportion of which are children, of whom roughly 50,000 die yearly because of complications of CD. *T cruzi* is found only in the Western Hemisphere and is transmitted to mammals through the infected feces of blood-sucking triatomine insects, popularly called "barbeiros." *T cruzi* can also be transmitted by blood transfusions. This means of transmission has been substantial in some Latin American countries [42]. *T cruzi* infection is directly related to poverty, because the barbeiros dwell in the modest homes of the rural areas of Latin America.

In human beings, *T cruzi* undergoes hematogenous spread to various organs, and the acute phase of the disease ensues within 2 weeks of inoculation. Approximately 3% of patients in this stage of the disease have fever, malaise, generalized lymph node enlargement, and the classic "Romaña sign" of unilateral swelling of the eyelids [44].

The chronic phases of CD usually begin approximately 2 months after infection and are classified as follows:

1. Indeterminate form in 60% to 70% of cases, which is symptom-free but can convert to other chronic forms in 2% to 5% of cases years later.
2. Gastrointestinal form in 10% of cases, which classically presents as chagasic megacolon or megaesophagus.
3. Cardiac form in 30% to 40% of cases. The most common clinically significant form of CD, it

affects patients decades after the primary infection [44,45]. The hallmark of this phase is congestive heart failure, but many patients present also or exclusively with electrocardiographic abnormalities, such as right bundle branch block, left anterior fascicular block, malignant arrhythmias, sudden death, or thromboembolic phenomena [34,45].

CD is a strong independent risk factor for all types of stroke, with an OR of 5.4 [46]. Although classic cardiovascular risk factors can also contribute to the elevated frequency of strokes in patients with CD, such risk factors are significantly less common in those with CD than in those without CD [34].

With chronic CD, patients with mild cardiac involvement have a low symptomatic stroke rate (1%), although autopsy studies have shown that the true incidence can be as high as 8.6%, which is significantly more frequent than in otherwise matched control groups [45,47]. Conversely, in patients with chronic CD and moderate to severe heart failure, cardiac thrombus is found in 36% to 76% of autopsies, with confirmed strokes in 17% of these [48,49].

Most ischemic strokes attributable to CD occur in the middle cerebral artery (MCA) territory (71%); 15% involve the basal ganglia or internal capsule. A little over half of CD strokes are cardioembolic, almost 10% are atherothrombotic, and 2% are lacunar [34].

Neurocysticercosis

NCC is the most common parasitic infection of the central nervous system (CNS) and is endemic in Latin America and other tropical regions of the world [50]. Human cysticercosis is transmitted by fecal-oral contamination with *Taenia solium* eggs of carriers, most commonly through water and vegetables. The infected individuals become intermediate hosts in the biologic cycle of *T solium*, and the ingested oncospheres cross the intestinal wall, enter the bloodstream, and are carried to other tissues, mainly muscles and the CNS.

Within the CNS, these viable cysticerci lodge preferentially in the subarachnoid space, brain tissue, and ventricles, causing local inflammation with leptomeningeal exudates and thickening. Viable cysticerci may remain in these compartments for years before they undergo degeneration, in which a second intense inflammatory process occurs, which is associated with multiple acute clinical manifestations. Depending on the number of cysticerci, this degeneration may occur episodically. Degenerated cysticerci may finally calcify and can be responsible for new-onset focal epileptic syndromes [11,51].

NCC is a variegated disease, with manifestations that include seizures (50%–80%), intracranial hypertension or hydrocephalus (20%–30%), focal signs and symptoms, acute or chronic meningitis, neuropsychiatric manifestations, dementia, and cranial

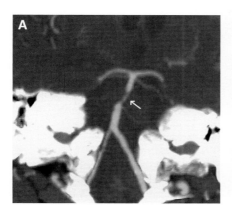
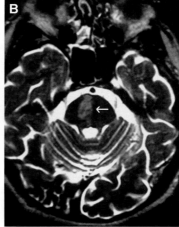

Fig. 2. (*A*) CT angiography, coronal maximum intensity projection view, demonstrates focal atherosclerotic stenosis of the midbasilar artery (*arrow*). (*B*) Axial T2-weighted MR imaging demonstrates the corresponding ischemic stroke in the medial right pons (*arrow*).

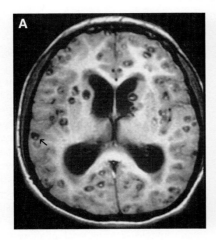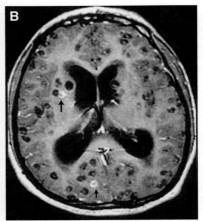

Fig. 3. Patient with intraparenchymal neurocysticercosis, predominantly in the vesicular stage. (*A*) Axial unenhanced T1-weighted MR imaging demonstrates multiple, diffuse, intraparenchymal viable cysts. Scolexes can be visualized inside the cysts (*arrow*). (*B*) Axial gadolinium-enhanced T1-weighted MR imaging. There is no significant enhancement of the viable cysts. Two colloidal cysts have prominent ring enhancement (*arrows*), however, demonstrating how cysticerci progress at different stages within the same patient.

nerve palsies [50,51]. Cerebral arteritis has been reported in up to 53% of patients with NCC [52]. Arteritis can involve small and large intracranial vessels; can be focal or diffuse; and may be accompanied by arterial occlusions, including that of the internal carotid artery.

Stroke has been reported in 6.5% of patients with any type of active NCC and in 21% to 53% of cases with active subarachnoid NCC [50,53]. In patients with stroke and NCC, those with focal arteritis have more acute symptomatic infarcts, headaches, and single infarcts. When the arteritis is diffuse, intracranial hypertension, multiple silent infarcts (deep and superficial), and abnormal cerebrospinal fluid (CSF) are present [50]. Lacunes are among the most frequent strokes attributable to NCC arteritis and can occur in up to 52% of cases, especially when associated with superimposed small vessel disease [50].

The neuroimaging findings of NCC depend on the location and stage of the cysticerci [54]. With respect to intraparenchymal NCC, four developmental stages of the cysticerci are recognized:

1. Viable cysts: on CT, these are small and rounded, nonenhancing, low-density foci, with an eccentric hyperdense nodular scolex internally. These cysts can be much better visualized on MR imaging, with a signal intensity corresponding to that of CSF (Figs. 3 and 4).
2. Colloidal cysts: this next phase in the cysticerci life cycle is characterized by surrounding edema and ring enhancement. In some severe

cases, the inflammatory pattern is diffuse, with profound edema and ventricular compression (Fig. 3B).
3. Granulomatous nodules: in this third phase of parenchymal NCC, the granulomatous nodules have surrounding edema and are moderately hyperdense on CT. On MR imaging, signal void can be seen on T1- and T2-weighted images.
4. Calcified NCC: this is the final stage of NCC, with markedly hyperdense lesions on CT.

In subarachnoid NCC, small cysts may be present within the cortical sulci; large, multilobulated, "racemose" cysts composed of various confluent cysts but typically with no live scolices are sometimes located in the basal cisterns and sylvian fissures, exerting mass effect on neighboring structures. Intraventricular NCC is another form of presentation that can be seen on CT or MR imaging by means of distortion of the ventricular system, because the NCC vesicles can have the same attenuation as CSF (Fig. 5) [54].

Sickle cell disease

Sickle cell disease (SCD) is an endemic disease in equatorial Africa as well as in some regions of North American and South America because of the miscegenation of their populations with African descendants. SCD is a genetically determined condition in which red blood cells have HbS hemoglobin. "Sickle cell anemia" occurs when there is homo-

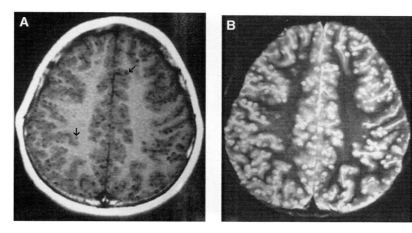

Fig. 4. Patient with intraparenchymal neurocysticercosis, vesicular phase. (*A*) Axial nonenhanced T1-weighted MR imaging demonstrates multiple, diffuse, intraparenchymal viable cysts, located mainly near the subarachnoid space (*arrows*). (*B*) Axial T2-weighted image demonstrates the same cysts, which are more conspicuous in this acquisition.

zygosity for HbS, but there are other SCDs, such as sickle cell hemoglobin C disease, and sickle-thalassemia disease.

Under normal homeostasis, HbS functions identically to common HbA. In the presence of infection, acidosis, or dehydration, however, HbS undergoes polymerization, causing elongation and increased density of red blood cells, ultimately leading to systemic microvascular occlusion and tissue hypoxia. This hemolytic anemia presents mainly with painful crises because of infarction of the affected tissue, principally the kidneys, lungs, bones, liver, and, of course, CNS [11,55,56].

The lifetime risk of stroke with SCD is 25% to 30% [57]. The prevalence of symptomatic stroke before the age of 19 years is 8.1%, and the overall prevalence of stroke on MR imaging is 17% [55,58]. Age-specific incidence of first stroke in SCD is low before 2 years of age, rising to greater than 1% at 2 to 5 years of age, and declining to 0.8% from 6 to 9 years of age. There is a second peak age-specific incidence over the age of 35 years [57]. The risk of recurrent stroke is as high as 67% [55].

Specific risk factors for ischemic stroke include previous transient ischemic attack (TIA), low hemoglobin levels, elevated systolic blood pressure, and

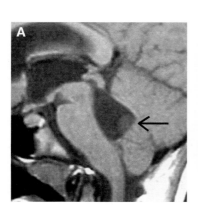
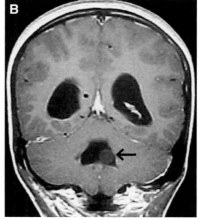

Fig. 5. Intraventricular neurocysticercosis. (*A*) Sagittal unenhanced T1-weighted MR imaging shows the cysticercosis of the fourth ventricle (*arrow*). (*B*) Coronal gadolinium-enhanced T1-weighted MR imaging demonstrates the same nonenhancing cysticercus in the fourth ventricle (*arrow*).

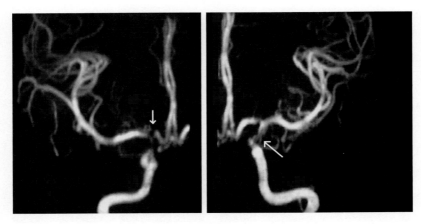

Fig. 6. Coronal projection MR angiograms of a patient with sickle cell disease. The arrows indicate focal stenosis of the distal portion of the intracranial internal carotid artery. (Courtesy of Gisele Sampaio Silva, MD, São Paulo, Brazil.)

recurrent acute chest pain. On transcranial Doppler (TCD), significantly elevated MCA (> 170 cm/s) or internal carotid artery (> 200 cm/s) velocities are associated with a relative risk for stroke of 44 [59]. Indeed, intracerebral TCD velocities greater than 200 cm/s are currently applied as a triage threshold for transfusion treatment of SCD anemia patients as a stroke preventative measure (Figs. 6 and 7) [60].

Silent ischemic strokes on brain MR imaging have been reported in 13% to 18% of sickle cell anemia patients [58,61,62]. Risk factors associated with the

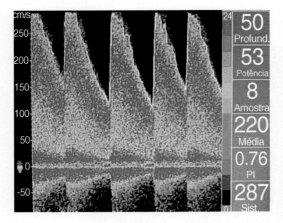

Fig. 7. TCD tracing of the same patient with sickle cell disease as in Fig. 6. The TCD reflects the waveform obtained at the M1-M2 portion of the MCA, with elevated flow velocities (220 cm/s). This patient would most likely be a candidate for prophylactic transfusion therapy for the prevention of stroke. (Courtesy of Gisele Sampaio Silva, MD, São Paulo, Brazil.)

presence of silent infarcts are a low rate of painful events (OR = 0.53 for every yearly painful event), seizures (OR = 14.4), low hemoglobin levels, and elevated leukocyte count (OR = 3.23) [61]. Silent infarcts are typically restricted to deep brain structures, particularly the basal ganglia and thalamus, whereas symptomatic infarcts occur in the cortex (mostly in the border zone regions of the frontal and parietal lobes) and deep white matter [56,58]. Ischemic lesions of the occipital lobes, cerebellum, and brain stem are infrequent [58].

Hemorrhagic stroke also occurs with SCD, commonly between the ages of 20 and 30 years. Risk factors include low hemoglobin, leukocytosis, and prior ischemic stroke [58]. Chronic large artery obstruction leads to moyamoya disease (see article on stroke in Asia in this issue), with the collateralized arteries predisposed to rupture [55].

Stroke in the young

There have been various reports on stroke in the young (age range: 15–50 years) in Latin America. Most have focused on the role of inherited thrombophilias (eg, protein S deficiency) and related racial differences with respect to these (eg, homozygosity for thermolabile methylenetetrahydrofolate reductase in Brazilian stroke sufferers of African descent) [20,21]. Young Brazilians have higher rates of ischemic stroke (86%) but lower rates of atherothrombotic disease than in otherwise matched groups. Up to 50% of those aged 15 to 29 years are classified as "other" with regard to stroke etiology [22,63]. In

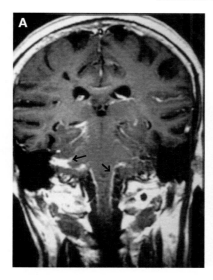

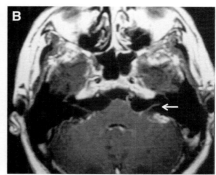

Fig. 8. Patient with neurotuberculosis. (*A*) Coronal gadolinium-enhanced T1-weighted MR imaging demonstrates leptomeningeal enhancement and thickening, mainly surrounding the brain stem and basal cisterns (*arrows*). (*B*) Axial gadolinium-enhanced T1-weighted MR imaging shows thickening and enhancement of the cranial nerves (*arrow*), which are commonly affected because of the basal meningeal inflammation of neurotuberculosis.

a case-control study of young Mexican women, migraine, oral contraceptive use, and smoking were significant risk factors for cardioembolic stroke [64]. Epidemiologic studies have not yet established if strokes in the young are more frequent in Latin America than in other geographic areas, however.

There are many other causes of arterial ischemic stroke relevant to Latin America that have not been discussed in this article, such as neurotuberculosis, infectious endocarditis, and malaria (Fig. 8). The interested reader is referred to the excellent review article by Del Brutto regarding cerebrovascular diseases in the tropics [11].

Venous infarcts

Cerebral venous thrombosis (CVT) is another not uncommon cause of stroke in the young of Latin America [65–67]. CVT is more common in the 25- to 40-year age range and is more common in women (female/male ratio: 1.3 to 2.5) [65,68–70].

CVT can present with multiple signs and symptoms, the most frequent of which are headache (70%–91%), focal deficits (motor deficits in 34%–79%), seizures (29%–63%), various levels of altered consciousness (26%–63%, most commonly with deep venous involvement), visual abnormalities (in 50% of CVT cases and in 80% of those associated with Behçet's disease, including papilledema, field

defects, loss of visual acuity, and diplopia), and aphasia [68,70–72]. These signs and symptoms can manifest acutely (<48 hours) in 28% to 54% of cases, subacutely (49 hours to 7 days), or chronically in up to 30% of cases [65,70,72].

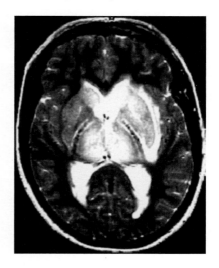

Fig. 9. Axial T2-weighted MR imaging of a patient with thrombosis of the deep cerebral venous system. This is a classic pattern of T2 hyperintense edema involving the bilateral basal ganglia and thalami, which can also progress to the frontobasal cortex and rostral midbrain. This pattern is typically caused by internal cerebral vein or basal vein of Rosenthal thrombosis.

Various CVT syndromes have been described, of which the most classic are pseudotumor syndrome, which occurs in 10% to 40% of cases and has an excellent prognosis; subacute encephalopathy, which is seen with CVT of the deep venous system; and a syndrome of focal deficits [72,73].

CVT has multiple causes, and an etiology is identified in up to 85% of cases [71]. One of the most important causes of CVT in Latin America is pregnancy and puerperium, as demonstrated in a large Mexican series [65]. Hereditary thrombophilias also figure dominantly as a cause of CVT in Latin America, particularly (1) hyperhomocystinemia, (2) G20210A prothrombin gene mutation, (3) factor V Leiden mutation, and (4) deficiencies of proteins C and S in specific ethnic groups [20,66,67,74]. As

occurs worldwide, the interaction between these inherited thrombophilias and oral contraceptive use significantly increases CVT risk [20,66,67,74]. Other causes of CVT that have been described in Latin America include antiphospholipid syndrome, parameningeal infection, and Behçet's disease [67].

On CT, signs of CVT may be direct (eg, high density in veins reflecting venous clot) or indirect (eg, findings of intracranial hypertension). No CT signs are specific for this disease, and CT scans may be normal in 10% to 50% of cases [75,76]. Among the direct signs of CVT, the classics are the "dense vessel" sign, "empty delta" sign, and "cord" sign. Nonspecific indirect signs of CVT are more common, including cerebral edema, which can be focal or diffuse (present in 60% of cases; Fig. 9); hemorrhagic

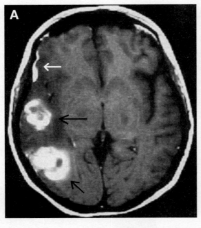
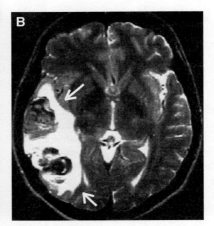
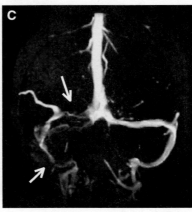

Fig. 10. Patient with hemorrhagic venous infarction attributable to right transverse sinus thrombosis. (*A*) Axial T1-weighted MR imaging shows multiple corticosubcortical hemorrhagic venous infarcts (*black arrows*), with surrounding edema, in the right temporal-parietal cortex. There is also an associated small subdural hemorrhage in the right temporal-frontal area (*white arrow*). (*B*) Axial T2-weighted MR imaging demonstrates the same hemorrhagic venous infarction with prominent hyperintense surrounding edema (*arrows*). (*C*) Coronal image from the MR venogram demonstrates partial occlusive filling defect of the right transverse and sigmoid sinuses (*arrows*), corresponding to the venous thrombosis.

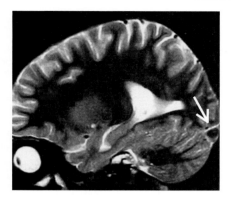

Fig. 11. Sagittal T2-weighted MR imaging of a patient with acute phase transverse sinus thrombosis. There is paramagnetic T2 hypointense thrombus (deoxyhemoglobin stage) in the transverse sinus (*arrow*).

venous infarcts, which are common in cortical-subcortical regions and are typically multiple and poorly defined (present in 10%–50% of cases; Fig. 10); and ischemic venous infarcts (present in 10%–40% of cases).

MR imaging can more sensitively reveal parenchymal abnormalities than CT (Figs. 11 and 12). Angiographic studies, CT angiography or MR angiography, can demonstrate the absence of contrast filling where thrombus is present (Fig. 10C) [77]. CT

venography, which is essentially intracranial CT angiography with a prolonged scan delay after contrast administration, is the most accurate method for actual venous clot detection [78,79].

Summary

Irrespective of socioeconomic problems, endemic disease, and regional tropical risk factors that differ from those in North America and Western Europe, the alarming recent increase in stroke incidence in Latin America is fundamentally attributable to the lack of public health initiatives to control risk factors, compounded by lack of awareness of the disease and its prevention by a significant portion of the population. Ignorance of stroke warning signs not only by patients and their families but by paramedics most certainly contributes to the delay of prompt treatment throughout most of Latin America [80].

Nonetheless, stroke units are being implemented in several Latin American centers, most notably at university-based or large private practice hospitals. This is particularly the case in major urban areas, where teams consisting of acute stroke neurologists, interventional neuroradiologists, and cerebrovascular neurosurgeons have been assembled, offering stroke victims timely and appropriate medical care [81–84].

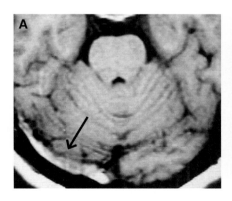

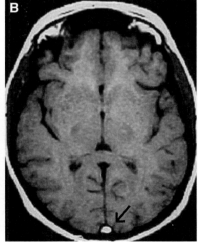

Fig. 12. Axial nonenhanced T1-weighted images of a patient with subacute CVT. (*A*) T1 hyperintense thrombosis (methemoglobin stage) of the right transverse sinus (*arrow*). (*B*) T1 hyperintense thrombosis of the superior sagittal sinus (*arrow*), not to be confused with bright "in plane" MR flow-related signal.

References

[1] Boden-Albala B, Sacco RL. The stroke prone individual. Rev Soc Cardiol Estado de São Paulo 1999;4: 501–8.

[2] Rothwell PM. The high cost of not funding stroke research: a comparison with heart disease and cancer. Lancet 2001;357(9268):1612–6.

[3] Bonita R, Beaglehole R. The enigma of the decline in stroke deaths in the United States: the search for an explanation. Stroke 1996;27(3):370–2.

[4] Whisnant JP. Effectiveness versus efficacy of treatment of hypertension for stroke prevention. Neurology 1996;46(2):301–7.

[5] Brown RD, Whisnant JP, Sicks JD, et al. Stroke incidence, prevalence, and survival: secular trends in Rochester, Minnesota, through 1989. Stroke 1996; 27(3):373–80.

[6] Sarti C, Rastenyte D, Cepaitis Z, et al. International trends in mortality from stroke, 1968 to 1994. Stroke 2000;31(7):1588–601.

[7] Saposnik G, Del Brutto OH. Stroke in South America: a systematic review of incidence, prevalence, and stroke subtypes. Stroke 2003;34(9):2103–7.

[8] Lessa I. Epidemiologia das doenças cerebrovasculares no Brasil. Rev Soc Cardiol Estado de São Paulo 1999; 4:509–18.

[9] Mansur AP, Souza MFM, Favarato D, et al. Stroke and ischemic heart disease mortality trends in Brazil from 1979 to 1996. Neuroepidemiology 2003;22(3): 179–83.

[10] Hauger-Klevene JH, Balossi EC. Coronary heart disease mortality and coronary risk factors in Argentina. Cardiology 1987;74(2):133–40.

[11] Del Brutto OH. Cerebrovascular disease in the tropics. Rev Neurol 2001;33(8):750–62.

[12] Jaillard AS, Hommel M, Mazetti P. Prevalence of stroke at high altitude (3380 m) in Cuzco, a town of Peru. A population-based study. Stroke 1995;26(4): 562–8.

[13] Cabral NL, Longo AL, Moro CH, et al. Epidemiology of cerebrovascular disease in Joinville, Brazil. An institutional study. Arq Neuropsiquiatr 1997;55(3A): 357–63.

[14] Del Brutto OH, Mosquera A, Sanchez X, et al. Stroke subtypes among Hispanics living in Guayaquil, Ecuador. Results from the Luis Vernaza Hospital Stroke Registry. Stroke 1993;24(12):1833–6.

[15] Nicoletti A, Sofia V, Giuffrida S, et al. Prevalence of stroke: a door-to-door survey in rural Bolivia. Stroke 2000;31(4):882–5.

[16] Freitas OC, Resende de Carvalho F, et al. Prevalence of hypertension in the urban population of Catanduva, in the State of Sao Paulo, Brazil. Arq Bras Cardiol 2001; 77(1):9–21.

[17] Martins IS, Marucci Mde F, Cervato AM, et al. Atherosclerotic cardiovascular disease, lipemic disorders, hypertension, obesity and diabetes mellitus in the population of a metropolitan area of southeastern

Brazil. II. Lipemic disorders. Rev Saude Publica 1996; 30(1):75–84.

[18] Del Brutto OH, Campos X, Tomala M, et al. Angiographic findings among Ecuadorian metis population with occlusive cerebrovascular disease of the anterior circulation. Rev Neurol 1997;25(137):40–3.

[19] Diaz V, Plate L, Erazo S, et al. Prevalence of carotid atherosclerosis in patients with cerebrovascular occlusive disease. Rev Med Chil 2001;129(2):161–5.

[20] Voetsch B, Damasceno BP, Camargo EC, et al. Inherited thrombophilia as a risk factor for the development of ischemic stroke in young adults. Thromb Haemost 2000;83(2):229–33.

[21] Barinagarrementeria F, Cantu-Brito C, De La Pena A, et al. Prothrombotic states in young people with idiopathic stroke. A prospective study. Stroke 1994;25(2): 287–90.

[22] Siqueira Neto JI, Santos AC, Fabio SR, et al. Cerebral infarction in patients aged 15 to 40 years. Stroke 1996;27(11):2016–9.

[23] Hernandez-Hernandez R, Armas-Padilla MC, Armas-Hernandez MJ, et al. Hypertension and cardiovascular health in Venezuela and Latin American countries. J Hum Hypertens 2000;14(Suppl 1):S2–5.

[24] Saposnik G, Caplan LR, Gonzalez LA, et al. Differences in stroke subtypes among natives and Caucasians in Boston and Buenos Aires. Stroke 2000;31(10): 2385–9.

[25] Nogales-Gaete J, Nunez L, Arriagada C, et al. Clinical characterization of 450 patients with cerebrovascular disease admitted to a public hospital during 1997. Rev Med Chil 2000;128(11):1227–36.

[26] Chizzola PR, Mansur AJ, da Luz PL, et al. Compliance with pharmacological treatment in outpatients from a Brazilian cardiology referral center. Sao Paulo Med J 1996;114(5):1259–64.

[27] Pittella JE, Duarte JE. Prevalence and pattern of distribution of cerebrovascular diseases in 242 hospitalized elderly patients, in a general hospital, autopsied in Belo Horizonte, Minas Gerais, Brazil, from 1976 to 1997. Arq Neuropsiquiatr 2002;60(1):47–55.

[28] Del Brutto OH, Sanchez J, Campos X, et al. Non-traumatic intracerebral hemorrhage in young adults living in Guayaquil, Ecuador (South America): analysis of 151 patients. Funct Neurol 1999;14(1):21–8.

[29] Saposnik G, Gonzalez L, Lepera S, et al. Southern Buenos Aires Stroke Project. Acta Neurol Scand 2001; 104(3):130–5.

[30] Lotufo PA, Bensenor IJ. Smoking and mortality from cerebrovascular disorders in Brazil: comparative study of capital cities of metropolitan regions, 1988. Arq Neuropsiquiatr 1995;53(2):238–44.

[31] Boden-Albala B, Sacco RL. Socioeconomic status and stroke mortality: refining the relationship. Stroke 2002;33(1):274–5.

[32] Nemes MI, Carvalho HB, Souza MF. Antiretroviral therapy adherence in Brazil. AIDS 2004;18(Suppl 3): S15–20.

[33] Dias JCP, Silveira AC, Schofield CJ. The impact of

Chagas' disease control in Latin America: a review. Mem Inst Oswaldo Cruz 2002;97:603–12.

[34] Carod-Artal FJ, Vargas AP, Melo M, et al. American trypanosomiasis (Chagas' disease): an unrecognised cause of stroke. J Neurol Neurosurg Psychiatry 2003; 74(4):516–8.

[35] Diaz V, Cumsille MA, Bevilacqua JA. Alcohol and hemorrhagic stroke in Santiago, Chile. A case-control study. Neuroepidemiology 2003;22(6):339–44.

[36] Hemphill III JC, Bonovich DC, Besmertis L, et al. The ICH score: a simple, reliable grading scale for intracerebral hemorrhage. Stroke 2001;32(4):891–7.

[37] Tellez-Zenteno JF, Negrete-Pulido O, Cantu C, et al. Hemorrhagic stroke associated with neurocysticercosis. Neurologia 2003;18(5):272–5.

[38] Kerrigan KR. Venomous snakebite in eastern Ecuador. Am J Trop Med Hyg 1991;44(1):93–9.

[39] Mosquera A, Idrovo LA, Tafur A, et al. Stroke following Bothrops spp. snakebite. Neurology 2003; 60(10):1577–80.

[40] Cole M. Cerebral infarct after rattlesnake bite. Arch Neurol 1996;53(10):957–8.

[41] Murthy JM, Kishore LT, Naidu KS. Cerebral infarction after envenomation by viper. J Comput Assist Tomogr 1997;21(1):35–7.

[42] Kirchhoff LV. Chagas' disease. American trypanosomiasis. Infect Dis Clin North Am 1993;7(3):487–502.

[43] Rey RC, Lepera SM, Kohler G, et al. Cerebral embolism of cardiac origin. Medicina (B Aires) 1992;52(3): 202–6.

[44] Umezawa ES, Stolf AM, Corbett CE, et al. Chagas' disease. Lancet 2001;357(9258):797–9.

[45] Bestetti R. Stroke in a hospital-derived cohort of patients with chronic Chagas' disease. Acta Cardiol 2000;55(1):33–8.

[46] Leon-Sarmiento FE, Mendoza E, Torres-Hillera M, et al. Trypanosoma cruzi-associated cerebrovascular disease: a case-control study in Eastern Colombia. J Neurol Sci 2004;217(1):61–4.

[47] Lopes ER, Marquez JO, da Costa Neto B, et al. Association of encephalic vascular accidents and Chagas' disease. Rev Soc Bras Med Trop 1991;24(2):101–4.

[48] Aras R, da Matta JA, Mota G, et al. Cerebral infarction in autopsies of chagasic patients with heart failure. Arq Bras Cardiol 2003;81(4):411–6.

[49] Samuel J, Oliveira M, Correa De Araujo RR, et al. Cardiac thrombosis and thromboembolism in chronic Chagas' heart disease. Am J Cardiol 1983;52(1): 147–51.

[50] Cantu C, Barinagarrementeria F. Cerebrovascular complications of neurocysticercosis. Clinical and neuroimaging spectrum. Arch Neurol 1996;53(3):233–9.

[51] Garcia HH, Gonzalez AE, Evans CA, et al. Taenia solium cysticercosis. Lancet 2003;362(9383):547–56.

[52] Barinagarrementeria F, Cantu C. Frequency of cerebral arteritis in subarachnoid cysticercosis: an angiographic study. Stroke 1998;29(1):123–5.

[53] Levy AS, Lillehei KO, Rubinstein D, et al. Subarachnoid neurocysticercosis with occlusion of the major intracranial arteries: case report. Neurosurgery 1995;36(1):183–8 [discussion: 188].

[54] Garcia HH, Del Brutto OH. Imaging findings in neurocysticercosis. Acta Trop 2003;87(1):71–8.

[55] Prengler M, Pavlakis SG, Prohovnik I, et al. Sickle cell disease: the neurological complications. Ann Neurol 2002;51(5):543–52.

[56] Adams RJ. Stroke prevention and treatment in sickle cell disease. Arch Neurol 2001;58(4):565–8.

[57] Ohene-Frempong K. Stroke in sickle cell disease: demographic, clinical, and therapeutic considerations. Semin Hematol 1991;28(3):213–9.

[58] Moser FG, Miller ST, Bello JA, et al. The spectrum of brain MR abnormalities in sickle-cell disease: a report from the Cooperative Study of Sickle Cell Disease. AJNR Am J Neuroradiol 1996;17(5):965–72.

[59] Adams R, McKie V, Nichols F, et al. The use of transcranial ultrasonography to predict stroke in sickle cell disease. N Engl J Med 1992;326(9):605–10.

[60] Adams RJ, McKie VC, Hsu L, et al. Prevention of a first stroke by transfusions in children with sickle cell anemia and abnormal results on transcranial Doppler ultrasonography. N Engl J Med 1998;339(1): 5–11.

[61] Kinney TR, Sleeper LA, Wang WC, et al. Silent cerebral infarcts in sickle cell anemia: a risk factor analysis. The Cooperative Study of Sickle Cell Disease. Pediatrics 1999;103(3):640–5.

[62] Bernaudin F, Verlhac S, Freard F, et al. Multicenter prospective study of children with sickle cell disease: radiographic and psychometric correlation. J Child Neurol 2000;15(5):333–43.

[63] Zetola VH, Novak EM, Camargo CH, et al. Stroke in young adults: analysis of 164 patients. Arq Neuropsiquiatr 2001;59(3-B):740–5.

[64] Barinagarrementeria F, Gonzalez-Duarte A, Miranda L, et al. Cerebral infarction in young women: analysis of 130 cases. Eur Neurol 1998;40(4):228–33.

[65] Cantu C, Barinagarrementeria F. Cerebral venous thrombosis associated with pregnancy and puerperium. Review of 67 cases. Stroke 1993;24(12):1880–4.

[66] Cantu C, Alonso E, Jara A, et al. Hyperhomocystinemia, low folate and vitamin B12 concentrations, and methylene tetrahydrofolate reductase mutation in cerebral venous thrombosis. Stroke 2004;35(8):1790–4.

[67] Camargo EC, Massaro AR, Bacheschi LA, et al. Ethnic differences in cerebral venous thrombosis. Cerebrovasc Dis 2005;19(3):147–51.

[68] Ferro JM, Canhao P, Stam J, et al. Prognosis of cerebral vein and dural sinus thrombosis: results of the International Study on Cerebral Vein and Dural Sinus Thrombosis (ISCVT). Stroke 2004;35(3):664–70.

[69] Bousser MG, Chiras J, Bories J, et al. Cerebral venous thrombosis—a review of 38 cases. Stroke 1985;16(2): 199–213.

[70] Ameri A, Bousser MG. Cerebral venous thrombosis. Neurol Clin 1992;10(1):87–111.

[71] Stam J. Thrombosis of the cerebral veins and sinuses. N Engl J Med 2005;352(17):1791–8.

[72] Bousser MG, Russell RR. Cerebral venous thrombosis. 1st edition. London: WB Saunders; 1997.

[73] Biousse V, Ameri A, Bousser MG. Isolated intracranial hypertension as the only sign of cerebral venous thrombosis. Neurology 1999;53(7):1537–42.

[74] Gadelha T, Andre C, Juca AA, et al. Prothrombin 20210A and oral contraceptive use as risk factors for cerebral venous thrombosis. Cerebrovasc Dis 2005; 19(1):49–52.

[75] Rao KC, Knipp HC, Wagner EJ. Computed tomographic findings in cerebral sinus and venous thrombosis. Radiology 1981;140(2):391–8.

[76] Chiras J, Bousser MG, Meder JF, et al. CT in cerebral thrombophlebitis. Neuroradiology 1985;27(2):145–54.

[77] Dormont D, Anxionnat R, Evrard S, et al. MRI in cerebral venous thrombosis. J Neuroradiol 1994;21(2): 81–99.

[78] Casey SO, Alberico RA, Patel M, et al. Cerebral CT venography. Radiology 1996;198(1):163–70.

[79] Ozsvath RR, Casey SO, Lustrin ES, et al. Cerebral venography: comparison of CT and MR projection venography. AJR Am J Roentgenol 1997;169(6): 1699–707.

[80] Leopoldino JF, Fukujima MM, Silva GS, et al. Time of presentation of stroke patients in Sao Paulo Hospital. Arq Neuropsiquiatr 2003;61(2A):186–7.

[81] Baruzzi AC, Knobel E, Cirenza C, et al. Use of tissue plasminogen activator factor for acute ischemic stroke. Arq Bras Cardiol 1997;68(5):347–51.

[82] Cabral NL, Moro C, Silva GR, et al. Study comparing the stroke unit outcome and conventional ward treatment: a randomized study in Joinville, Brazil. Arq Neuropsiquiatr 2003;61(2A):188–93.

[83] Kihara EN, Andrioli MS, Zukerman E, et al. Endovascular treatment of carotid artery stenosis: retrospective study of 79 patients treated with stenting and angioplasty with and without cerebral protection devices. Arq Neuropsiquiatr 2004;62(4):1012–5.

[84] Trabuco CC, Pereira de Jesus PA, Bacellar AS, et al. Successful thrombolysis in cardioembolic stroke from Chagas' disease. Neurology 2005;64(1):170–1.

ELSEVIER
SAUNDERS

Neuroimag Clin N Am 15 (2005) 297 – 324

NEUROIMAGING
CLINICS OF
NORTH AMERICA

Brainstem Vascular Stroke Anatomy

Kathleen M. Burger, DO[a], Stanley Tuhrim, MD[a], Thomas P. Naidich, MD[b,c],*

[a]*Department of Neurology, Mount Sinai Medical Center, New York, NY, USA*
[b]*Department of Radiology, Mount Sinai Medical Center, New York, NY, USA*
[c]*Department of Neurosurgery, Mount Sinai Medical Center, New York, NY, USA*

Stroke is a leading cause of death and disability in the United States and throughout the world. Each year, 150,000 Americans die of cerebral infarction [1,2]. More than 4 million live with stroke-induced disability [3]. Ischemic vertebrobasilar strokes account for 23% of all first episodes of ischemic brain strokes [4,5]. Because half (48%) of these affect the brainstem [5], ischemic brainstem strokes constitute 11% of all first ischemic brain strokes [4,5]. First ischemic vertebrobasilar strokes involve the pons (27%) more commonly than the medulla (14%) or midbrain (7%). They affect the cerebellum in 7% of cases, the posterior cerebral artery (PCA) territory in 36%, and multiple sites in 9% [5–8].

The most common mechanisms of brainstem stroke include embolism from the heart or large arteries (artery-to-artery embolism), large artery atherosclerosis (by directly obstructing small vessel ostia or by hemodynamic compromise), and lipohyalinosis (causing lacunar infarcts) [9]. Stenoses and occlusions of the posterior circulation vessels are most commonly found within the extracranial vertebral arteries (VAs; 32%), the intracranial VAs (32%), and the basilar artery (BA; 27%) [10]. Arterial dissections cause 20% to 30% of medullary strokes [11], are exceptionally rare causes of pontine strokes [6,12], and account for up to 4.8% of mesencephalic strokes [7].

Ischemic medullary strokes most commonly result from hypoperfusion secondary to stenoses of the intracranial VAs (73%) and arterial dissections (26%) and are rarely caused by cardiac emboli [11]. Ischemic pontine strokes most frequently result from stenoses or occlusions of the BA [10]: specifically, atherosclerosis of the ostia of BA branches (39%), small artery disease (21%), and large artery (vertebrobasilar) disease (18%). Cardioembolism accounts for only 8% of pontine ischemic strokes, because the emboli usually pass beyond the pons to lodge more distally [6]. No cause for the pontine stroke is found in 11% of cases [6]. Ischemic mesencephalic infarcts arise from large artery disease (39%), small artery disease (13%–24%), cardiogenic and artery-to-arterial emboli (20%–46%), in situ thrombosis (2%–23%), arterial dissection (0%–5%), and "unknown causes" (up to 10%) [7].

Approach to clinical localization of brainstem strokes

Brainstem strokes commonly cause hemiparesis, hemisensory loss, paralysis of the tongue, diplopia, dysphagia, and vertigo. Quadriparesis or sensory loss involving all four limbs occurs occasionally. Disparity between the side of the face and the side of the body affected by hemiparesis or hemianalgesia ("crossed sensory or motor signs") strongly suggests brainstem localization of the stroke. Clinically, neurologists first localize a lesion to the medulla, pons, or midbrain by identifying the cranial nerve nuclei

* Corresponding author. Department of Radiology, Mount Sinai Medical Center, One Gustave Levy Place, Box 1234, New York, NY, 10029.
  E-mail address: thomas.naidich@mountsinai.org (T.P. Naidich).

and fascicles affected. They then determine whether that lesion lies ventral versus dorsal and medial versus lateral by the specific cranial nerve nuclei and fiber tracts affected and spared. Thus, lower cranial nerve (CN) nuclei 9 through 12 (glossopharyngeal, vagus, accessory, and hypoglossal nerves) lie within the medulla. CN nuclei 5 through 8 (trigeminal, abducens, facial, and vestibulocochlear nerves) lie within the pons, and CN nuclei 3 and 4 (oculomotor and trochlear nerves) lie within the midbrain. Further, CN nuclei 3, 4, 6, and 12, the corticospinal tracts, the medial lemnisci, and the medial longitudinal fasciculi all lie medially within the brainstem, so involvement of these structures indicates a medial lesion. Conversely, CN nuclei 5, 7, 8, and 9 and the spinothalamic tracts all lie laterally within the stem, so involvement of these structures indicates a lateral lesion Together, these anatomic features provide a good first approximation of the site of the infarct (Table 1). Correlations with the known vascular patterns of brainstem blood supply and the imaging appearance of the lesion then refine the localization and provide a specific diagnosis of the brainstem stroke present (Table 2).

Vascularization of the brainstem

The vascularization of the brainstem consists of large, often variable, extrinsic vessels that bring the blood to the surface of the brainstem and small intrinsic vessels that penetrate the stem to supply defined vascular compartments within each part of the stem [13,14]. The extrinsic vessels include the VA, anterior spinal artery (ASA), posterior spinal artery (PSA), BA, posterior inferior cerebellar artery (PICA), anterior inferior cerebellar artery (AICA), and superior cerebellar artery (SCA). The uppermost brainstem also receives supply from the posterior medial choroidal artery, PCA, collicular arterial branches of the PCA, and the anterior choroidal artery. The major branches carrying this extrinsic arterial supply to the surface of the stem vary along the length of the stem from caudal to cranial. A great many variations of extrinsic arterial supply may be encountered. Ultimately, however, whichever extrinsic artery is nearby conveys blood supply to the adjacent portion of the brainstem, regardless of the vascular variation that brought it into proximity with the stem.

Table 1
Quick guide to brainstem localization

Part of brainstem	Cranial nerves	Structures	
		Medial[a]	Lateral[a]
Medulla	9–12	Corticobulbar tract	Inferior olive
	Part of 5	Corticospinal tract	Spinal nucleus/tract of 5
	Part of 8	Medial lemniscus	Spinothalamic tract
		Medial longitudinal fasciculus	Sympathetic tract
		Cranial nerve 12 nucleus	Nucleus ambiguus
			Inferior cerebellar peduncle
			Vestibular nuclei
Pons	5–8	Corticobulbar tract	Motor nucleus of 5
		Corticospinal tract	Principle nucleus of 5
		Corticopontine fibers	Spinal nucleus/tract of 5
		Medial lemniscus	Spinothalamic tract
		Medial longitudinal fasciculus	Middle cerebellar peduncle
		Cranial nerve 6 nucleus/paramedian	Sympathetic tract
		pontine reticular formation	Cranial nerve 7 nucleus
			Cranial nerve 8 nucleus
Midbrain	3 and 4	Corticobulbar tract	Sympathetic tract
	Part of 5	Corticospinal tract	Spinothalamic tract
		Substantia nigra	
		Red nucleus	
		Medial longitudinal fasciculus	
		Cranial nerve nuclei 3 and 4	
		Colliculi	
		Superior cerebellar peduncle	

[a] Listed from ventral to dorsal.

Table 2
Localization of key structures in the brainstem

Structure	Deficit	Part of brainstem	Intrinsic vascular territory			
			AM	AL	Lateral	Dorsal
Corticospinal tract	Contralateral hemiparesis/hemiplegia	Mid-Pons-Med	●	●		
Corticobulbar tract	Dysarthria	Mid-Pons-Med	●●			
Medial lemniscus	Contralateral loss position sense, vibration, and deep sensation	Mid-Pons-Med	●	●		
Spinal nucleus and tract of cranial nerve 5	Ipsilateral loss facial pain, temperature sensation	Mid-Pons-Med			●●	
Spinothalamic tract	Contralateral loss body pain, temperature sensation	Mid-Pons-Med			●●	
Inferior cerebellar peduncle	Ipsilateral or trunkal ataxia	Med				●
Vestibular nuclei	Contralateral ataxia, nausea, and vomiting	Pons-Med				●
Coclear nuclei	Ipsilateral hearing loss	Pons				●
Cranial nerve 12 nucleus/fascicle	Ipsilateral tongue weakness	Med	●			
Nucleus ambiguus	Dysarthria, dysphagia, hoarsness	Med			●	
Sympathetic Tract	Ipsilateral Horner's syndrome	Mid-Pons-Med			●	
Medial longitudinal fasciculus	Ipsilateral internuclear ophthalmoplegia	Mid-Pons-Med	●●			
Cranial nerve 6 fascicle	Contralateral lateral gaze palsy	Pons	●●			
Cranial nerve 6 nucleus/paramedian pontine reticular formation	Ipsilateral gaze palsy	Pons	●			
Cranial nerve 7 nucleus/fascicle	Ipsilateral facial palsy	Pons	●●			●
Middle cerebellar peduncle	Contralateral ataxia	Pons				●
Reticular formation	Lethargy	Mid-Pons-Med	●●	●	●	●
Red nucleus	Contralateral coarse tremor or choreathetosis	Mid	●●●			
Cranial nerve 3 fascicle	Ipsilateral superior, inferior, and medial rectus, inferior oblique palsies, ptosis, and pupil enlargement	Mid	●●			
Cranial nerve 3 nucleus	As above with additional contralat superior rectus, palsy, and ptosis	Mid				
Cranial nerve 4 nucleus	Contralateral superior oblique palsy	Mid				
Superior cerebellar peduncle	Contralateral ataxia	Mid				
Superior and inferior colliculi	Vertical gaze abnormalities	Mid				●

Abbreviations: AL, anterolateral; AM, anteromedial; Med, medulla; Mid, midbrain.

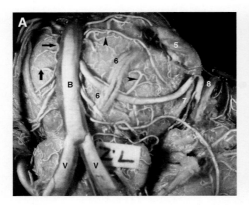
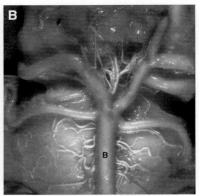

Fig. 1. Brainstem perforators. Gross anatomic specimens of the anterior surfaces of the upper medulla, pons, and midbrain after opacification of the major branches with micropulverized barium. (*A*) Upper medulla and pons. The vertebral arteries (V) of each side join to form the basilar artery (BA) (B) at the pontomedullary junction. Paramedian perforating branches (*horizontal arrow*) penetrate the brainstem immediately adjacent to the BA to supply the anteromedian arterial territory. Short circumflex arteries (*vertical arrow*) extend a short distance laterally before entering the stem to supply the anterolateral arterial territory. Long circumflex arteries (*arrowheads*) arise directly from the BA or from larger traversing branches, such as the anterior inferior cerebellar artery (AICA) (A), to supply the lateral arterial territory. Note that the AICA passes between fascicles of cranial nerve (CN) 6 (6) and then extends laterally to run along the anterior surface of CN 7 (7), loop over CN 7, nearly touch CN 5 (5), and then return toward the surface of the stem along the anterior surface of CN 8 (8). (*B*) Upper pons and midbrain.

When the extrinsic supply reaches the stem, it is apportioned into distinct, substantially constant intrinsic vascular territories designated anteromedial (synonym: paramedian), anterolateral, lateral, and (at some levels) dorsal territories. Anteromedial perforating branches arise from the major arteries near the midline and immediately penetrate into the anteromedial stem to supply the anteromedial zone of the brainstem (Fig. 1). Short circumflex (anterolateral) arteries arise from the major vessels and travel a short distance around the stem before penetrating it to supply the anterolateral zone of the brainstem. Long circumflex arteries arise from the major vessels in the midline or the large laterally directed branches like the AICA and SCA. These vessels nearly circumscribe the brainstem before penetrating it to supply the lateral territory of the brainstem [15]. Posterior perforating arteries arise from PSA branches of the VA and PICA inferiorly and from the PCAs and their posterior medial choroidal and collicular branches superiorly. These penetrate the posterior surface of the stem to supply the posterior compartment.

Medulla

The medulla oblongata, or myelencephalon, extends from the rostral end of the spinal cord caudally to the pontomedullary junction superiorly.

Anatomy of medullary structures

The intrinsic arterial territories of the medulla are considered in four zones: a large anteromedial, small anterolateral, large lateral, and small dorsal arterial zone (Figs. 2–4) [13]. From ventral to dorsal, the medulla comprises the following:

Anteromedial
The anteromedial medullary structures include medial portions of the pyramids, the medial lemnisci, the medial longitudinal fasciculi, and the nuclei and fibers of the hypoglossal nerve (CN 12).

Anterolateral
The anterolateral medullary structures include the lateral portions of the pyramids, ventral portions of the hypoglossal nerve fascicles (CN 12), and ventrolateral portions of the inferior olivary nuclei.

Lateral
The lateral medullary structures include the dorsolateral portions of the inferior olivary nuclei; the spinothalamic tracts; the ambiguus nuclei; fibers of the vagal nerves; the spinal nuclei and tracts of CN 5; the inferior cerebellar peduncles; ventral portions of the gracile, medial cuneate, and lateral cuneate nuclei; the dorsal motor vagal nuclei; the solitary nuclei and tracts; and the medial vestibular nuclei.

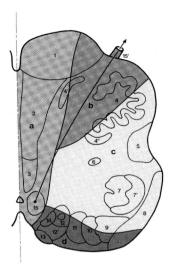

Fig. 2. Intrinsic arterial territories of the lower medulla. Shaded areas displayed clockwise from anterior to posterior: anteromedial (a), anterolateral (b), lateral (c), and posterior (d) medullary vascular territories. Numbered structures include corticospinal tract (1), medial lemniscus (2), medial longitudinal fasciculus (3), inferior olivary nucleus (4), medial accessory olivary nucleus (4′), spinothalamic tract (5), nucleus ambiguous (cranial nerve [CN] 9, 10, and 11) (6), spinal nucleus (7) and tract (7′) of the trigeminal system (receiving CN 5, 7, 9, and 10), inferior cerebellar peduncle (8), lateral cuneate nucleus (9), medial cuneate nucleus (10), gracile nucleus (11), nucleus of the solitary tract (receiving CN 7, 9, and 10) (12), area postrema (13), dorsal motor nucleus of the vagus (CN 10) (14), hypoglossal nucleus (CN 12) (15), and hypoglossal nerve (CN 12) (15′) (see Figs. 5 and 6). (*From* Duvernoy HM. The human brain stem and cerebellum. Vienna: Springer-Verlag; 1995. Fig. 90A, p. 126–7; with permission.)

Dorsal

The dorsal medullary structures include dorsal portions of the spinal nuclei and tracts of CN 5; the dorsal motor vagal nuclei; the solitary nuclei and tracts; the gracile, medial cuneate, and lateral cuneate nuclei; the areas postremae; and the inferior cerebellar peduncles. The precise structures in each arterial territory vary from low to high along the axis of the medulla, so the same structure may exist in two different compartments at different levels.

Arterialization: zones

The blood supply of the medulla derives primarily from the paired VAs, their anterior and PSA branches, and the PICA. The low BA contributes supply to the rostrolateral portion of the medulla.

Anteromedial

The anteromedial zone is supplied by anteromedial medullary perforators arising from the ASA inferiorly and from the ASA and VA further superiorly. These penetrate the medulla at the anteromedian sulcus.

Anterolateral

The anterolateral zone is supplied by anterolateral medullary perforators arising from the ASA and PICA inferiorly and from the ASA and VA superiorly. These penetrate the medulla at the pyramids and the preolivary sulci.

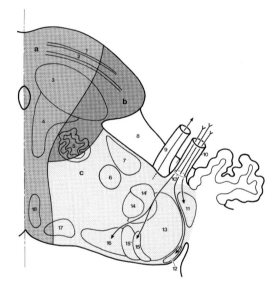

Fig. 3. Intrinsic arterial territories of the pontomedullary junction. Shaded areas displayed clockwise from anterior to posterior: anteromedial (a), anterolateral (b), and lateral (c) medullary vascular territories. Numbered structures include pontocerebellar fibers (1), pontine nuclei (2), corticospinal tract (3), medial lemniscus (4), superior portion of the inferior olivary nucleus (5), facial nucleus (CN 7) (6), spinothalamic tract (7), pontomedullary sulcus (8), facial nerve (CN 7) (9), vestibulocochlear nerve (CN 8) (10 and 10′), ventral cochlear nucleus (CN 8) (11), dorsal cochlear nucleus (CN 8) (12), inferior cerebellar peduncle (13), spinal nucleus (14) and tract (14′) of the trigeminal system (receiving CN 5, 7, 9, and 10), inferior vestibular nucleus (15), descending vestibular root (15′), medial vestibular nucleus (16), nucleus prepositus (17), and medial longitudinal fasciculus (18). (*From* Duvernoy HM. The human brain stem and cerebellum. Vienna: Springer-Verlag; 1995. Fig. 92A, p. 130–1; with permission.)

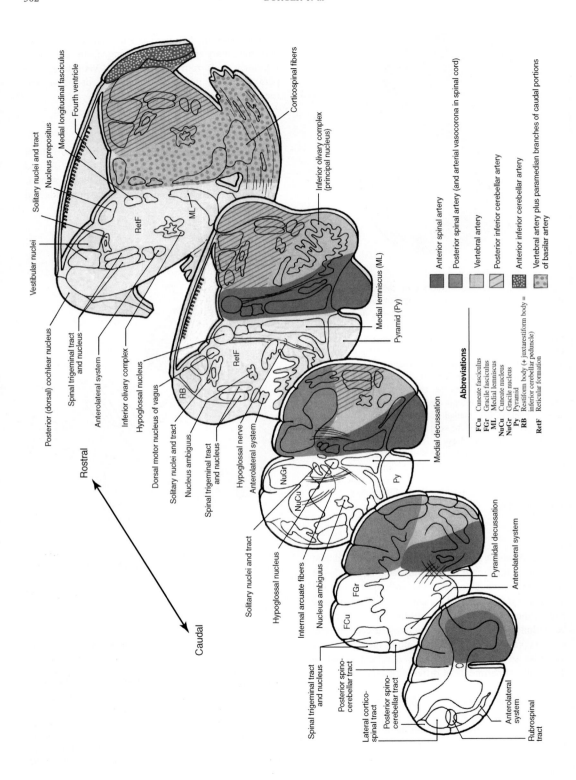

Rostral

Caudal

Medial longitudinal fasciculus
Nucleus prepositus
Solitary nuclei and tract
Fourth ventricle

Corticospinal fibers

Inferior olivary complex
(principal nucleus)

Vestibular nuclei

Posterior (dorsal) cochlear nucleus
Spinal trigeminal tract and nucleus
Anterolateral system
Inferior olivary complex
Hypoglossal nucleus
Dorsal motor nucleus of vagus
Solitary nuclei and tract
Nucleus ambiguus
Spinal trigeminal tract and nucleus
Hypoglossal nerve
Anterolateral system

RetF

ML

RetF

RB

Medial lemniscus (ML)
Pyramid (Py)

Medial decussation

Solitary nuclei and tract
Hypoglossal nucleus
Internal arcuate fibers
Nucleus ambiguus

NuGr
NuCu

Py

Pyramidal decussation
Anterolateral system

Spinal trigeminal tract and nucleus
Posterior spino-cerebellar tract
Lateral cortico-spinal tract
Posterior spino-cerebellar tract

FCu
FGr

Anterolateral system
Rubrospinal tract

Anterior spinal artery
Posterior spinal artery (and arterial vasocorona in spinal cord)
Vertebral artery
Posterior inferior cerebellar artery
Anterior inferior cerebellar artery
Vertebral artery plus paramedian branches of caudal portions of basilar artery

Abbreviations

FCu	Cuneate fasciculus
FGr	Gracile fasciculus
ML	Medial lemniscus
NuCu	Cuneate nucleus
NuGr	Gracile nucleus
Py	Pyramid
RB	Restiform body (+ juxtarestiform body = inferior cerebellar peduncle)
RetF	Reticular formation

Lateral

The lateral zone is supplied by perforators arising from the PICA inferiorly, from the VA in the middle, and from the low BA and AICA superiorly. These penetrate the medulla in the lateral medullary fossa.

Dorsal

The dorsal zone is supplied by perforators arising from PSA branches of the VA and PICA inferiorly and from the PICA superiorly.

Function

The clinical functions of the medulla are usually considered in two broad medial and lateral compartments rather than the four intrinsic compartments. Medially, the ventromedial pyramids contain motor fibers of the corticospinal tracts and the corticobulbar tracts. These motor fibers are organized somatotopically as medial corticobulbar fibers, midposition upper extremity fibers, and lateral lower extremity fibers. At least 75% of the corticospinal fibers decussate in the lowermost medulla and descend within the contralateral cord as the lateral corticospinal tracts. This decussation is orderly, with fibers destined for the cervical cord crossing first. The remaining uncrossed fibers continue directly into the ipsilateral spinal cord as the anterior corticospinal tracts or descend ipsilaterally to join the crossed fibers of the other side in the lateral corticospinal tract. The uncrossed fibers typically innervate the most proximal muscles of the extremities, whereas the crossed fibers innervate more distal musculature, including the hands. The dorsomedial sensory columns are also organized somatotopically with lower extremity fibers in the medial fasciculus gracilis and upper extremity fibers in the more lateral fasciculus cuneatus. Fibers responsible for coordination of the upper extremities pass further laterally to enter the accessory cuneate nuclei. The ascending sensory fibers of the dorsal columns synapse in the nuclei gracilis and cuneatus. In turn, these nuclei give rise to internal arcuate fibers, which course ventromedially around the central gray matter and central canal to the ventral midline. There, the internal arcuate fibers from both sides decussate in the great sensory decussation and emerge on the opposite sides, just lateral to the midline, as the paired medial lemnisci.

The medial lemnisci are also organized somatotopically, with lower extremity fibers filling in the ventral portion of the medial lemnisci from foot to groin, followed further dorsally by the upper extremity fibers filling in from fingers to axilla. The hypoglossal nuclei provide motor innervation for the tongue. The medial longitudinal fasciculi (MLF) are best known for interconnecting CN nuclei 3 and 6 to coordinate horizontal gaze. At the medullary level, however, the MLF mostly carry vestibular connections to CN 3 and 6. These help to maintain conjugate gaze during movements of the head and body.

Laterally, the inferior olivary nuclei receive fibers from the ipsilateral red nuclei via the central tegmental tracts, and project excitatory fibers completely across the medulla to the contralateral inferior cerebellar peduncles and cerebellum to assist in the control of voluntary movements. The spinothalamic tracts carry pain and temperature sensation from the contralateral body, excluding the face. The spinal nuclei and tracts of CN 5 convey pain and temperature sensation from the ipsilateral face. The nuclei ambigui provide parasympathetic motor fibers to CN 9, 10, and 11 for the laryngeal and pharyngeal musculature [16]. The ventral and dorsal spinocerebellar tracts convey fibers for fine coordination and posture of the ipsilateral lower extremity. The dorsal spinocerebellar fibers ascend through the ipsilateral spinal cord, medulla, and inferior cerebellar peduncles to reach the ipsilateral cerebellum. These fibers do not cross the midline, so their functions and deficits are ipsilateral. The ventral spinocerebellar fibers course rostrally through the superior cerebellar peduncles to reach the contralateral cerebellum. These fibers cross the midline twice, once in the spinal cord near to their origin and again in the superior cerebellar peduncle. Therefore, the functions and deficits observed for the ventral spinocerebellar tract within the brainstem are theoretically contralateral. The cuneocerebellar fibers convey fibers for fine coordination and posture of the ipsilateral upper extremity and neck. The inferior cerebellar peduncles (synonym: restiform bodies) carry uncrossed fibers from the dorsal spinocerebellar tracts, accessory cuneate nuclei, and vestibular nuclei to the ipsilateral cerebellum to coordinate motor function of the extremities and trunk. The inferior and medial vestibular nuclei (CN 8) assist in equilibrium and

---

Fig. 4. Intrinsic arterial territories of the medulla (multiple levels). (Note that the diagram is oriented with ventral to the bottom.) The usual external arterial supply to each zone is given as a list of vessels in the lower right corner. (*From* Haines DE. Neuroanatomy. An atlas of structures, sections and systems. 6th edition. Philadelphia: Lippincott Williams & Wilkins; 2004. Figs. 5–14, p. 111; with permission.)

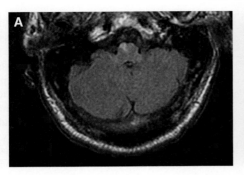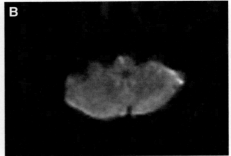

Fig. 5. Anteromedial medullary stroke. A 64-year-old-man with left hemiparesis. Axial fluid-attenuated inversion recovery (*A*) and diffusion-weighted (*B*) images. Increased signal in the pyramid reaching to the median raphe indicates an acute anteromedial medullary infarction (see Figs. 2 and 3).

spatial orientation. The nuclei of the solitary tract receive fibers from CN 7, 9, and 10 that convey taste innervation from the anterior two thirds of the tongue (CN 7), the posterior third of the tongue (CN 9), and the pharynx (CN 10). A complex multisynaptic pathway carries descending sympathetic fibers from the hypothalamus through the lateral brainstem and cervical spinal cord to synapse in the upper thoracic cord. These fibers later ascend to the orbit in a complex fashion to innervate pupillary dilators and the superior tarsal muscle (Mueller's muscle). Dorsomedially, between the vestibular nuclei laterally and the hypoglossal nuclei medially, the dorsal motor nuclei of the vagi (CN 10) provide parasympathetic innervation to the thoracic and abdominal viscera.

Infarctions of the medulla

Epidemiology of medullary infarcts

Medullary infarcts represent 7% of all ischemic brainstem strokes [5–8]. Lateral medullary strokes are approximately five times more frequent than medial medullary strokes [11]. Isolated dorsal medullary strokes are rare, although the dorsal medulla may be included in conjunction with cerebellar strokes. Medial medullary strokes are usually caused by occlusions of the ASAs that supply the inferior medial medulla or the VAs that supply the superior medial medulla. Lateral medullary strokes are usually caused by large artery disease of the VA (67%) or the PICA (10%) [17]. The most common risk factors for medullary infarcts are increasing age and diabetes mellitus [11]. Arterial dissections cause 20% to 30% of medullary strokes [11]. Men are affected more commonly than women by medial medullary strokes (M/F ratio = 3.6:1) and lateral medullary strokes (M/F ratio = 2.7:1) [11].

Medial. (Fig. 5 and Table 3). Medial medullary infarcts cause dysfunction of the medial medullary structures injured, including contralateral hemiparesis from the pyramids; theoretic ipsilateral loss of vibration and position sense from the dorsal sensory columns of the fasciculi gracilis and cuneatus, their nuclei gracilis and cuneatus, and the internal arcuate fibers; bilateral loss of vibration and position sense from decussation of the medial lemniscus; contralateral loss of vibration and position sense from the medial lemnisci; paresis of the ipsilateral tongue from the hypoglossal nucleus and fibers; and occasional nystagmus or skew deviation of the eyes from the medial longitudinal fasciculus.

Lateral. (Fig. 6 and Table 3). Lateral medullary infarcts cause dysfunction of the lateral medullary structures injured, including late-onset palatal myoclonus from the inferior olive; hypalgesia of the contralateral trunk and extremities from the spinothalamic tract; loss of facial pain and temperature sensation from the spinal tract and nucleus of CN 5; paralysis of the ipsilateral palate, pharynx, and larynx with dysphagia, dysarthria, hoarseness, and, rarely, respiratory arrest (Ondine's curse) [18] from the nucleus ambiguus; ipsilateral ataxia from the restiform body, dorsal spinocerebellar tract, or cerebellum; vertigo, nausea, and vomiting from the vestibular nuclei, restiform bodies, cerebellum, or area postrema; ipsilateral Horner's syndrome (ptosis, miosis, and anhydrosis) attributable to unopposed parasympathetic tone from the descending sympathetic tract; and, rarely, autonomic instability (labile heart rate) from the dorsal motor nucleus of the vagus. In addition, there may be skew deviation of the eyes with diplopia from the MLF [19]. Theoretically, contralateral ataxia may occur from injury to the segment of

Table 3
Medullary stroke syndromes

Medullary stroke syndromes	Artery involved	Ventral; dorsal; medial; lateral	Structure involved	Signs and symptoms	Eponym/other designation
Medial medullary	Verteberal artery and/or anterior spinal artery	Medial–ventral	Corticospinal tract	Contralateral arm/leg hemiparesis/hemiplegia	Dejerine's anterior bulbar syndrome
			Cranial nerve 12 nucleus/fascicle	Ipsilateral tongue paresis	
			Medial lemniscus	Contralateral loss of joint position sense	
Lateral medullary	Intracranial vertebral artery and/or posterior inferior cerebellar artery	Lateral–dorsal	Spinal trigeminal nucleus/tract	Ipsilat absent corneal reflex	Wallenberg syndrome
				Ipsilateral facial numbness	
			Lateral spinothalamic tract	Contralateral arm/trunk/leg numbness	
			Inferior cerebellar peduncle	Ipsilateral ataxia	
			Vestibular nuclei	Vertigo, nausea, and vomiting	
			Sympathetic fibers	Ipsilateral Horner's syndrome	
			Nucleus ambiguus	Dysphagia, dysarthria, hoarse voice	

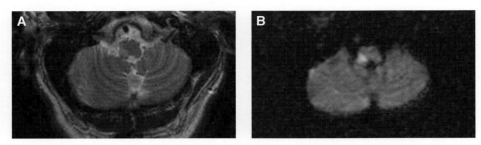

Fig. 6. Lateral medullary stroke. A 52-year-old-man with dysarthria, dysphagia, vertigo, right-sided ataxia, left hemisensory deficit, and right Horner's syndrome. Axial T2 (*A*) and diffusion-weighted (*B*) images. Increased signal in the restiform body reaching to the lateral pial surface but sparing the posterolateral portion of the restiform body indicates an acute lateral medullary infarction (see Fig. 2).

the ventral spinocerebellar tract that has not yet recrossed in the superior cerebellar peduncle.

Clinically, the triad of ipsilateral Horner's syndrome, ipsilateral ataxia, and contralateral hemisensory findings defines the lateral medullary syndrome of Wallenberg [20]. This syndrome is one of the few causes of disparate loss of pain and temperature,

sense, with a "crossed pattern" affecting the ipsilateral face and contralateral body. The crossed pattern occurs because the spinothalamic tract carrying pain and temperature sensation for the body decussates within the spinal cord just two to three vertebral levels above its innervation in the body, whereas the trigeminothalamic tracts carrying tri-

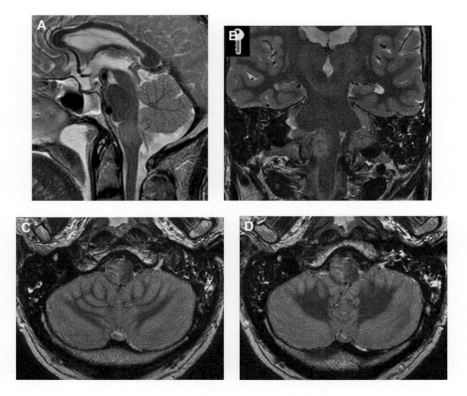

Fig. 7. Hemimedullary stroke. A 72-year-old man who presented with vertigo, vomiting, right facial weakness, right Horner's syndrome, and right ataxia. Hours later, he developed numbness of the left arm and leg. Sagittal T2 (*A*), coronal T2 (*B*), and axial T2 (*C* and *D*) images. Increased signal in the right half of the medulla from the median raphe to the lateral pial surface indicates a hemimedullary infarction, with sharply delimited sparing of the posterior arterial zone in some sections (*D*) (see Fig. 2).

geminal fibers for pain and temperature sensation from the face decussate cephalic to the trigeminal nucleus at the midpontine level (see Table 3).

Hemimedullary. (Fig. 7). Hemimedullary infarcts cause dysfunction of the medial and lateral medullary structures simultaneously, with contralateral hemiparesis, contralateral hemisenory loss, ipsilateral Horner's syndrome, ipsilateral ataxia, ipsilateral facial sensory loss, ispilateral tongue paresis, dysarthria, nausea, and vomiting [21]. Such hemimedullary syndromes account for 3% of medullary infarcts [11] and are attributable to occlusion of the ipsilateral VA proximal to the PICA and its ASA branches.

Pons

The pons, or metencephalon, extends from the pontomedullary junction caudally to the pontomes-

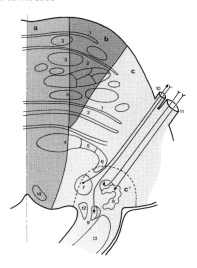

Fig. 9. Intrinsic arterial territories of the midpons. Shaded areas displayed clockwise from anterior to posterior: anteromedial (a), anterolateral (b), and lateral (c) pontine vascular territories. Numbered structures include pontocerebellar fibers (1), pontine nuclei (2), corticospinal tract (3), medial lemniscus (4), spinothalamic tract (5), lateral lemniscus (6), motor trigeminal nucleus (CN 5) (7), principal sensory trigeminal nucleus (CN 5) (8), mesencephalic trigeminal nucleus (CN 5) (9), fibers of the motor root of CN 5 (10), fibers of the sensory root of CN 5 (11), superior vestibular nucleus (CN 8) (12), superior cerebellar peduncle (13), and medial longitudinal fasciculus (14). (*From* Duvernoy HM. The human brain stem and cerebellum. Vienna: Springer-Verlag; 1995. Fig. 94A, p. 134–5; with permission.)

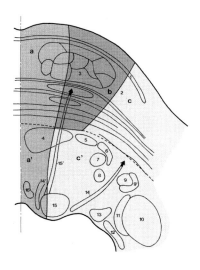

Fig. 8. Intrinsic arterial territories of the low pons. Shaded areas displayed clockwise from anterior to posterior: anteromedial (a), anterolateral (b), and lateral (c) pontine vascular territories. Numbered structures include pontocerebellar fibers (1), pontine nuclei (2), corticospinal tract (3), medial lemniscus (4), spinothalamic tract (5), lateral lemniscus (6), superior olivary nucleus (7), facial nucleus (CN 7) (8), spinal nucleus (9) and tract (9′) of the trigeminal system (receiving CN 5, 7, 9, and 10), inferior cerebellar peduncle (10), lateral vestibular nucleus (CN 8) (11), superior vestibular nucleus (CN 8) (12), medial vestibular nucleus (CN 8) (13), fibers of the facial nerve (CN 7) (14 and 14′), abducens nucleus (CN 6) (15), fibers of the abducens nucleus (CN 6) (15′), and medial longitudinal fasciculus (16). (*From* Duvernoy HM. The human brain stem and cerebellum. Vienna: Springer-Verlag; 1995. Fig. 93A, p. 132–3; with permission.)

encephalic junction rostrally (Figs. 8–11). It is subdivided into the basis pontis ventrally and the pontine tegmentum dorsally by an arbitrary coronal line drawn through the two medial lemnisci [13].

Anatomy of pontine structures

The arterial territories of the pons are considered in four zones: a large anteromedial, smaller anterolateral, large to extremely large lateral, and (in the rostral pons only) a small dorsal arterial zone (Figs. 8–12) [13]. From ventral to dorsal, the pons comprises the following:

Anteromedial

The anteromedial pontine structures include the medial pontine nuclei and pontocerebellar fibers, medial portions of the corticospinal tracts intermixed with corticopontocerebellar and corticobulbar fibers, medial portions of the medial lemnisci, fibers of the facial nerve (CN 7), small medial wedges of the abdu-

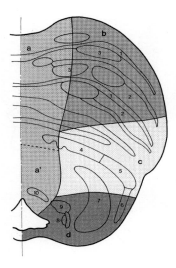

Fig. 10. Intrinsic arterial territories of the upper pons. Shaded areas displayed clockwise from anterior to posterior: anteromedial (a), anterolateral (b), lateral (c), and posterior (d) pontine vascular territories. Numbered structures include pontocerebellar fibers (1), pontine nuclei (2), corticospinal tract (3), medial lemniscus (4), spinothalamic tract (5), lateral lemniscus (6), superior cerebellar peduncle (7), mesencephalic trigeminal nucleus (CN 5) (8), locus ceruleus (nucleus coeruleus) (9), and medial longitudinal fasciculus (10). (*From* Duvernoy HM. The human brain stem and cerebellum. Vienna: Springer-Verlag; 1995. Fig. 96A, p. 138–9; with permission.)

cens nuclei (CN 6) and some emerging sixth nerve fascicles, the paramedian pontine reticular formation (PPRF; horizontal gaze center), and the MLF.

Anterolateral

The anterolateral pontine structures include the lateral pontine nuclei and pontocerebellar fibers, lateral portions of the corticospinal tracts intermixed with corticopontocerebellar and corticobulbar fibers, sixth nerve fascicles (lower pons), and small mid-lateral portions of the medial lemnisci (variable). Depending on the specific caudorostral level along the axis of the pons, the anterolateral zone may terminate ventral to the medial lemnisci or extend into the medial lemnisci. It typically does not extend further dorsally into the pontine tegmentum. The anterolateral zones do not extend far enough laterally to involve the spinothalamic tracts [13].

Lateral

The lateral pontine structures are comprised of two separate pontine regions (the upper and lower). In the large lateral zone of the low to midpons, lateral pontine infarctions include the lateral pontine nuclei

and pontocerebellar fibers, rostral portions of the inferior cerebellar peduncles (low pons only), middle cerebellar peduncles (low and mid pons), lateral portions of the medial lemnisci and lateral spinothalamic tracts, lateral lemnisci, facial nuclei and fascicles, the trigeminal complex (including the spinal nuclei and tracts, motor nuclei and fascicles, and principal sensory nuclei and fascicles of CN 5), the vestibular complex (including the medial, superior, and lateral vestibular nuclei), and most of the abducens nuclei and their fascicles. At these levels, the fascicles of CN 7 arise from the laterally situated facial nuclei and course dorsomedially to the medial aspects of the abducens nuclei (CN 6). The facial fibers then recurve ventrolaterally around the rostral poles of the abducens nuclei to course ventrolaterally to their exits at the supraolivary fossettes. In the smaller lateral zone of the upper pons, lateral pontine structures include the lateral pontine nuclei and pontocerebellar fibers, lateral portions of the medial lemnisci and lateral spinothalamic tracts, lateral lemnisci, and a ventral portion of the superior cerebellar peduncle (uppermost pons only).

Dorsal

The dorsal pontine structures are present in the upper pons only. No separate dorsal zones are found in the low to midpontine levels. Dorsal pontine structures include portions of the lateral lemnisci, portions of the superior cerebellar peduncles, the loci cerulei, and the mesencephalic nuclei of CN 5. The precise structures in each arterial territory vary from the low to high pons, so structures that extend along

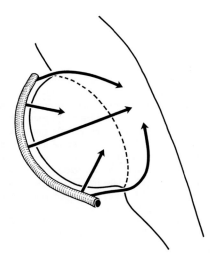

Fig. 11. Vascularization of the basis pontis and pontine tegmentum (see text).

the length of the pons may exist in different vascular compartments at different pontine levels.

Arterialization: zones

The blood supply to the pons derives primarily from the uppermost VAs, the BA, and the AICA and SCA branches of the BA:

Anteromedial

The anteromedial zone is supplied by anteromedial pontine perforators arising from the BA and entering (1) the foramen cecum at the midline pontomedullary junction inferiorly, (2) along the median sulcus of the pons in the middle, and (3) at the interpeduncular fossa superiorly (see Fig. 11) [13]. These perforators follow different courses for the basis pontis and the pontine tegmentum. The perforators for the basis pontis pass directly posteriorly from the BA into the basis pontis. The perforators for the tegmentum arise in three major groups: (1) perforators for the inferior tegmentum pass from the BA into the foramen cecum at the pontomedullary junction and then ascend to supply the inferior pontine tegmentum; (2) perforators for the midtegmentum arise from the BA and pass directly posteriorly through the basis pontis to supply the midpontine tegmentum; and (3) perforators for the superior tegmentum arise from the interpeduncular branches of the BA, enter the stem via the interpeduncular fossa, and then descend to supply the superior pontine tegmentum.

Anterolateral

The anterolateral zone is supplied by anterolateral pontine perforators arising directly from the BA.

Lateral

The lateral zone is supplied by lateral pontine perforators that arise directly from the BA, from the AICA, or from the SCA. The inferior lateral pontine artery arises directly from the BA to supply the middle cerebellar peduncle. The superior lateral pontine artery arises directly from the BA to penetrate the lateral pons in the region of the entrance or exit zone of CN 5. Lateral pontine branches of the AICA and SCA may similarly irrigate the lateral zone.

Dorsal

Where present rostrally, the dorsal zone is supplied by posterior pontine perforators that arise from the SCA to supply the superior cerebellar peduncles.

External to the brainstem, the AICAs also supply the fibers of CN 6 in the prepontine cistern, the fibers

of CN 7 and 8 in the cerebellopontine angles, and the petrous surfaces of the cerebellum (see Fig. 1). Internal auditory artery branches of the BA or AICA often supply the fibers of CN 7 and 8 within the porus acusticus. Occlusion of the internal auditory artery may cause ipsilateral hearing loss.

Function of the pontine structures

The functions of the pons are usually considered in terms of their intrinsic arterial territories.

Anteromedial

The medial corticobulbar tracts contain motor fibers that cross in the upper pons to reach the bulbar nuclei to assist in movements of the eyes, face, pharynx, and tongue. Just lateral to these, the corticospinal tracts contain motor fibers for the upper extremities en route to the spinal cord. The corticopontocerebellar tracts receive fibers from the motor cortex and send fibers to the cerebellar nuclei via the middle cerebellar peduncles to assist with motor control. The medial portions of the medial lemnisci convey ascending fibers for vibration, proprioception, and deep sensation from the contralateral upper extremities. The fascicles of the facial nerve provide motor innervation to the ipsilateral face. The abducens nuclei and fascicles provide motor innervation to the lateral recti. The PPRF lies adjacent to the abducens nucleus and assists in horizontal gaze in the ipsilateral direction. At the lower pontine level, the MLF contain predominantly vestibulocervical spinal cord fibers to coordinate gaze with head motion, whereas at the upper pontine level, the MLF contain predominantly fibers that extend between CN nuclei 3 and 6 to coordinate horizontal gaze.

Anterolateral

The lateral corticopontine nuclei connect extrapyramidal fibers from the cortex with the contralateral cerebellum to assist in motor control. Lateral portions of the corticospinal tracts contain predominantly motor fibers traveling to the contralateral lower extremity. Sixth nerve fascicles innervate the ipsilateral lateral rectus muscle to provide ipsilateral monocular abduction. Lateral portions of the medial lemnisci provide contralateral vibration and position sense, especially for the lower extremities.

Lateral

The lateral pontine nuclei and pontocerebellar fibers make up a small portion of the lateral territory. The rostral portions of the inferior cerebellar peduncles in the lower pons convey inflow tracts to

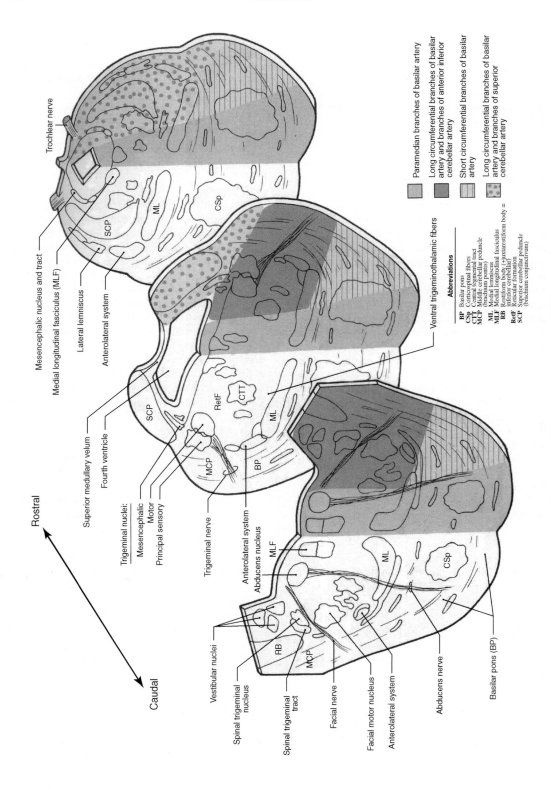

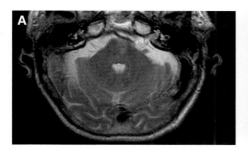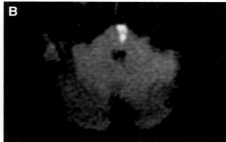

Fig. 13. Anteromedial pontine stroke. A 93-year-old-woman with dysarthria and right hemiparesis. Axial T2 (*A*) and diffusion-weighted (*B*) images. The narrow band of increased signal in the midpons reaching to the median raphe indicates an anteromedial medullary infarction (see Fig. 8).

the cerebellum to assist in motor control. The middle cerebellar peduncles in the midpons carry cortico-pontine fibers from the pons to the cerebellum to assist in control of movement. Lateral portions of the medial lemnisci receive contralateral fibers concerned with joint position sense and vibratory sense from the contralateral upper and lower extremities. The spino-thalamic tracts carrypain and temperature sensation from the contralateral body and extremities, excluding the face. The lateral lemnisci carry multisynaptic auditory input from the cochlear nuclei to the inferior colliculi. The facial nuclei and fascicles provide motor innervation to the ipsilateral facial muscles. The spinal nuclei and tracts of CN 5 carry pain and temperature sensation from the ipsilateral face. The motor nucleus of CN 5 provides innervation to the ipsilateral muscles of mastication (temporalis, masseter, medial and lateral pterygoid, tensor veli palatini, and tensor tympani muscles). The principal sensory nucleus of CN 5 receives ipsilateral light touch sensation from the face and subserves the corneal reflex. The pontine vestibular complex (medial, superior, and lateral vestibular nuclei) assists in maintaining equilibrium. The abducens nuclei and their fascicles innervate the lateral rectus for ipsilateral gaze. The facial fibers provide ipsilateral motor innervation to the facial muscles.

Dorsal

The lateral lemnisci convey auditory fibers from the contralateral trapezoid body to the inferior colliculus. Portions of the superior cerebellar peduncles represent outflow tracts from the cerebellum to assist in motor control. The mesencephalic nuclei of CN 5

receive proprioceptive information from the muscles of mastication.

Infarction of the pons

Epidemiology of pontine infarcts

Isolated pontine infarcts make up 3% of all ischemic strokes and 12% of posterior circulation strokes [6]. Most pontine strokes result from hemo-dynamic effects of BA stenoses or occlusions or from atherosclerotic lesions that occlude the origins of small perforating arteries to the brainstem. Emboli account for fewer than 10% of ischemic strokes of the pons because emboli usually travel beyond the pons to lodge at the top of the BA. Dissections rarely cause ischemic pontine infarcts. Risk factors for pontine stroke include hypertension (73%), hypercholesterolemia (32%), diabetes mellitus (30%), and smoking (21%) [6]. Pontine infarctions affect men (53%) slightly more frequently than women (47%) [6].

Kumral and colleagues [6] divided pontine ischemic lesions into five possible syndromes: anteromedial pontine infarcts constitute 58% of pontine strokes, followed by the anterolateral pontine infarcts (17%), tegmental infarcts (10%), bilateral infarcts (11%), and multiple pontine infarcts (4%). Lateral pontine infarcts are uncommon (1 of 150 cases [0.7%]) [6]. These clinical groupings do not correspond directly with the vascular territories delineated by Duvernoy [13].

Anteromedial. (Fig. 13 and Table 4). Anteromedial pontine infarcts cause dysfunction of the anterome-

Fig. 12. Intrinsic arterial territories of the pons (multiple levels). (Note that the diagram is oriented with ventral to the bottom). The usual external arterial supply to each zone is given as a list of vessels in the lower right corner. (*From* Haines DE. Neuroanatomy. An atlas of structures, sections and systems. 6th edition. Philadelphia: Lippincott Williams & Wilkins; 2004. Figs. 5–21, p. 125; with permission.)

Table 4
Pontine stroke syndromes

Pontine stroke syndromes	Artery involved	Ventral; dorsal; medial; lateral	Structure involved	Signs and symptoms	Eponym/other designation
Anteromedial	Anteromedial artery (aka paramedian perforating artery)	Medial–ventral	Corticospinal tract	Contralateral hemiparesis/hemiplegia	Pure motor stroke
				Contralateral ataxia	Ataxic hemiparesis/hemiplegia
			Corticobulbar tract	Dysarthria	Clumsy-hand dysarthria
			Medial longitudinal fasciculus	Internuclear ophthalmoplegia	Raymond syndrome: Ipsilateral cranial nerve 6 palsy and contralateral hemiparesis/hemiplegia
			Cranial abducens nerve fascicle	Ipsilateral lateral rectus palsy	Millard-Gubler syndrome—ipsilateral cranial nerves 6 and 7 palsies with contralateral hemiparesis/hemiplegia
			Paramedian pontine reticular formation	Ipsilateral horizontal gaze paresis	
			Cranial facial nerve fascicles	Ipsilateral facial weakness	
Anterolateral	Anterolateral artery (aka short circumflex artery)	Lateral–ventral	Corticospinal tract	Contralateral hemiparesis/hemiplegia	Pure motor stroke
				Contralat ataxia	Ataxic hemiparesis/hemiplegia
			Spinothalamic tract	Contralat numbness	Sensorimotor stroke

Location	Artery	Position	Structure	Sign/symptom	Syndrome
Lateral or dorsolateral	Caudal pons—anterior inferior cerebellar artery short or long circumflex arteries	Lateral–dorsal	Lateral corticospinal tract	Contralateral hemiparesis leg > arm	Foville syndrome—ipsilateral gaze paresis, ipsilateral facial paralysis, contralateral hemiparesis/hemiplegia
			Spinal nucleus/tract of cranial nerve 5	Ipsilateral facial numbness	
			Cranial nerve 7 fasciculus/nucleus	Ipsilateral facial weakness	
			Cranial nerve 8	Hearing loss	
			Cerebellum	Ipsilateral ataxia	
			Spinothalamic tract	Contralateral numbness	Marie-Foix syndrome—ipsilateral ataxia, contralateral sensory loss to pinprick sensation and temperature, contralateral hemiparesis/hemiplegia
	Rostral pons—superior cerebellar artery or long circumflex arteries	Lateral–dorsal	Sympathetic tract	Horner's syndrome	
			Superior cerebellar peduncle	Contralateral ataxia (may be ipsilateral)	
			Spinothalamic tract	Contralateral body numbness	
Bilateral	Basilar artery	Bilateral–ventral	Corticospinal tract	Quadriplegia	Locked in syndrome
			Corticobulbar tract	Aphonia/dysphagia	
			Paramedian pontine reticular formation	Bilateral horizontal gaze paresis	
			Cranial facial nerve fascicles/nucleus	Bilateral facial weakness	
			Reticular formation	Transient lethargy	

dial structures injured: hemiplegia or hemiparesis from the corticospinal tracts; contralateral ataxia or pathologic laughter [22] from the corticopontine tracts; dysarthria, dysphagia, or contralateral facial palsy from the corticobulbar tracts; rare contralateral loss of proprioception from the medial lemnisci; ipsilateral facial palsy from the nuclei or fibers of CN 7; ipsilateral sixth nerve palsy from the fascicles of CN 6; and paresis of ipsilateral horizontal gaze from the PPRF or the nucleus of CN 6. Injury of the MLF leads to internuclear ophthalmoplegia (INO) with disconjugate lateral gaze. The ipsilateral eye is unable to adduct as it attempts to look to the contralateral side, whereas the contralateral eye abducts normally but shows horizontal nystagmus as it gazes to the contralateral side. The INO seen with pontine infarcts characteristically spares convergence. Pure motor strokes that involve the face, the arm, and the leg equally are the most common presentation of anteromedial pontine infarcts. By the somatotopic organization of motor fibers within the corticospinal tracts, however, extremely medial pontine infarcts may cause pure motor plegias of the arm and face out of proportion to leg weakness [23]. Because the corticospinal, corticopontine, and corticobulbar tracts lie together in the ventral pons, paresis or paraplegia may occur in conjunction with ataxia as part of the ataxic-hemiparesis syndrome or in conjunction with dysarthria as part of the clumsy-hand dysarthria syndrome. Pure sensory strokes and combined sensory-motor strokes are other possible presentations of the anteromedial syndrome. It must be noted that lacunar strokes of the internal capsule may cause the same clinical findings as pontine strokes, including pure motor stroke, ataxic hemiparesis, sensorimotor stroke, and clumsy-hand dysarthria, because the internal capsule is the one other site at which all these fibers converge [24].

Three named but rare syndromes arise from the anteromedial arterial distribution (see Table 4):

1. *Raymond syndrome* is a ventromedial pontine syndrome in which infarction causes ipsilateral paresis of the lateral rectus muscle (from the fascicles of CN 6) and contralateral hemiplegia (from the corticospinal tract).
2. *Millard-Gubler syndrome* is a ventrocaudal pontine syndrome in which the infarction causes ipsilateral abducens palsy (from the fascicles of CN 6), ipsilateral facial palsy (from the nucleus or fascicles of CN 7), and contralateral hemiparesis of arm and leg (from the corticospinal tract). This syndrome may be regarded as a larger version of the Raymond syndrome.
3. *Cheiro-oral syndrome* is a pure sensory stroke of the midpons in which infarction involving the medial portion of the medial lemniscus and the ventral trigeminothalamic tract causes sensory loss in the perioral region and the contralateral hand [25,26].

Anterolateral. (Fig. 14 and Table 4). Anterolateral pontine infarcts cause dysfunction of the anterolateral structures injured, including plegia or paresis from the corticospinal tracts, ataxia or pathologic laughter from the corticopontine tracts, and vibration or proprioceptive loss from the medial lemnisci. Because the anterolateral zone of the pons contains the lateral portions of the same structures found in the anteromedial zone, the major clinical features of anterolateral pontine infarcts are similar to those of anteromedial pontine infarcts. Therefore, anterolateral infarcts may also present with pure motor stroke, ataxic hemiparesis, hypesthetic ataxic hemiparesis, clumsy-hand dysarthria, or sensorimotor stroke. Pontine infarctions may also involve the anteromedial

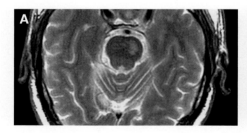
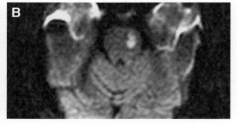

Fig. 14. Anterolateral pontine stroke. A 65-year-old-man with new right hemiparesis. Axial T2 (*A*) and diffusion-weighted (*B*) images. The paramedian band of increased signal in the midpons not reaching to the median raphe or the lateral pial surface indicates an anterolateral medullary infarction (see Fig. 10).

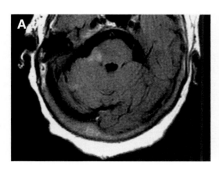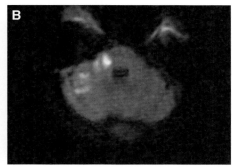

Fig. 15. Lateral pontine stroke. An 85-year-old-woman with slurred speech and weakness of the left face, arm, and leg. Axial fluid-attenuated inversion recovery (*A*) and diffusion-weighted (*B*) images. The posterolateral band of increased signal in the midpons with concurrent anterolateral cerebellar involvement indicates a lateral pontine infarction in association with an anterior inferior cerebellar artery infarction (see Fig. 9).

and anterolateral zones in continuity. At times, however, subtle features may suggest that a pontine infarct is purely anterolateral. Because the lateral zones of the corticospinal tracts contain predominantly motor fibers to the lower extremities and the lateral zones of the medial lemnisci contain predominantly sensory fibers from the lower extremities, more severe weakness and loss of position sense in the lower extremities could theoretically signify anterolateral involvement. Further, because the anterolateral zones contain the spinothalamic tracts, loss of pain and temperature sensation from the contralateral trunk and extremities may also signify anterolateral zone infarction. Rare extension of the infarct into the tegmentum might present as conjugate gaze paralysis, vertigo, skew deviation, or INO.

Lateral. (Fig. 15 and Table 4). Lateral pontine infarcts in the large lateral pontine zone of the low to midpons cause dysfunction of the lateral pontine structures injured, including ataxia from the inferior cerebellar peduncles, pontocerebellar fibers, and middle cerebellar peduncles; loss of pain and temperature sensation in the contralateral upper and lower extremities and trunk from the lateral spinothalamic tracts; tinnitus, reduced auditory acuity on either side, and abnormal sound lateralization from the lateral lemnisci [27–29]; ipsilateral motor deficits of the face from the facial nuclei and fascicles; loss of facial sensation, paresis of the ipsilateral muscles of mastication, and loss of the ipsilateral corneal reflex from the trigeminal complex; vertigo, nausea, and vomiting from the vestibular complex; and lateral rectus palsy from the abducens nuclei.

Infarctions in the smaller lateral pontine zone of the rostral pons cause dysfunction of the lateral pontine structures injured, including ataxia from the

pontocerebellar fibers, the middle cerebellar peduncles, and the superior cerebellar peduncles; loss of pain and temperature sensation in the contralateral upper and lower extremities and trunk from the lateral spinothalamic tracts; reduced auditory acuity and sound localization from the lateral lemniscus; and ipsilateral loss of jaw movement and facial sensation from the motor and sensory nuclei and fascicles of the trigeminal complex. These infarcts lie rostral to the nuclei and fascicles of CN 6, 7, and 8, so the patients do not display palsies of those cranial nerves.

Dorsolateral. (See Table 4). Dorsolateral pontine infarcts (at the same rostral level) cause dysfunction of the dorsolateral pontine structures, including reduced auditory acuity and sound localization from the lateral lemniscus or cochlear nucleus, ataxia from the superior cerebellar peduncles, theoretic parkinsonian symptoms from the loci cerulei, and decreased ipsilateral jaw jerk from the mesencephalic nuclei of CN 5. One small case series indicates that these lesions may manifest as sensorimotor or pure motor infarctions and often involve the leg more than the arm or face [30].

Three named but rare syndromes arise from infarcts in the (dorso)lateral arterial distribution (see Table 4):

1. *Marie-Foix syndrome* is a lateral pontine syndrome characterized by ipsilateral ataxia (from the middle cerebellar peduncle), contralateral hemiparesis (from the corticospinal tracts), and contralateral hypesthesia to pain and temperature (from the spinothalamic tract).
2. *Foville syndrome* is a dorsal caudal pontine infarct involving the PPRF, the nucleus and

fascicles of CN 7, and the corticospinal tract; it is characterized by ipsilateral horizontal gaze paresis, ipsilateral peripheral facial palsy, and contralateral hemiparesis.

3. *Raymond-Cestan-Chenais syndrome* is a rostral dorsal pontine infarct characterized by ataxia (from the cerebellum), contralateral loss of facial and body sensation (from the medial lemniscus and spinothalamic tracts), and contralateral hemiparesis (from the corticospinal tracts).

Tegmental. Tegemental pontine infarcts are characterized by predominant localization of the infarct to the dorsal (tegmental) portion of the pons. Clinically, tegmental infarcts exhibit prominent cranial nerve deficits and ataxia that are out of proportion to the motor findings. The overall picture may resemble other pontine syndromes but with more frequent diplopia, skew deviation of the eyes, abducens (CN 6) palsy, and vertigo.

Bilateral. Bilateral pontine infarcts of the ventral pons disrupt the corticospinal, corticopontine, and corticobulbar fibers on both sides; the fascicles of the abducens nerve on both sides; the PPRF on both sides; and the reticular formation. These lesions typically present as acute or subacute onset of quadriplegia, aphonia, bilateral facial paralysis, and horizontal gaze paresis. Involvement of the reticular formation reduces consciousness initially, but consciousness returns later. Variable injury to the spinothalamic tracts may cause loss of pain and temperature sensation in the body and extremities (but not the face), or not. In severe cases, affected patients may be left with vertical gaze movements as their sole remaining motor function ("locked-in syndrome"). Overall outcome of vertebrobasilar steno-occlusion has traditionally been poor, with a mortality of 50% to 90% [31], although more recent data suggest the potential for good outcome in 71% of cases, residual severe disability in 23%, and death in 2.3% [32]. Those with locked-in syndrome, however, rarely have a meaningful recovery [33].

Hemipontine syndrome usually results from pontine hemorrhage but may be seen with ischemic pontine stroke secondary to occlusion of the BA or multiple BA branches [34]. The major manifestations include ipsilateral gaze paresis, ipsilateral facial weakness, contralateral hemiparesis, contralateral hemisensory loss of the face and extremities, contralateral ataxia, and dysarthria.

Midbrain

The midbrain, or mesencephalon, extends from the pontomesencephalic junction to the diencephalon. It is subdivided into three regions. The basis mesencephali is formed by the cerebral peduncles. The tegmentum lies between the basis mesencephali and the aqueduct. The tectum lies dorsal to the cerebral aqueduct and is formed predominantly by the superior and inferior colliculi.

Anatomy of the structures

The arterial territories of the midbrain are considered in four zones: a prominent anteromedial, large anterolateral, small lateral, and small dorsal arterial zone (Figs. 16–18) [13]. From ventral to dorsal, the midbrain comprises the following:

Anteromedial mesencephalic

Anteromedial mesencephalic structures include small, extremely medial portions of the cerebral pe-

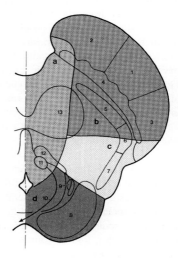

Fig. 16. Intrinsic arterial territories of the lower midbrain (level of the inferior colliculus). Shaded areas displayed clockwise from anterior to posterior: anteromedial (a), anterolateral (b), lateral (c), and posterior (d) mesencephalic vascular territories. Numbered structures include corticospinal tract (1), frontopontine tract (2), parietotemporopontine tract (3), dorsal substantia nigra (pars compacta) (4), medial lemniscus (5), spinothalamic tract (6), lateral lemniscus (7), inferior colliculus (8), mesencephalic trigeminal nucleus (CN 5) (9), fibers of the trochlear nerve (CN 4) (10), trochlear nucleus (CN 4) (11), medial longitudinal fasciculus (12), and superior cerebellar peduncle (13). (*From* Duvernoy HM. The human brain stem and cerebellum. Vienna: Springer-Verlag; 1995. Fig. 97A, p. 140–1; with permission.)

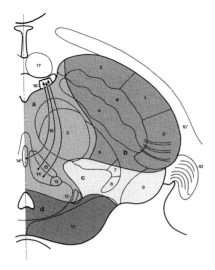

Fig. 17. Intrinsic arterial territories of the upper midbrain (level of the superior colliculus). Shaded areas displayed clockwise from anterior to posterior: anteromedial (a), antero-lateral (b), lateral (c), and posterior (d) mesencephalic vascular territories. Numbered structures include corticospinal tract (1), frontopontine tract (2), parietotemporopontine tract (3), dorsal substantia nigra (pars compacta) (4), ventral substantia nigra (pars reticulata) (4'), red nucleus (5), medial lemniscus (6), spinothalamic tract (7), lateral lemniscus (8), medial genicu-late body (audition) (9), lateral geniculate body (vision) (10), optic tract (10'), superior colliculus (11), mesencephalic trigeminal nucleus (CN5) (12), Edinger-Westphal (accessory oculomotor) nucleus (CN 3) (13), principal oculomotor nu-cleus (CN 3) (14), nucleus of Perlia (14'), medial longitudinal fasciculus (15), fibers of CN 3 (16 and 16'), and mammillary body (17). (*From* Duvernoy HM. The human brain stem and cerebellum. Vienna: Springer-Verlag; 1995. Fig. 98A, p. 142–3; with permission.)

duncles, extremely medial portions of the substantiae nigrae, the interpeduncular nucleus, the red nuclei, superior cerebellar peduncles and their decussation, a small medial portion of the medial lemniscus, the me-dial longitudinal fasciculi, nuclei and fibers of CN 3, nuclei and short segments of the fibers of CN 4, and the mesencephalic nucleus of CN 5 (rostrally).

Anterolateral mesencephalic

Anterolateral mesencephalic structures include the descending corticopontocerebellar, corticospinal, and corticobulbar fibers of the cerebral peduncles; the pars compacta (ventrally) and pars reticulata (dor-sally) of the substantiae nigrae; the ascending medial lemnisci; lateral portions of the superior cerebellar peduncles; and ventral portions of the ascending spinothalamic tracts. The optic tracts hug the ventral surfaces of the cerebral peduncles as they course

posterolaterally from the chiasm to the lateral geniculate bodies, so they are listed here, although technically they fall outside the brainstem.

Lateral structures of the low midbrain

Lateral structures of the low midbrain include the most posterolateral portions of the cerebral peduncles, posterior portions of the spinothalamic tracts, the lateral lemnisci, extremely small lateral portions of the MLF, and a small ventrolateral wedge of the inferior colliculi. The lateral structures of the high midbrain include posterior portions of the medial lemnisci, posterior portions of the spinothala-mic tracts, and the lateral lemnisci. The medial geniculate bodies (technically metathalami structures) are appended to the midbrain in the lateral zone.

Dorsal structures of the low midbrain

Dorsal structures of the low midbrain include the nuclei of CN 4, the mesencephalic nuclei of CN 5, the periaqueductal gray matter, and the inferior colliculi. The dorsal structures of the high midbrain include the superior colliculi and the midline posterior com-missure immediately dorsal to the cephalic ostium of the aqueduct.

Arterialization: zones

The distal BA terminates by bifurcating into the paired SCAs and PCAs. These give rise to most of the mesencephalic blood flow. The internal carotid arteries provide additional flow via the anterior cho-roidal arteries.

Anteromedial

The anteromedial zone is supplied by groups of perforators that arise in the middle of the interpedun-cular fossa. Of these, the more medial perforators enter just off the midline to pass to the trochlear nuclei (CN 4) inferiorly and to the oculomotor nuclei (CN 3) superiorly, whereas the more lateral perfo-rators enter the root exit zone of CN 3 to reach the superior cerebellar peduncle inferiorly and the red nuclei superiorly. On occasion, a single common trunk may supply the paramedian mesencephalon bilaterally [35].

Anterolateral

The anterolateral zone is supplied by anterolateral perforators, which arise in ascending order along the stem from the collicular artery, posteromedial cho-roidal artery, PCA, and anterior choroidal artery. The lateral zone is supplied by a group of lateral me-sencephalic arteries, which arise in ascending order

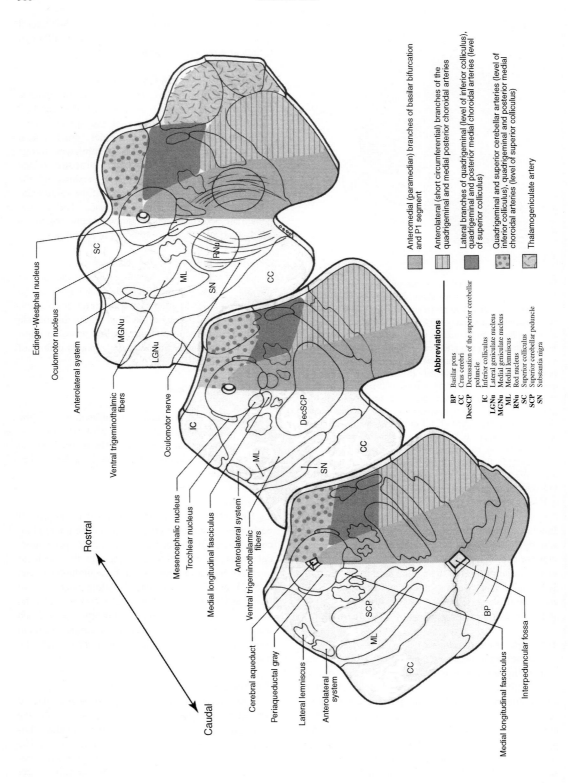

Rostral

Caudal

Edinger-Westphal nucleus

Oculomotor nucleus

Anterolateral system

Ventral trigeminothalmic fibers

Oculomotor nerve

Mesencephalic nucleus

Trochlear nucleus

Medial longitudinal fasciculus

Anterolateral system

Ventral trigeminothalmic fibers

Cerebral aqueduct

Periaqueductal gray

Lateral lemniscus

Anterolateral system

Medial longitudinal fasciculus

Interpeduncular fossa

SC

RNu

ML

SN

MGNu

LGNu

CC

IC

DecSCP

ML

SN

CC

SCP

ML

BP

CC

Abbreviations

BP	Basilar pons
CC	Crus cerebri
DecSCP	Decussation of the superior cerebellar peduncle
IC	Inferior colliculus
LGNu	Lateral geniculate nucleus
MGNu	Medial geniculate nucleus
ML	Medial lemniscus
RNu	Red nucleus
SC	Superior colliculus
SCP	Superior cerebellar peduncle
SN	Substantia nigra

Anteromedial (paramedian) branches of basilar bifurcation and P1 segment

Anterolateral (short circumferential) branches of the quadrigeminal and medial posterior choroidal arteries

Lateral branches of quadrigeminal (level of inferior colliculus), quadrigeminal and posterior medial choroidal arteries (level of superior colliculus)

Quadrigeminal and superior cerebellar arteries (level of inferior colliculus), quadrigeminal and posterior medial choroidal arteries (level of superior colliculus)

Thalamogeniculate artery

along the stem from the collicular artery, postero-medial choroidal artery, and PCA. These penetrate the stem at the lateral mesencephalic sulcus. The posterior zone is supplied by a posterior group of mesencephalic arteries, which arise in ascending order along the stem from the SCA, collicular artery, and posteromedial choroidal artery. These form a dense vascular plexus over the colliculi.

Function of the midbrain structures

The functions of the midbrain are usually consid-ered in terms of their intrinsic arterial territories.

Anteromedial

The substantiae nigra contain the dopaminergic cells of the partes compactae, important for smooth motor control. The red nuclei receive fibers from the dentate nuclei via the superior cerebellar peduncles and project fibers to the inferior olives via the central tegmental tracts (Molleret's triangle) to aid in the precision of voluntary movements. Cerebellar fibers traverse the superior cerebellar peduncles to synapse in the contralateral red nuclei to assist in motor con-trol. The MLF carries fibers that interconnect CN 3 with CN 6 to achieve conjugate lateral gaze. The third nerve nuclear complex is composed of multiple subnuclei for the levator palpebrae, medial recti, and superior recti muscles medially and the inferior recti and inferior oblique muscles laterally. The Edinger-Westphal nuclei send parasympathetic pupillary fibers for accommodation and pupillary constriction to bright light. These fibers course along the super-ficial aspect of the occulomotor nerve fascicles as they pass ventrally through the red nuclei to exit into the interpeduncular fossa just medial to the cerebral peduncles.

Anterolateral

The descending corticopontine fibers carry extra-pyramidal fibers from the cortex to the corticopontine nuclei to assist in motor control. The medial cortico-spinal tracts carry motor fibers that pass predomi-nantly to the upper extremities and less so to the lower extremities. The partes compactae (ventrally) and the partes reticulatae (dorsally) of the substantiae nigrae facilitate smooth motor movement and mini-mize excess movement. The ascending medial lem-

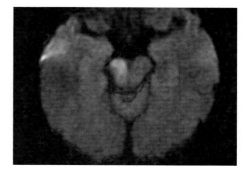

Fig. 19. Anteromedial mesencephalic stroke. A 34-year-old-man with hypertension, hypercholesterolemia, new onset of right gaze paresis, right facial weakness, and left hemipare-sis attributable to basilar artery occlusion. Axial diffusion-weighted image. The curvilinear band of increased signal in the midbrain reaching to the median raphe indicates an anteromedial mesencephalic infarction. The lateral extent of the signal abnormality suggests possible extension to the anterolateral territory as well (see Fig. 16).

nisci convey position sense, vibration, and deep sensation upward to the ventroposterolateral (VPL) nuclei of the thalami. The lateral portions of the superior cerebellar peduncles carry output fibers of the cerebellum to assist in motor control. The ventral portions of the ascending spinothalamic tracts carry pain and temperature sensory fibers primarily from the contralateral upper extremity and trunk. The optic tracts carry visual fibers, which arise in the ipsilateral temporal retina and the contralateral nasal retina from the optic chiasm to the lateral geniculate bodies.

Lateral

The posterolateral cerebral peduncles carry de-scending motor fibers for the lower extremities predominantly. The posterior portions of the spino-thalamic tracts carry ascending pain and sensory fibers from the contralateral lower extremity. The lateral lemnisci carry auditory fibers for acuity and sound localization to the inferior colliculi. The medial geniculate bodies receive and process auditory input for acuity and spatial localization. The descending sympathetic fibers assist in pupillary dilatation and opening the palpebral fissures.

Fig. 18. Intrinsic arterial territories of the midbrain (multiple levels). (Note that the diagram is oriented with ventral to the bottom). The usual external arterial supply to each zone is given as a list of vessels in the lower right corner. (*From* Haines DE. Neuroanatomy. An atlas of structures, sections and systems. 6th edition. Philadelphia: Lippincott Williams & Wilkins; 2004. Figs. 5–27, p. 137; with permission.)

Table 5
Midbrain stroke syndromes

Midbrain syndromes	Artery involved	Ventral; dorsal; medial; lateral	Structures involved	Signs and symptoms	Eponym/other designation
Anteromedial	Paramedian or thalamoperforating artery	Ventral–medial	Corticospinal tract	Contralateral hemiparesis/hemiplegia	Pure motor stroke
			Corticobulbar tract	Contralateral ataxia	Ataxic hemiparesis/hemiplegia
				Dysarthria	
			Red nucleus	Contralateral choreoathetosis	Benedikt syndrome—ipsilateral cranial nerve lesion, and contralateral choreoathetosis/tremor
				Contralateral coarse tremor	
			Decussation of superior cerebellar peduncle	Contralateral ataxia	Weber syndrome—ipsilateral cranial nerve 3 lesion and contralateral hemiparesis/hemiplegia
			Cranial nerve 3 fascicle	Ipsilateral cranial nerve 3 palsy	Claude syndrome—ipsilateral cranial nerve 3 lesion and contralateral ataxia
Anterolateral	Short circumflex arteries from the posterior cerebral artery	Ventral–lateral	Corticospinal tract	Contralateral hemiparesis/hemiplegia	Pure motor stroke (lower extremity > upper extremity)
			Medial spinothalamic tract	Contralateral sensory (pain and temperature) loss in extremities	Ataxic hemiparesis/hemiplegia
			Portions of superior cerebellar peduncle	Contralateral ataxia	Sensorimotor stroke

Lateral	Long circumflex arteries	Dorsal–lateral	Descending sympathetic fibers	Ipsilateral Horner's syndrome	Often predominantly sensory syndromes
			Lateral spinothalamic tract	Contralateral sensory (pain and temperature) loss	
Dorsal	Long circumflex artery, superior cerebellar peduncle, anterior and posterior choroidal arteries, and collicular arteries[a]	Dorsal	Superior/inferior colliculi	Vertical gaze palsies	Parinaud syndrome[a]—convergence retraction nystagmus, abnormal accommodation, eyelid retraction, loss of upward gaze
			Posterior commissure	Loss of accomodation
Loss of pupillary light reflex	
			Cranial nerve 3 nucleus	Ipsilateral cranial nerve 3 lesion
Contralateral paresis of upward gaze, and bilateral ptosis	
			Cranial nerve 4 nucleus	Contralateral superior oblique weakness	
Bilateral	Basilar artery	Midline	Midbrain	Vertical gaze palsies and cranial nerve 3 palsies	Top of the basilar syndrome
			Thalamus	Sensory findings and inattention	
			Medial temporal lobes	Memory disturbance and aphasias	
			Occipital lobes	Visual field deficits	

[a] This syndrome is usually due to compression from diencephalon and not from vascular lesions.

Dorsal

The trochlear nuclei and fascicles provide motor innervation to the contralateral superior oblique muscles to intort and depress the eyes. CN 4 is the only cranial nerve that wholly decussates to innervate a contralateral structure (the superior oblique muscle). The mesencephalic nuclei of CN 5 assist in proprioception of the masticatory muscles and subserve the "jaw jerk" reflex. The periaqueductal gray matter contains pretectal nuclei and pupillary fibers en route to both Edinger-Westphal nuclei to assist in pupillary constriction. The inferior colliculi are relay nuclei for audition, whereas the superior colliculi are relay nuclei for vision.

Infarctions of the mesencephalon

Epidemiology of mesencephalic infarcts

Isolated mesencephalic infarcts account for only 0.9% of brainstem infarcts [7]. More frequently, midbrain infarctions accompany infarcts in the PCA territories (3%). The most common cause of isolated midbrain infarction is small artery disease. The most common causes of all midbrain infarcts are large artery disease [including artery-to-artery embolism; (39%), small vessel disease with lacunar infarction (24%), and cardioembolism (20%)]. Dissections cause approximately 5% of ischemic midbrain infarcts [7]. The most common risk factor for midbrain infarctions is hypertension, followed by diabetes, smoking, atrial fibrillation, hyperlipidemia, and atherosclerotic ischemic heart disease. Men are affected more frequently than women (by a ratio of approximately 3:2) [7].

Anteromedial. (Fig. 19 and Table 5). Anteromedial mesencephalic infarcts cause dysfunction of the anteromedial structures injured, including dysarthria or dysphagia from the corticobulbar tracts, contralateral facial and upper extremity weakness from the

medial corticospinal tracts, contralateral choreoathetosis or tremor from the red nuclei, contralateral ataxia from the superior cerebellar peduncles, and INO from the MLF. The INO seen with mesencephalic infarcts characteristically impairs convergence, whereas the INO resulting from pontine infarcts characteristically spares convergence. Infarctions of the nuclei or fascicles of CN 3 manifest as deviation of the ipsilateral eye downward and laterally, with pupillary dilatation and ptosis of the lid. Pure motor hemiparesis and ataxic hemiparesis rarely occur in the midbrain. Lacunar infarcts of the cerebral peduncle may occasionally cause contralateral pure motor hemiparesis and ataxic hemiparesis, however [36].

Three named syndromes arise from infarcts in the anteromedial arterial distribution (see Table 5):

1. *Weber's syndrome* involves the third nerve fascicles and cerebral peduncle, causing ipsilateral third nerve palsy with contralateral hemiparesis.
2. *Benedikt's syndrome* affects the third nerve fascicles and red nucleus posterior to Weber syndrome, causing ipsilateral third nerve palsy with contralateral chorea, tremor, or athetosis.
3. *Claude's syndrome* involves the superior cerebellar peduncle and fascicles of CN 3, causing an ipsilateral third nerve palsy and contralateral ataxia [37].

Anterolateral. (See Table 5). Anterolateral mesencephalic infarcts cause dysfunction of the anterolateral structures injured, including contralateral ataxia from the descending corticopontine fibers and the superior cerebellar peduncles, contralateral hemiparesis affecting the upper and lower extremities predominantly from the corticospinal tracts, loss of contralateral vibration and joint position sense from the medial lemnisci, and loss of pain and temperature sense in the trunk and extremities from the ascending

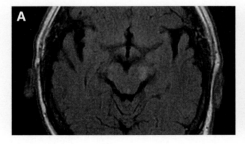 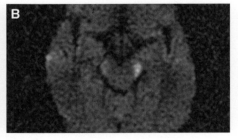

Fig. 20. Lateral mesencephalic stroke. A 58-year-old-man with diabetes mellitus, hypertension, hypercholesterolemia, and right ataxic hemiparesis from a basilar artery occlusion. Axial fluid-attenuated inversion recovery (*A*) and diffusion-weighted (*B*) images. The crescentic band of increased signal in the lateral midbrain indicates a lateral mesencephalic infarction (see Fig. 17).

spinothalamic tracts. Infarctions involving the optic tracts manifest as contralateral incongruous homonymous hemianopsia.

Lateral. (Fig. 20 and Table 5). Lateral mesencephalic infarcts cause dysfunction of the lateral structures injured, including contralateral hemiparesis predominantly affecting the lower extremities from the cerebral peduncles, loss of pain and temperature sensation in the contralateral trunk and extremities from the ascending spinothalamic tracts, ipsilateral or contralateral hearing loss from the lateral lemnisci (rare), and Horner's syndrome (ptosis, miosis, and anhydrosis) from the descending sympathetic tracts. Infarcts that involve the medial geniculate bodies may rarely cause auditory abnormalities [38].

Dorsal mesencephalic infarcts. (See Table 5). Dorsal mesencephalic infarcts cause dysfunction of the dorsal structures injured, including extorsion of the eye, slight elevation of the eye (hypertropia), and diplopia from CN 4 palsy; vertical gaze abnormalities from the periaqueductal gray matter; and tinnitus, hyperacusis, and, rarely, loss of auditory acuity from the inferior colliculi [38,39].

Compressive dorsal midbrain lesions may give rise to Parinaud's syndrome, characterized by loss of upward gaze, eyelid retraction, convergence nystagmus, and loss of accommodation. Because this portion of the brainstem has a rich vascular supply that protects against infarctions, dorsal mesencephalic compressive lesions are actually more frequent than ischemic lesions in this location.

The "top of the basilar (artery) syndrome" may result when emboli arising in the heart or proximal vertebrobasilar system lodge in the distal BA and infarct the bilateral midbrain, thalamus, and temporal and occipital lobes. These infarctions cause vertical gaze palsy, convergence disorders, semi-nonreactive pupils, peduncular hallucinosis, delirium, hemianopia or cortical blindness, motor deficits, and sensory deficits [40].

Hemimesencephalic syndrome is expected to combine the features of all the affected zones but is exceptionally rare (see Fig. 20).

Venous structures

The venous territories of the brainstem are similar to the arterial territories, level-by-level, but with subtle, often significant, variations. These are detailed in reference [13].

Summary

Thorough understanding of the organization of the brainstem and its intrinsic vascular compartments enables the physician (1) to plan an adequate imaging examination on the basis of the patient's symptoms and neurologic deficits, (2) recognize the patterns of ischemic infarction displayed on the images, and (3) predict patient signs and symptomatology from the structures shown to be involved.

Acknowledgments

The authors thank Joel Mindel, MD, for his assistance with this article.

References

[1] Brown RD, Whisnant JP, Sicks JD, et al. Stroke incidence, prevalence, and survival: secular trends in Rochester, Minnesota, through 1989. Stroke 1996; 27(3):373–80.

[2] Broderick J, Brott T, Kothari R, et al. The Greater Cincinnati/Northern Kentucky Stroke Study: preliminary first-ever and total incidence rates of stroke among blacks. Stroke 1998;29(2):415–21.

[3] Morris D, Schroeder E. Stroke epidemiology. Available at: http://www.uic.edu/com/ferne/pdf/strokeepi0501.pdf.

[4] Turney TM, Garraway WM, Whisnant JP. The natural history of hemispheric and brainstem infarction in Rochester, Minnesota. Stroke 1984;15(5):790–4.

[5] Bogousslavsky J, Van Melle G, Regli F. The Lausanne Stroke Registry: analysis of 1,000 consecutive patients with first stroke. Stroke 1988;19(9):1083–92.

[6] Kumral E, Bayulkem G, Evyapan D. Clinical spectrum of pontine infarction. Clinical-MRI correlations. J Neurol 2002;249(12):1659–70.

[7] Kumral E, Bayulkem G, Akyol A, et al. Mesencephalic and associated posterior circulation infarcts. Stroke 2002;33(9):2224–31.

[8] Martin PJ, Chang HM, Wityk R, et al. Midbrain infarction: associations and aetiologies in the New England Medical Center Posterior Circulation Registry. J Neurol Neurosurg Psychiatry 1998;64(3):392–5.

[9] Bogousslavsky J, Regli F, Maeder P, et al. The etiology of posterior circulation infarcts: a prospective study using magnetic resonance imaging and magnetic resonance angiography. Neurology 1993;43(8):1528–33.

[10] Caplan LR, Wityk RJ, Glass TA, et al. New England Medical Center Posterior Circulation registry. Ann Neurol 2004;56(3):389–98.

[11] Kameda W, Kawanami T, Kurita K, et al. Lateral and medial medullary infarction: a comparative analysis of 214 patients. Stroke 2004;35(3):694–9.

[12] Bassetti C, Bogousslavsky J, Barth A, et al. Isolated infarcts of the pons. Neurology 1996;46(1):165–75.

[13] Duvernoy HM. The human brain stem and cerebellum surface, structure, vascularization and three-dimensional sectional anatomy with MRI. Wien (NY): Springer-Verlag; 1995.

[14] Haines DE. Neuroanatomy: An atlas of structures, sections, and systems. 6th edition. Baltimore: Lippincott Williams & Wilkins; 2004.

[15] Brazis PW, Masdeu JC, Biller J. Localization in clinical neurology. 4th edition. Philadelphia: Lippincott Williams & Wilkins; 2001.

[16] Carpenter MB. Core text of neuroanatomy. 4th edition. Baltimore: William & Wilkins; 1996.

[17] Kim JS. Pure lateral medullary infarction: clinical-radiological correlation of 130 acute, consecutive patients. Brain 2003;126(Pt 8):1864–72.

[18] Bogousslavsky J, Khurana R, Deruaz JP, et al. Respiratory failure and unilateral caudal brainstem infarction. Ann Neurol 1990;28(5):668–73.

[19] Brazis PW. Ocular motor abnormalities in Wallenberg's lateral medullary syndrome. Mayo Clin Proc 1992;67(4):365–8.

[20] Sacco RL, Freddo L, Bello JA, et al. Wallenberg's lateral medullary syndrome. Clinical-magnetic resonance imaging correlations. Arch Neurol 1993;50(6):609–14.

[21] Mossuto-Agatiello L, Kniahynicki C. The hemimedullary syndrome: case report and review of the literature. J Neurol 1990;237(3):208–12.

[22] Parvizi J, Anderson SW, Martin CO, et al. Pathological laughter and crying: a link to the cerebellum. Brain 2001;124(Pt 9):1708–19.

[23] Kataoka S, Hori A, Shirakawa T, et al. Paramedian pontine infarction. Neurological/topographical correlation. Stroke 1997;28(4):809–15.

[24] Fisher CM. Lacunar strokes and infarcts: a review. Neurology 1982;32(8):871–6.

[25] Shintani S, Tsuruoka S, Shiigai T. Pure sensory stroke caused by a pontine infarct. Clinical, radiological, and physiological features in four patients. Stroke 1994;25(7):1512–5.

[26] Shintani S, Tsuruoka S, Shiigai T. Pure sensory stroke caused by a cerebral hemorrhage: clinical-radiologic correlations in seven patients. AJNR Am J Neuroradiol 2000;21(3):515–20.

[27] Furst M, Aharonson V, Levine RA, et al. Sound lateralization and interaural discrimination. Effects of brainstem infarcts and multiple sclerosis lesions. Hear Res 2000;143(1–2):29–42.

[28] Cho TH, Fischer C, Nighoghossian N, et al. Auditory and electrophysiological patterns of a unilateral lesion of the lateral lemniscus. Audiol Neurootol 2005;10(3):153–8.

[29] Sato K, Nitta E. A case of ipsilateral ageusia, sensorineural hearing loss and facial sensorimotor disturbance due to pontine lesion [in Japanese]. Rinsho Shinkeigaku 2000;40(5):487–9.

[30] Kataoka S, Miaki M, Saiki M, et al. Rostral lateral pontine infarction: neurological/topographical correlations. Neurology 2003;61(1):114–7.

[31] Devuyst G, Bogousslavsky J, Meuli R, et al. Stroke or transient ischemic attacks with basilar artery stenosis or occlusion: clinical patterns and outcome. Arch Neurol 2002;59(4):567–73.

[32] Voetsch B, DeWitt LD, Pessin MS, et al. Basilar artery occlusive disease in the New England Medical Center Posterior Circulation Registry. Arch Neurol 2004;61(4):496–504.

[33] Mellado P, Sandoval P, Tevah J, et al. [Intra-arterial thrombolysis in basilar artery thrombosis. Recovery of two patients with locked-in syndrome]. Rev Med Chil 2004;132(3):357–60 [in Spanish].

[34] Kushner MJ, Bressman SB. The clinical manifestations of pontine hemorrhage. Neurology 1985;35(5):637–43.

[35] Savoiardo M, Bracchi M, Passerini A, et al. The vascular territories in the cerebellum and brainstem: CT and MR study. AJNR Am J Neuroradiol 1987;8(2):199–209.

[36] Gorman MJ, Dafer R, Levine SR. Ataxic hemiparesis: critical appraisal of a lacunar syndrome. Stroke 1998;29(12):2549–55.

[37] Seo SW, Heo JH, Lee KY, et al. Localization of Claude's syndrome. Neurology 2001;57(12):2304–7.

[38] Hausler R, Levine RA. Auditory dysfunction in stroke. Acta Otolaryngol 2000;120(6):689–703.

[39] Musiek FE, Charette L, Morse D, et al. Central deafness associated with a midbrain lesion. J Am Acad Audiol 2004;15(2):133–51 [quiz: 172–3].

[40] Mehler MF. The rostral basilar artery syndrome: diagnosis, etiology, prognosis. Neurology 1989;39(1):9–16.

ELSEVIER
SAUNDERS

Neuroimag Clin N Am 15 (2005) 325–339

NEUROIMAGING
CLINICS OF
NORTH AMERICA

An Introduction to MR Imaging-Based Stroke Morphometry

Nikos Makris, MD, PhD[a,b,*], Verne S. Caviness, MD, DPhil[a,b,c],
David N. Kennedy, PhD[a,b,d]

[a]Department of Neurology, Harvard Medical School, Charlestown, MA, USA
[b]Center for Morphometric Analysis, Massachusetts General Hospital, Charlestown, MA, USA
[c]Pediatric Neurology, Massachusetts General Hospital, Charlestown, MA, USA
[d]Division of Health Sciences and Technology, Harvard–Massachusetts Institute of Technology, Cambridge, MA, USA

Thromboembolic stroke is a principal cause of morbidity and death in middle and late life [1,2], but it may occur at any moment in the human life cycle [1–3]. Inferences from the anatomy of the stroke lesion are central to the clinical diagnosis and treatment of stroke and to investigations of the underlying pathophysiology of the disease. Reestablishment of blood flow after occlusion and increase in tissue tolerance to ischemia are principal strategies for the treatment of stroke [1,4–6]. MR imaging allows approximate evaluation of stroke topography and size and, when combined with diffusion and perfusion studies, can provide a view of the evolution of stroke contours in relation to a perimeter of relative hypoperfusion [7–9]. Quantitative applications remain a work in progress but represent a vast, untapped source of biologically relevant information [9–11]. MR technologies have introduced a new set of tools for capturing features of normal brain anatomy and pathology in living humans. In doing so, these tools have begun to revolutionize the way we view the brain—literally and figuratively—

and our expectations for future diagnostic and investigative possibilities.

Protons are the most commonly used nuclei for MR in medical imaging. Through the use of radio-frequency pulses and manipulations of static and dynamic magnetic fields, signals can be received and localized from protons in the body [12,13]. These signals are turned into spatial images that characterize the contribution from each "voxel" (volume element). Much of the utility of MR imaging arises from the array of properties that this signal can be made to highlight. These include the intrinsic magnetic properties of tissue, such as relaxation times (T1, T2) and proton density [12,13]. The macroscopic and microscopic movements of protons can also be detected, providing the basis for depiction of circulation, including angiography [14] and tissue perfusion parameters such as blood flow and blood volume [4,15,16], and diffusion characteristics [17–19]. Because the MR signal is modulated by the local magnetic field that the protons experience, tissue properties that alter the local magnetic field can be detected, including variations in blood oxygenation state [20] and the chemical composition of tissue (eg, protons that are contained in water experience a different local magnetic field from protons that are contained in fat) [21–23]. These MR signal sensitivities can be used to create images that reveal distinctive characteristics of tissue. New or revised imaging protocols that are sensitive to additional properties of brain tissue are continually being developed; these imaging protocols have a growing repertoire of potential clinical and research applications. In this article, we discuss a

This work was supported by National Institutes of Health Grants PO1 NS27950 and DA 09467, by Human Brain Project Grant NS34189, and by grants from the Fairway Trust and the Giovanni Armenise Harvard Foundation for Advanced Scientific Research.

* Corresponding author. Center for Morphometric Analysis, Massachusetts General Hospital, MGH-East Building, 149 13th Street, Charlestown, MA 02129.

E-mail address: nikos@cma.mgh.harvard.edu (N. Makris).

set of quantitative anatomic descriptions applied to the study of patients who have had stroke.

Methodology

The quantification of morphometric properties is a valuable adjunct in the interpretation of MR images in the clinical domain. This approach takes advantage of the digital nature of the MR image and its utility for computerized image analysis. There are many morphometric properties of normal and pathologic structures that can be perceived by the human observer. To this end, quantification of properties, such as volume (size), shape, location, and intensity characteristics within a region, have found utility for many classes of structural analysis [24].

Structures are observed in an image based on regions of intensity, homogeneity, and similarity. Different contrast mechanisms for MR images result in the identification of different types of structures. For example, in images with T1 contrast, image intensity provides good differentiation (ie, contrast) between the gray matter, white matter, and cerebrospinal fluid compartments of the brain. This anatomic structure-based contrast makes these types of images useful for the quantification of anatomic structure. Other MR images (eg, those with T2 contrast) often show markedly contrasting signal intensity differences in the transition between normal tissue and tissue that is diseased or damaged (eg, some tumors, infarction, and infections). Such images are particularly suitable for the quantitative characterization of the volumetric extent of the pathologic process.

Segmentation

Segmentation is the process of delimiting homogeneous regions. Segmentation, as a topic in imaging science, radiology, and computer vision, has a long and rich literature. A number of comprehensive reviews provide a detailed overview of this topic [25,26]. Segmentation is a necessary precursor to quantitative regional morphometric treatments. The procedures used for segmentation depend on the nature of the image intensity information. In addition to the input image, segmentation procedures typically take advantage of derived features, such as edge information, textures, and spatial variation in illumination [27]. Segmentation may also depend in part on manual or automated knowledge-based judgments regarding interstructural boundaries [28,29]. User

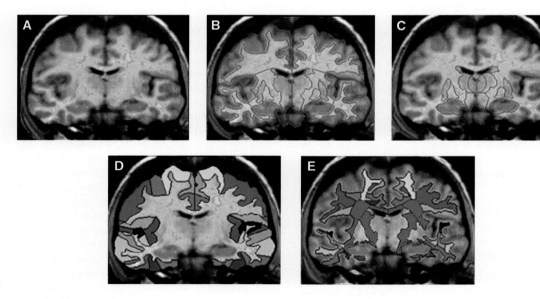

Fig. 1. (*A*) Results of morphometric procedures in an exemplar T1-weighted MR imaging coronal section. (*B*) Results of general segmentation procedure. The cortical ribbon, the subcortical gray structures, and the white matter are segmented as individual entities in their globality and are outlined in green. (*C*) Results of subcortical parcellation. The subcortical gray structures are parcellated further in more than one PUs and are outlined in green. (*D*) Cortical parcellation results. The cortical ribbon is subdivided into 48 PUs, each of which has a different color. (*E*) White matter parcellation results. The subcortical white matter is subdivided into two broad sectors (superficial and deep), which are parcellated into several more fine-grained PUs.

input is often required for segmentation to provide training data, to establish parameters, or to verify or modify the resultant regions.

Methodologies have been developed that allow brain segmentation based on many types of neuro-anatomic description. Typical anatomic divisions include the forebrain, brainstem, and cerebellum. The forebrain can further be segmented by standard algorithms into cerebral cortex, cerebral white matter, caudate, putamen, pallidum, thalamus, hippocampus, and amygdala [30,31]. Dedicated software allows the principal cerebral cortical gyri to be parcellated by a semi-automated method into 48 parcellation units (PUs) per hemisphere, with reference to a set of anatomic landmarks and the course of fissures (Fig. 1) [32,33].

For the delineation of a stroke lesion, the location of the border of the infarction must be identified, and this feature is dependent upon the imaging modality used. Thresholding techniques can be used to segment the region of lesion represented by image intensity alteration from normal expectation. Frank cavitation and a surrounding rim of altered signal in-

tensity can be readily distinguished from adjacent brain tissue. It is important to estimate the premorbid condition to characterize the tissue destroyed or at risk. Because premorbid imaging studies are rarely available, prestroke contours of structures destroyed within the stroke perimeter can be estimated by reference to corresponding undamaged structures in the opposite hemisphere. Although there is error in this approximation, it is expected to be relatively small compared with the substantial total volume of the stroke itself. Using the image segmentation tools and a comprehensive neuroanatomic system for general segmentation and cortical parcellation, we can analyze a stroke lesion in terms of its volume and location. Fig. 2 illustrates the method used for a stroke lesion analysis.

Morphometric descriptors

Once the desired segmentation is achieved, the determination of other morphometric parameters can follow. Volumetric determinations have been among

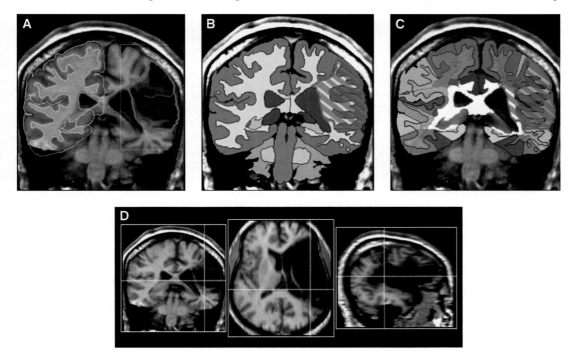

Fig. 2. Procedure and results of stroke morphometric analysis. (*A*) A T1-weighted MR imaging coronal section shows a stroke lesion in the left hemisphere that extends from the hemispheric surface to the lateral ventricle. (*B* and *C*) Location of the stroke lesion shown by overlaying the cortical parcellation (*B*) and white matter parcellation (*C*) outlines on top of the lesion. This detailed analysis produces a precise localization of the lesion and the volumetric estimate of anatomic structure that has been damaged in the brain due to stroke. (*D*) A cross-referential procedure using cross-hair projection lines that allows navigation throughout the brain across its three cardinal views.

Box 1. Cortical territories of the cerebral arteries shown as lists of cortical parcellation units using the cortical parcellation scheme

ACA

>   Frontal pole
>   Superior frontal gyrus
>   Juxtaparacentral cortex
>   Superior parietal lobule
>   Paracingulate cortex
>   Frontal medial cortex
>   Subcallosal cortex
>   Cingulate gyrus, anterior
>   Cingulate gyrus, posterior
>   Precuneus

PCA

>   Lateral occipital cortex, superior
>   Lateral occipital cortex, inferior
>   Occipital pole
>   Cuneal cortex
>   Supracalcarine cortex
>   Intracalcarine cortex
>   Lingual gyrus
>   Parahippocampal gyrus, anterior
>   (choroidal artery)
>   Parahippocampal gyrus, posterior
>   (choroidal artery)
>   Occipital fusiform gyrus

MCA (superior division)

>   Middle frontal gyrus
>   Inferior frontal gyrus, pars triangularis
>   Frontal orbital cortex
>   Precentral gyrus
>   Postcentral gyrus
>   Supramarginal gyrus, anterior
>   Supramarginal gyrus, posterior
>   Frontal operculum
>   Central operculum
>   Parietal operculum
>   Insula

MCA (inferior division)

>   Angular gyrus
>   Temporal pole
>   Superior temporal gyrus, anterior

>   Superior temporal gyrus, posterior
>   Middle temporal gyrus, anterior
>   Middle temporal gyrus, posterior
>   Inferior temporal gyrus, anterior
>   Inferior temporal gyrus, posterior
>   Temporal fusiform, anterior
>   Middle temporal gyrus, temporooccipital
>   Inferior temporal gyrus, temporooccipital
>   Temporooccipital fusiform gyrus
>   Planum polare
>   Heschl's gyrus
>   Planum temporale

This box represents an approximation, especially in the areas supplied by more than one artery or branch of the middle cerebral artery. (*Data from* Caviness Jr VS, Meyer JW, Makris N, et al. MRI-based topographic parcellation of the human neocortex: an anatomically specified method with estimate of reliability. J Cogn Neurosci 1996;8:566–87.)

the most frequent of such applications. The volume of a segmented region is obtained by summation of the volume of all voxels assigned to it by segmentation [31].

Location can be characterized in a number of ways. Location is described relative to a "coordinate" system that is typically defined in relation to specific anatomic landmarks. The most commonly used coordinate system is the Talairach proportional coordinate system [34,35], which uses a set of anatomic landmarks in the brain to define the transformation of that brain into a "standard" space. The Talairach space transformation is piece-wise linear and is quick and relatively simple to achieve, but a substantial amount of anatomic variability is not accounted for. Higher-order spatial deformations between images (including deformation to a "standard" brain) are also being widely developed [29,36,37]. An alternate form of anatomic localization is provided by the observation of an "anatomic description hierarchy" within the individual subject. The use of a standard, comprehensive, taxonomic definition of anatomic structure, matched to the types of features that are available within the MR image, provides a valuable basis for establishing where a region is within the coordinate system [32,38]. An anatomic structure, given a specified set of definitions and nomenclature, provides a comprehensive location in the neuroanatomic (ie, what it is part of and what it is comprised of) and neurofunctional systems hierarchy.

Implications for cerebral vascular territories

Because of its neuroanatomic design, the gyral-based cortical parcellation system allows the inference of relationships between gyral regions and the typical vascularization pattern in the normal human brain. Box 1 and Fig. 3 show the relationships between the cerebral parcellation units and the cerebral arteries. From the anatomic building blocks, we can devise representations of various important classes of tissue. For example, we distinguish a "superficial" compartment corresponding to the perfusion territory of the leptomeningeal branches (M2–M4) of the middle cerebral artery (MCA) (cortex and subjacent white matter radiata [39,40]) and a "deep" compartment (basal ganglia, thalamus, amygdala, and white matter of the capsules and commissures) corresponding to the perfusion territory of the M1 division of the MCA system [41–46].

Survey of sample morphometric applications in stroke

Application A: volumetric assessment

We have performed a comprehensive assessment of the topographic and volumetric distribution of infarcts with respect to neuroanatomic structures, perfusion compartments, and tissue types in 21 brains. The segmentation and cortical parcellation procedure is shown in Figs. 1 and 2. Details on subject demographic information and clinical profiles have been presented previously [47]. In summary, there were 21 subjects (10 men and 11 women, age range 34–75 years, mean 57.5 ± 12.5 years), mostly right handed, with no clinically recognized prior stroke or other cerebral disorder. In all subjects, dysphasic disturbance was of acute onset and was considered to be consequent to MCA territory embolus of the language-dominant hemisphere. The median interval between the acute stroke and imaging was 16 months. A principal infarction was located in the central Sylvian region in each of the 21 brains.

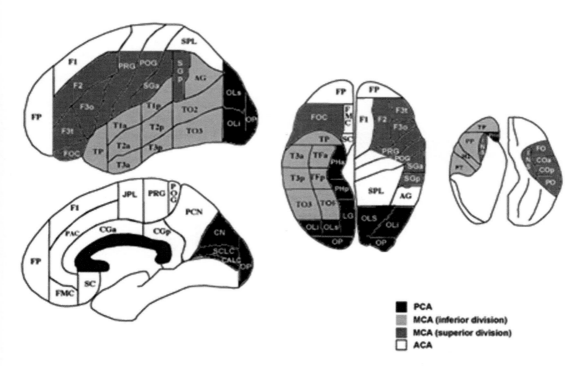

Fig. 3. The cortical territories of the cerebral arteries are depicted on templates using the cortical parcellation scheme. This is an approximation, especially in the areas supplied by more than one arteries or branches of the MCA. PUs supplied mainly by the ACA are white. PUs supplied by the PCA are black. PUs supplied by the two divisions of the MCA are gray. The inferior MCA division territory is shaded in lighter gray, and the superior MCA division territory is shaded in darker gray.

Stroke and vascular topography

Of the principal infarctions, 17 were within the left (15 right handed, one left handed, one handedness not determined), and four were within the right hemisphere (all right handed). In all but three, these fell exclusively within the classically accepted territory of perfusion of the middle cerebral artery [48]. In three cases, infarctions also involved the accepted territories of perfusion of the anterior (the medial frontal and cingulate cortical fields) or the posterior (the medial occipital and occipital polar fields) cerebral arteries.

In the collective set of infarctions, all cerebral regions within the M2 to M4 perfusion territory were involved (Fig. 4). There was an emphasis on the insular and adjacent opercular region (M2 and M3 territories) and the cortical regions supplied by the precentral, central, and anterior parietal branches of the M4 system. With reference to the subdivisions of the MCA [48], we distinguish by case number four general patterns of distribution of infarction. Infarc-

tion may be (1) limited to the M1 territory, (2) limited to the M2 to M4 territory, (3) distributed within the M1 and M2 to M4 territories where the tissue volumes involved are continuous, and (4) distributed within the M1 and M2 to M4 territories where the tissue volumes involved are discontinuous. Patterns 1 and 2 illustrate the commonplace occurrence where infarction occurs independently in the deep nuclear and capsular (M1 alone) regions or in the superficial cortical territories of the MCA (M2–M4 alone).

Stroke volume and brain topography

The total volumes of the infarctions were distributed over a two order of magnitude range (3–256 mL), with a mean of 103 mL (left 105 mL, right 96 mL). The volumes of individual infarctions spread over a relatively uniform distribution. Approximately 60% and 20% of total stroke volume are assigned to cortex and radiate white matter, respectively.

Gyral PUs within the classical territory of MCA perfusion were infarcted in 19 of the 21 brains (90%)

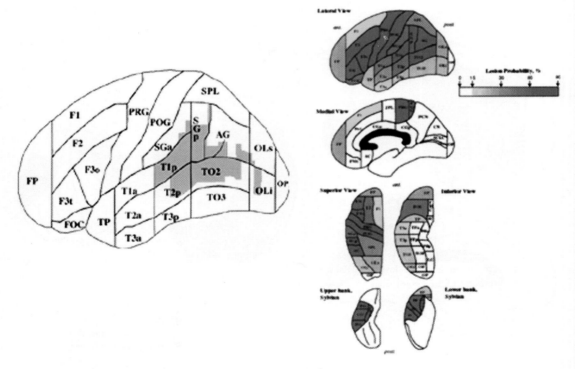

Fig. 4. The stroke cortical topography is shown in the cerebral template on the left side of the figure. The distribution of the infarction is mapped on the surface of the hemisphere as reconstructed from a series of T1-weighted MR imaging coronal slices. On the right, the probability of infarction for the MCA PU is represented as intensity of shading; intensity of shading represents the probability that the PU was lesioned by > 10% of its volume in the full series of 21 cases published previously by our group [47].

(Box 1). A small number of PUs (three subjects) was excluded because infarction was judged to extend into the territories of anterior cerebral artery (ACA) or posterior cerebral artery (PCA) perfusion. For this subset of 19 brains, the probability that one of the MCA PUs would be involved ranged from 0.84 to 0.16 (Fig. 4), with a mean of 0.54. For 19 (63%) of the PUs (specifically those of the insula, opercular, paracentral, inferior frontal, and the junction of the temporal/parietal/occipital regions), this probability was at least 0.5. For six MCA PUs (principally at the inferior and posterior temporal and superior frontal regions), this probability was less than 0.3. The mean volume of tissue destroyed in the MCA PU ranged from 0.4 to 10.5 mL, corresponding to a range from 30.6% to 88.3% of the individual PUs, with mean of 57.6%.

In 15 brains where stroke involved the deep perfusion compartment, putamen, pallidum, and caudate were involved with probabilities of 1.0, 0.80, and 0.87, respectively. The average fraction of nucleus damaged was 53%, 67%, and 48%, respectively, for the three nuclei. That is, the putamen was involved in all, and the other two in most of the cases included the M1 compartment. In all 15 cases, there was injury to the deep white matter of the capsules. The ventral diencephalon was involved in only one case, the thalamus and amygdala in two cases each, and the accumbens nucleus in three cases. The fractional damage to both diencephalic structures was approximately 20%; the fractional damage to accumbens and amygdala was approximately 50% each. In each of these brains, the patterns of neocortical PU involvement indicated that there had been associated infarction in the ACA or PCA territories.

Application B: Integration of three magnetic resonance modalities

In application B, we illustrate the integration of T1 morphometric analysis with diffusion tensor (DT) MR imaging and MR spectroscopy to demonstrate (1) the topography of a stroke lesion, (2) the secondary degeneration of a cerebral fiber tract (specifically the superior longitudinal fasciculus [SLF]), and (3) the metabolic alterations of cortical regions remote but connected to the lesioned cortical areas. The subject was a 65-year-old, right-handed, English-speaking man [18]. The patient suffered an embolic infarction of the left inferior parietal lobule (parietal operculum, lower portion of supramarginal gyrus adjacent to the parietal operculum, dorsal portion of the supramarginal gyrus posterior to the sylvian fissure, and higher portion of the angular gyrus) and

presented with conduction aphasia. The DT-MR imaging pattern observed in this patient showed remarkable reduction in preferred diffusion orientation for the left SLF, as compared with the patient's right hemisphere and as compared with normal control subjects (Fig. 5), suggesting damage to this structure [18]. In addition to DT imaging, spectroscopic analysis was performed using an NAA-based technique for cerebral metabolism. We then applied the cortico-cortical anatomic connection map (see below) for the SLF to assess its predictive value for identifying abnormal metabolism of cortical regions connected by this bundle after SLF damage. Hypometabolism was observed in the inferior parietal lobule and the inferior frontal gyrus (Fig. 5)—areas interconnected by the SLF. The potential clinical relevance of this quantitative characterization of fiber pathway variability is that lesioned pathways may correlate with functional deficits, whereas spared fiber tracts may predict the nature and extent of recovery.

Application C: Integration of magnetic resonance imaging and positron emission tomography

In application C, we integrated T1 morphometric MR imaging and positron emission tomography (PET) to localize the stroke lesion and to evaluate the metabolic pattern of cortical regions remote from but connected to the lesioned areas in two subjects affected by embolic stroke. Both patients presented with embolic infarction of the caudal temporal lobe (Fig. 6). Hypometabolic activity of the rostral temporopolar cortex was demonstrated using PET in patient 2 only. Presumably, this was due to damage of the stem portion of the inferior longitudinal fasciculus (ILF), which interconnects the caudal temporal lobe with the temporopolar cortex (Fig. 6). In contrast, in patient 1, who presented a similar cortical lesion that did not extend deeply enough to damage the stem of the inferior longitudinal fasciculus, hypometabolism was not observed (Fig. 6).

Application D: Alterations in subcortical regions after cortical insult

Using T1 morphometric MR imaging, we performed volumetric analyses of subcortical structures to evaluate changes in volume of the thalamus, basal ganglia, hippocampus, and amygdala and the brainstem and pons [49]. We studied the remote effects of cortical damage in 19 patients and subcortical damage in two patients affected by stroke due to embolic occlusion of the left middle cerebral artery

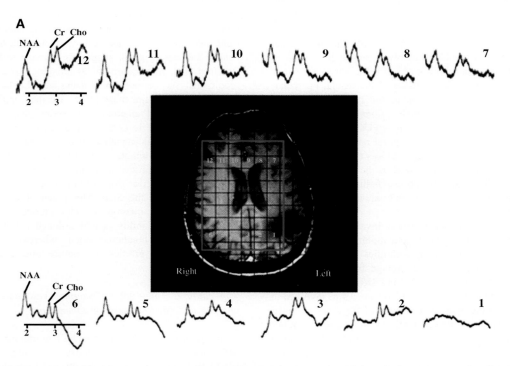

Fig. 5. Data from a stroke case. (*A*) Localized proton spectroscopy in this patient demonstrates regional alterations in metabolite concentrations. Spectra 1 through 6 are representative of the posterior portion of this slice through the lesion. These spectra indicate absence of discernible peaks within the lesion and a normalization of the spectra as one moves to the contralateral, normal hemisphere. Spectra 7 through 12 represent a series of spectra from the anterior portion of this slice. Although all metabolite peaks are present, the ipsilateral spectra demonstrate a marked diminution of the metabolite concentrations relative to the contralateral hemisphere. (*B*) T1-MR imaging axial slice cutting through the genu and splenium of the corpus callosum. Dotted red lines represent the trajectory of the SLF in this axial level. Note how areas of the parietal gyrus would connect with lateral frontal cortices through the SLF. This axial slice is identical to the one in (*A*). (*C*) Mapping of cortical lesion on a template derived from the cortical parcellation system indicating a lesion (*gray*) involving the inferior portion of the anterior supramarginal and the superior portions of the posterior supramarginal and angular parcellation units of the inferior parietal lobule. This stroke lesion involved parietal lobe cortical parcellation units SGa, SGp, PO, and angular gyrus (AG) of the cortical parcellation system of Rademacher and colleagues [32]. The blue rectangular area shows the approximate location of a hypometabolic area located mainly in the inferior frontal gyrus (F3) corresponding to voxel 7 in (*A*) and the left frontal area in (*B*). Arrows indicate the level of coronal slice shown in (*D*). (*D*) Diffusion primary eigenvector map image of Application B. The arrows show the superior longitudinal fasciculus and the cingulum bundle in both hemispheres. Note the reduction in number of the pixels indicating anterior-posterior orientation (*green*) for the superior longitudinal fasciculus (*two adjacent arrows*) on the patient's left. CB, cingulum bundle. (*E*) SLF$_{MAC}$. A representation of the connections of SLF is presented, derived from anatomic studies in the human and the experimental material [39] (*dark blue*). Frontal lobe parcellation units F3t, F3o, and FO and temporal lobe parcellation units T1a and T1p are connected to parietal lobe cortical parcellation units supramarginal gyrus, anterior (SGa); supramarginal gyrus, posterior (SGp); PO, and AG. F1, superior frontal gyrus; F2, middle frontal gyrus; F3o, inferior frontal gyrus, pars opercularis; F3t, inferior frontal gyrus, pars triangularis; FOC, frontal orbital cortex; FP, frontal pole; OLi, lateral occipital cortex, inferior; OLs, lateral occipital cortex, superior; OP, occipital pole; POG, postcentral gyrus; PP, planum polare; PRG, precentral gyrus; SPL, superior parietal lobule; T1a, superior temporal gyrus, anterior; T1p, superior temporal gyrus, posterior; T2a, middle temporal gyrus, anterior; T2p, middle temporal gyrus, posterior; T3a, inferior temporal gyrus, anterior; T3p, inferior temporal gyrus, posterior; TO2, middle temporal gyrus, temporooccipital; TO3, inferior temporal gyrus, temporooccipital; TP, temporal pole.

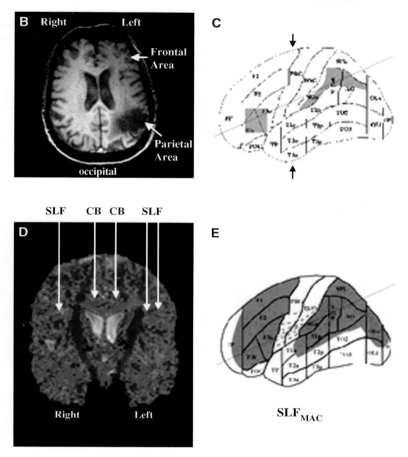

Fig. 5 (*continued*).

[47]. We hypothesized that damage of cortical gray matter would result in decreased volumes of subcortical structures, such as the thalamus or the corpus striatum, that are remote but connected to these cortical regions.

We observed volumetric reduction of subcortical gray structures in the 19 stroke patients who had cortical damage, most notably ipsilateral to their lesions. The raw data for the thalamus provide a representative example of our findings. In our normal control young adults, the mean value of the right thalamus was 7.4 mL with a standard deviation of 0.6 mL, whereas in the stroke patients the right thalamus was 6.5 ± 1.4 mL. This mildly reduced volume ($P < .02$) presumably represents an effect of age and disease. In contrast, the left thalamic volumes in the normal subjects (7.34 ± 0.62 mL) versus the patients (5.22 ± 1.3 mL) differed significantly ($P < 6.2 \times 10^{-7}$). The asymmetry of this effect is presumably due to a disease-related volumetric alteration on the side ipsilateral to the lesion. Similar observations in the corpus striatum, hippocampus, and amygdala lend additional evidence for systematic alterations of these deep gray structures in response to cortical insults [50]. This connectivity likely reflects diaschisis.

Related neuroscience themes

We have illustrated how lesions of stroke patients can be segmented, measured, and localized by means of anatomic and vascular topographic mapping using T1-weighted MR images. Our methods for morphometric analysis can be integrated with other imaging modalities, such as DT-MR imaging, MR spectroscopy, and PET. This allows for quantitative measurement and statistical analyses correlating alterations in

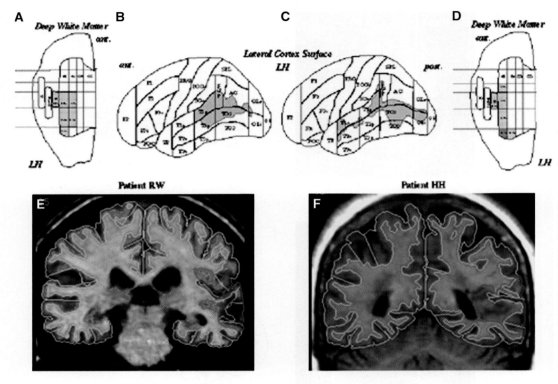

Fig. 6. Metabolic PET maps in two individuals affected by stroke. (*A–F*) The anatomic (cortical and subcortical white matter) lesion as determined from T1-weighted volumetric imaging for two cases (*A, B,* and *E* for case RW; *C, D,* and *F* for case HH). These cases show a similar pattern of cortical involvement but a substantially greater involvement of white matter in case HH, particularly in the regions of deep white matter of the temporal lobe. Each of these cases had PET FDG imaging performed to assess cerebral metabolism. (*G* and *H*) Axial images from the PET scan for cases RW and HH, respectively. The degree of temporal lobe metabolic asymmetry noted in these cases is markedly different in that case HH shows considerable asymmetry compared with case RW. This effect is presumably due to damage of the ILF produced by the deeper white matter lesion in case HH. (*I*) Illustration of MACs for the ILF, as inferred from the human and experimental nonhuman primate, is indicated by the shaded cortical areas [39]. AG, angular gyrus; F1, superior frontal gyrus; F2, middle frontal gyrus; F3o, inferior frontal gyrus, pars opercularis; F3t, inferior frontal gyrus, pars triangularis; FOC, frontal orbital cortex; FP, frontal pole; OLi, lateral occipital cortex, inferior; OLs, lateral occipital cortex, superior; OP, occipital pole; POG: postcentral gyrus; PP: planum polare; PRG: precentral gyrus; SGa: supramarginal gyrus, anterior; SGp, supramarginal gyrus, posterior; SPL, superior parietal lobule; T1a, superior temporal gyrus, anterior; T1p, superior temporal gyrus, posterior; T2a, middle temporal gyrus, anterior; T2p, middle temporal gyrus, posterior; T3a, inferior temporal gyrus, anterior; T3p, inferior temporal gyrus, posterior; TO2, middle temporal gyrus, temporooccipital; TO3, inferior temporal gyrus, temporooccipital; TP, temporal pole. (*From* Caviness Jr VS, Meyer JW, Makris N, et al. MRI-based topographic parcellation of the human neocortex: an anatomically specified method with estimate of reliability. J Cogn Neursci 1996;8:566–87; with permission.)

cerebral anatomy and physiology within a comprehensive framework of neural systems biology.

Stroke volume and vascular topography

In the discussion of application A, we observed that the overall volume of tissue destroyed by MCA infarction in the superficial perfusion compartment was considerably larger than that destroyed in the deep perfusion compartment. This disproportion in the topographic distribution of post-stroke encepha-

lomalacic change reflects the volume of the MCA perfusion territories inasmuch as the volume of the perfused M2 to M4 MCA subdivisions is far greater than the volume of the perfused M1 MCA subdivisions. These topographic patterns are consistent with the fact that the deep structures of the hemisphere—namely, the caudate, putamen, globus pallidus, and capsules but not the thalamus and amygdala—are within the M1 perfusion territory [48].

For strokes caused by embolic occlusive disease within the MCA system, there is an over-

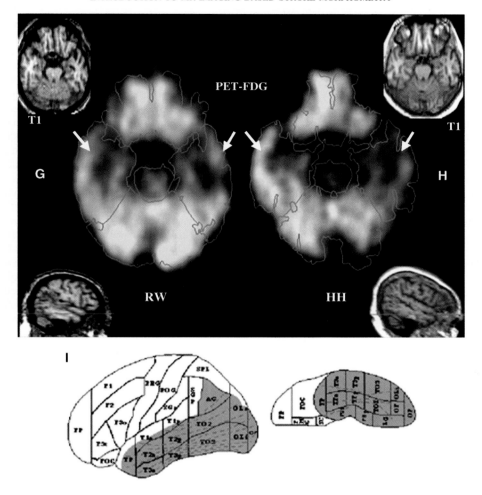

Fig. 6 (*continued*).

representation of gray- compared with white-matter lesions. Most notably, our analysis specifies putamen and caudate as the deep tissues most sensitive to M1 occlusion. The likelihood of deep infarction in the putamen was 100%, and in the caudate it was nearly as high. Moreover, preexisting infarction in the putamen, as identified by CT, has been proposed as a sensitive index of the hemorrhagic risk when tPA is given for lysis of M1 clot [51,52].

The comprehensive, statistical analysis of stroke distribution patterns presented here goes beyond that usually undertaken for diagnostic and therapeutic purposes in individual patients. We have analyzed neuroanatomic structure quantitatively (ie, volumetrically) and in great detail with respect to the distinction between superficial and deep perfusion compartments and between gray and white matter tissue types.

We envision two broad applications for this system of anatomic analysis: (1) as a tool for anatomic studies of forebrain tissue infarction with respect to vascular territories, tissue compartments, and tissue types within given vascular territories; and (2) for real-time management of acute and chronic stroke. This methodology is being extended to the study of early phases of stroke evolution with MR and CT imaging. With the addition of perfusion and diffusion-type data, morphometric analysis might help to, automatically or semi-automatically, distinguish "irreversibly infarcted core" from "potentially salvageable penumbral" tissue. This could facilitate more rational therapeutic choices regarding thrombolysis, other aggressive endovascular treatments, or tissue protective agents (if and when these become available). Eventually, this approach, aided by automated or semi-automated image analysis technology and correlated with studies of neurologic outcome and adaptation, may increase the power of admission imaging to predict long-range outcome in response to various stroke treatments [53].

Multimodal imaging

Although morphometric methods may be sufficient for investigations focused on precise volumetric changes of detailed brain anatomy over time, the integration of morphometry with other imaging modalities has opened a novel window in neuroscience, allowing investigation of the living human brain under normal and pathologic conditions [22]. For example, after an ischemic insult, white matter changes due to axonal degeneration result in modified water diffusivity and hence alterations in fractional anisotropy. DT-MR imaging is sensitive in depicting these changes, facilitating mapping of degenerating fiber tracts after stroke. Thus, the combination of morphometry with DT-MR imaging offers a unique opportunity to study white matter fiber tract anatomy in addition to cortical and subcortical gray matter structure. The combined use of T1-MR imaging morphometry, DT-MR imaging, MR spectroscopy, and PET are important assets for the clinico-anatomic correlation studies of structure-function relationships.

Clinico-anatomic correlations

The DT-MR imaging technique has been used to study secondary degeneration of the SLF in a patient with conduction aphasia, identifying a twofold reduction in preferred diffusion orientation of the SLF ipsilateral to the lesion [18]. The remarkable recovery of this patient's language function has to be emphasized and can likely be attributed to the partial sparing of the damaged SLF. Therefore, it seems that the DT-MR imaging technique is a sensitive instrument for detailed evaluation of normal and damaged fiber pathways and could be applied in other clinical conditions to predict clinical outcome and to assess recovery of function [54].

Structure-function relationships, anatomic connectional map, and "remote effect of disconnection"

Knowledge of anatomic connections is critical for lesion studies and for analysis of functional neuroimaging data. It has been demonstrated that a stroke lesion can lead to decreased cerebral metabolism in remote, anatomically interconnected cortical areas (so-called "diaschisis") (Fig. 5) [55].

The lesion shown in Fig. 5 is situated in the map of anatomic connection (MAC) of the superior longitudinal fasciculus (SLF$_{MAC}$). In this case, the lesion has compromised the inferior portion of the anterior supramarginal gyrus and the superior portions of the posterior supramarginal and angular gyri within the inferior parietal lobule. This corresponds approximately to Brodmann's cytoarchitectonic areas 40 and 39, respectively. In the nonhuman primate, these cortical regions are connected through cortico-cortical associational connections with frontal (areas 46, 45, 44, and 8; middle frontal gyrus, pars triangularis, pars opercularis, and frontal operculum of the inferior frontal gyrus) and temporal (area 22, superior temporal gyrus) Brodmann's architectonic areas [56,57] and to the superior, middle, and inferior frontal gyri via the superior longitudinal fasciculus [39]. Based on secondary degeneration and neuroanatomic postmortem studies in the human and in experimental monkey work, it is reasonable to postulate that these connections exist in the human. Therefore, the described lesion involves the fiber systems underlying the aforementioned cortical areas of the parietal lobe (which could include the more superficially located U-fibers and axonal systems of corticothalamic, cortico-striatal, and corticopontine projections).

As demonstrated by DT imaging [18], the SLF has been reduced significantly, probably due to secondary degeneration. Presumably, remote frontal and temporal neurons that had been connected bi-directionally via fibers of this tract before their disruption now fail to receive or deliver their usual input-output, leading to changes in their metabolism. We call this the "remote effect of disconnection" (RED) (disconnection being a partial interruption of a connection, as opposed to a complete interruption, which would be a transection). RED was confirmed in this case by the hypometabolic pattern involving territories of SLF, such as the inferior parietal lobule and inferior frontal gyrus areas, in the cortical metabolic map (Fig. 6). Hypometabolic activity of the rostral temporopolar cortex, as demonstrated by PET, was also observed (Fig. 6) in another patient with embolic infarction of the caudal temporal lobe with presumed damage to the ILF. Hypometabolism was not observed in a third patient, with a similar cortical lesion that does not extend deeply enough to damage the stem of the ILF.

Integrated magnetic resonance neuro-examination

DT-MR imaging may prove to be an important part of a comprehensive functional neuro-MR imaging examination. Quantitative assessment of (1) anatomic volume as measured by morphometric MR imaging [33], (2) fiber pathway anisotropy and size by DT imaging, (3) metabolic state by MR spectroscopy, and (4) functional state by fMR imaging provides a multidimensional data space for the elucidation of structural, functional, behavioral, and clinical correlates. For example, the relative contributions of each of these imaging modalities can be assessed for any developmental, aging, or degenerative process using principal component analysis. This leads to an optimized, temporally efficient, MR imaging neuro-examination that captures the salient features of the structural, metabolic, and functional states as they change over time. Monitoring these manifestations could elucidate the neurobiologic underpinnings of normal brain development and aging and the end points of etiology, natural history, and therapeutic intervention in disease states [22].

Secondary degeneration

The neuron is an anatomic and physiologic unit; a lesion of one of its parts has repercussions to the remainder. After a cortical ischemic event that damages the neuronal bodies within different cortical layers, neurons can degenerate following different spatial-temporal patterns.

Corticofugal, or Wallerian, degeneration is observed with recent lesions. Corticopetal or retrograde degeneration occurs as the lesion becomes older. A third type of degeneration, relating to lesions of early childhood or to very old lesions, is encountered that involves second- and third-order neurons and may lead to secondary or tertiary atrophy [58]. In general, a cortical lesion produces degeneration of all fiber systems that originate or terminate within the lesioned cortex. These systems include (1) projection fibers connecting the cortical area with the thalamus, basal ganglia, pons, amygdala, and hippocampus; (2) commissural fibers of the corpus callosum, the anterior commissure, and the dorsal hippocampal commissure; and (3) cortico-cortical fibers of different lengths, such as short intragyral U-fibers, medium-range intralobar fibers, and long-range interlobar fibers.

Summary

This article addresses the quantitative morphometric study of stroke, the integration of different imaging modalities in stroke lesion analysis, and the evaluation of the distributed consequences of the pathologic insult. It elaborates on the classes of information that are readily available in the MR image and methods for extracting quantitative results and presents sample applications of these types of techniques to stroke. These applications emphasize tissue and anatomic-based contrasts regarding the nature of stroke, a system for the characterization of structural and vascular brain topography of stroke lesions, and the broad repercussions of stroke lesions within the brain. The results underscore our capability to study changes in the volume of brain structures—quantitatively and in vivo—after damage to remote but connected brain regions. The different classes of analyses described may lead to a comprehensive model and to further understanding of human cerebral anatomic connectivity.

Acknowledgments

We thank Dr. Bruce Jenkins for his assistance with magnetic resonance spectroscopy.

References

[1] Brott T, Bogousslavsky J. Treatment of acute ischemic stroke. N Engl J Med 2000;343:710–22.

[2] Camarata PJ, Heros RC, Latchaw RE. "Brain attack": the rationale for treating stroke as a medical emergency. Neurosurgery 1994;34:144–57 [discussion: 57–8].

[3] du Plessis AJ, Volpe JJ. Perinatal brain injury in the preterm and term newborn. Curr Opin Neurol 2002;15:151–7.

[4] Aksoy FG, Lev MH. Dynamic contrast-enhanced brain perfusion imaging: technique and clinical applications. Semin Ultrasound CT MR 2000;21:462–77.

[5] Jones TH, Morawetz RB, Crowell RM, et al. Thresholds of focal cerebral ischemia in awake monkeys. J Neurosurg 1981;54:773–82.

[6] Barber PA, Darby DG, Desmond PM, et al. Prediction of stroke outcome with echoplanar perfusion- and diffusion-weighted MRI. Neurology 1998;51:418–26.

[7] Beaulieu C, de Crespigny A, Tong DC, et al. Longitudinal magnetic resonance imaging study of perfusion and diffusion in stroke: evolution of lesion volume and correlation with clinical outcome. Ann Neurol 1999;46:568–78.

[8] Lev MH, Nichols SJ. Computed tomographic angiography and computed tomographic perfusion imaging of hyperacute stroke. Top Magn Reson Imaging 2000;11: 273–87.

[9] Schellinger PD, Fiebach JB, Jansen O, et al. Stroke magnetic resonance imaging within 6 hours after onset of hyperacute cerebral ischemia. Ann Neurol 2001; 49:460–9.

[10] Schwamm LH, Koroshetz WJ, Sorensen AG, et al. Time course of lesion development in patients with acute

stroke: serial diffusion- and hemodynamic-weighted magnetic resonance imaging. Stroke 1998;29:2268–76.

[11] Pineiro R, Pendlebury ST, Smith S, et al. Relating MRI changes to motor deficit after ischemic stroke by segmentation of functional motor pathways. Stroke 2000;31:672–9.

[12] Haacke EM. Magnetic resonance imaging: physical principles and sequence design. New York: J. Wiley & Sons; 1999.

[13] Hinshaw WS, Lent AH. An introduction to NMR imaging: from the Bloch equation to the imaging equation. Proc IEEE 1983;71.

[14] Caputo GR, Kondo C, Higgins CB. Magnetic resonance angiography and blood flow quantification. Am J Card Imaging 1993;7:233–42.

[15] Rosen BR, Belliveau JW, Aronen HJ, et al. Susceptibility contrast imaging of cerebral blood volume: human experience. Magn Reson Med 1991;22:293–9 [discussion: 300–3].

[16] Sudikoff S, Banasiak K. Techniques for measuring cerebral blood flow in children. Curr Opin Pediatr 1998;10:291–8.

[17] Basser PJ, Mattiello J, LeBihan D. Estimation of the effective self-diffusion tensor from the NMR spin echo. J Magn Reson B 1994;103:247–54.

[18] Makris N, Worth AJ, Sorensen AG, et al. Morphometry of in vivo human white matter association pathways with diffusion-weighted magnetic resonance imaging. Ann Neurol 1997;42:951–62.

[19] Pierpaoli C, Basser PJ. Toward a quantitative assessment of diffusion anisotropy. Magn Reson Med 1996;36:893–906.

[20] Ogawa S, Tank DW, Menon R, et al. Intrinsic signal changes accompanying sensory stimulation: functional brain mapping with magnetic resonance imaging. Proc Natl Acad Sci USA 1992;89:5951–5.

[21] Guimaraes AR, Baker JR, Jenkins BG, et al. Echoplanar chemical shift imaging. Magn Reson Med 1999;41:877–82.

[22] Jenkins BG, Chen YI, Kuestermann E, et al. An integrated strategy for evaluation of metabolic and oxidative defects in neurodegenerative illness using magnetic resonance techniques. Ann N Y Acad Sci 1999;893:214–42.

[23] Ross B, Michaelis T. Clinical applications of magnetic resonance spectroscopy. Magn Reson Q 1994;10:191–247.

[24] Kennedy D, Caviness V, Makris N. Structural morphometry in the developing brain. In: Thatcher RW, Lyon GR, Rumsey J, Krasnegor N, editors. Developmental neuroimaging: mapping the development of brain and behavior. New York: Academic Press; 1996.

[25] Clarke LP, Velthuizen RP, Camacho MA, et al. MRI segmentation: methods and applications. Magn Reson Imaging 1995;13:343–68.

[26] Viergever MA, Maintz JB, Niessen WJ, et al. Registration, segmentation, and visualization of multimodal brain images. Comput Med Imaging Graph 2001;25:147–51.

[27] Wells WM, Grimson WEL, Kikinis R, et al. Adaptive segmentation of MRI data. IEEE Trans Med Img 1996;15:429–42.

[28] Collins D, Holmes C, Peters T, et al. Automatic 3-D model-based neuroanatomical segmentation. Hum Brain Mapp 1995;3:190–208.

[29] Thompson PM, MacDonald D, Mega MS, et al. Detection and mapping of abnormal brain structure with a probabilistic atlas of cortical surfaces. J Comput Assist Tomogr 1997;21:567–81.

[30] Filipek PA, Richelme C, Kennedy DN, et al. The young adult human brain: an MRI-based morphometric analysis. Cerebr Cort 1994;4:344–60.

[31] Kennedy DN, Filipek PA, Caviness Jr VS. Anatomic segmentation and volumetric calcuations in nuclear magnetic resonance imaging. IEEE Trans Med Imaging 1989;8:1–7.

[32] Rademacher J, Galaburda AM, Kennedy DN, et al. Human cerebral cortex: localization, parcellation and morphometry with magnetic resonance imaging. J Cogn Neurosci 1992;4:352–74.

[33] Caviness Jr VS, Meyer JW, Makris N, et al. MRI-based topographic parcellation of the human neocortex: an anatomically specified method with estimate of reliability. J Cogn Neurosci 1996;8:566–87.

[34] Talairach J, Szikla G, Tournoux P. Atlas d'anatomie stereotaxique du telencephale. Paris: Masson; 1967.

[35] Talairach J, Tournoux P. Co-planar stereotaxic atlas of the human brain. New York: Thieme Medical Publishers; 1988.

[36] Fischl B, Sereno MI, Dale AM. Cortical surface-based analysis. II: inflation, flattening, and a surface-based coordinate system. Neuroimage 1999;9:195–207.

[37] Fischl B, Sereno MI, Tootell RB, et al. High-resolution intersubject averaging and a coordinate system for the cortical surface. Hum Brain Mapp 1999;8:272–84.

[38] Rademacher J, Caviness VSJ, Steinmetz H, et al. Topographical variation of the human primary cortices: implications for neuroimaging, brain mapping and neurobiology. Cereb Cort 1993;3:313–29.

[39] Makris N, Meyer JW, Bates JF, et al. MRI-based topographic parcellation of human cerebral white matter and nuclei. I: rationale and applications with systematics of cerebral connectivity. Neuroimage 1999;9:17–45.

[40] Meyer J, Makris N, Bates J, et al. MRI-Based topographic parcellation of the human cerebral white matter. I: technical foundations. Neuroimage 1999;9:1–17.

[41] Van den Bergh R. Centrifugal elements in the vascular pattern of the deep intracerebral blood supply. Angiology 1969;20:88–94.

[42] Vander Eecken HM, Adams RD. The anatomy and functional significance of the meningeal arterial anastomoses of the human brain. J Neuropathol Exp Neurol 1953;12:132–57.

[43] Moody DM, Bell MA, Challa VR. Features of the cerebral vascular pattern that predict vulnerability to perfusion or oxygenation deficiency: an anatomic study. AJNR Am J Neuroradiol 1990;11:431–9.

[44] De Reuck J. The human periventricular arterial blood supply and the anatomy of cerebral infarctions. Eur Neurol 1971;5:321–34.

[45] de Groot JC, de Leeuw FE, Oudkerk M, et al. Cerebral white matter lesions and cognitive function: the Rotterdam Scan study. Ann Neurol 2000;47:145–51.

[46] Bogousslavsky J, Regli F. Borderzone infarctions distal to internal carotid artery occlusion: prognostic implications. Ann Neurol 1986;20:346–50.

[47] Caviness VS, Makris N, Montinaro E, et al. Anatomy of stroke, part I: an MRI-based topographic and volumetric System of analysis. Stroke 2002;33:2549–56.

[48] Gibo H, Carver CC, Rhoton Jr AL, et al. Microsurgical anatomy of the middle cerebral artery. J Neurosurg 1981;54:151–69.

[49] Makris N, Hodge SM, Albaugh MD, et al. Pontine consequences of cerebral stroke as revealed by MRI-based morphometry. Hum Brain Mapping 2003.

[50] Makris N, Sahin NT, Bates JF, et al. MRI-based volumetric analysis of anatomical consequences of stroke. Hum Brain Mapping 2001;13:S813.

[51] Beauchamp Jr NJ, Barker PB, Wang PY, et al. Imaging of acute cerebral ischemia. Radiology 1999;212:307–24.

[52] Fiorelli M, Bastianello S, von Kummer R, et al. Hemorrhagic transformation within 36 hours of a cerebral infarct: relationships with early clinical deterioration and 3-month outcome in the European Cooperative Acute Stroke Study I (ECASS I) cohort. Stroke 1999;30:2280–4.

[53] Fischl B, Salat DH, Busa E, et al. Whole brain segmentation: automated labeling of neuroanatomical structures in the human brain. Neuron 2002;33:341–55.

[54] Pierpaoli C, Barnett A, Pajevic S, et al. Water diffusion changes in Wallerian degeneration and their dependence on white matter architecture. Neuroimage 2001; 13:1174–85.

[55] Kosslyn SM, Daly PF, McPeek RM, et al. Using locations to store shape: an indirect effect of a lesion. Cereb Cortex 1993;3:567–82.

[56] Petrides M, Pandya DN. Projections to the frontal cortex from the posterior parietal region in the rhesus monkey. J Comp Neurol 1984;288:105–16.

[57] Petrides M, Pandya DN. Association fiber pathways to the frontal cortex from the superior temporal region in the rhesus Monkey. J Comp Neurol 1988;273:52–66.

[58] Dejerine J. Anatomie des centres nerveux. Paris: Rueff et Cie; 1895.

ELSEVIER
SAUNDERS

Neuroimag Clin N Am 15 (2005) 341–350

NEUROIMAGING
CLINICS OF
NORTH AMERICA

Positron Emission Tomography Imaging of Cerebral Ischemia

Colin P. Derdeyn, MD[a,b,*]

[a]Mallinckrodt Institute of Radiology, Washington University School of Medicine, St. Louis, MO, USA
[b]Departments of Neurology and Neurological Surgery, Washington University School of Medicine, St. Louis, MO, USA

Positron emission tomography (PET) provides in vivo regional measurement of several important physiologic parameters in living humans, including cerebral blood flow (CBF) and oxygen metabolism. PET studies have advanced our understanding of normal human brain physiology and, as detailed in this article, our understanding of human cerebrovascular pathophysiology. This article focuses on knowledge gained from PET regarding acute ischemic stroke and chronic oligemia from arterial occlusive disease. The author first discusses the basic principles of PET. Next, he reviews normal cerebral hemodynamics and metabolism. He then reviews the responses of the brain and its vasculature to reduced perfusion pressure, primarily autoregulatory vasodilatation and increased oxygen extraction fraction (OEF). This section is followed by a review of the use of PET to investigate the effects of chronic hemodynamic compromise. Finally, the author reviews the knowledge we have gained using PET to study the pathophysiology of acute ischemic stroke.

Positron emission tomography basics

PET imaging requires three components: a radiotracer, a system to detect and measure the quantity of

radiation, and a mathematical model relating the physiologic process under study to the detected radiation. One method for the measurement of CBF, for example, uses a bolus injection of oxygen-15 (^{15}O)-labeled water. The PET camera measures the counts in the head during the circulation of the water through the brain. Finally, the PET image of raw counts is converted into a map of regional quantitative CBF using computer programs that require measurements of arterial blood counts and incorporate models and assumptions regarding the transit of water through the cerebral circulation. Radiotracers are radioactive molecules administered in such small quantities that they do not affect the physiologic process under study. PET radiotracers may be separated into two broad categories: normal biologic molecules, such as ^{15}O-labeled water, and nonbiologic elements attached to organic molecules as radiolabels, such as fluorine-18–labeled deoxyglucose (^{18}F-FDG). By definition, these tracers decay by positron emission. Their half-lives range from a few minutes to a few hours. The most commonly used radiotracers, ^{18}F and ^{15}O, require a linear accelerator or cyclotron for production.

The PET imaging detection system uses the phenomenon of annihilation radiation to localize and to quantify physiologic processes in the brain. PET radionuclides decay by emission of a positively charged electron (a positron). The positron may travel a few millimeters within the tissue losing energy before encountering an electron. This encounter results in the annihilation of both the positron and electron and the consequent generation of two gamma photons of equal energy. These two photons are emitted in

This article was supported by grants NINDS R01 NS39864, P01 NS35966, and R01 NS39526.

* Mallinckrodt Institute of Radiology, Washington University School of Medicine, 510 South Kingshighway Boulevard, St. Louis, MO 63110.

E-mail address: derdeync@wustl.edu

characteristic 180° opposite directions. A pair of detectors positioned on either side of the source of the annihilation photons detects them simultaneously. This method allows localization of the point source of the radiation. The spatial resolution of a pair of annihilation coincidence detectors is nearly uniform for most of the region found between detectors. After the correction for attenuation, the data from the detector pairs are used to construct a series of projections, each representing the distribution of regional radioactivity viewed from a different angle. These projections are then combined by a computer to produce a two-dimensional reconstruction of the regional radioactivity within the combined field of view of all the detector pairs. Scanners with multiple rings of detectors are capable of generating several reconstructed slices of the imaged volume simultaneously, each depicting a different level of the brain and together providing a three-dimensional image.

The most important limitations of PET imaging of physiologic processes relate to the phenomenon of full width, half maximum (FWHM) and a related phenomenon of partial-volume averaging. Detected radiation is observed over a larger area than the actual source. The spread or distribution of activity is approximately Gaussian for a point source of radiation, with the maximum located at the original point. The FWHM describes the degree of smearing of radioactivity in a reconstructed image. The ability of a PET scanner to discriminate between two small adjacent structures or accurately measure the activity in a small region will depend on the FWHM of the system as well as on the amount and distribution of activity within the region of interest and the surrounding areas. *Because of the smearing or redistribution of detected radioactivity, any given region in the reconstructed image will not contain all the activity actually within the region. Some of the activity will spill over into adjacent areas.* Similarly, activity in the surrounding tissue or structures will also be redistributed into the region of interest. This phenomenon is known as the partial volume effect. An important consequence of this principle is that PET will always measure a gradual change in activity where an abrupt change actually exists, such as in an infarct or hemorrhage or at the border of different structures, such as brain and cerebrospinal fluid or gray and white matter. Measurements made at the borders of such structures will not be accurate.

In the third step, the externally measured tissue concentration of the positron-emitting radiotracer (PET counts) is quantitatively related to the physiologic variable under study by a mathematical model. The PET scanner measures the total counts in a volume of tissue. The models calculate how that measured activity reflects the physiologic parameter under study. These calculations account for several factors related to the tracer biomechanics and metabolism. These factors include the mode of tracer delivery to the tissue, the distribution and metabolism of the tracer within the tissue, the egress of the tracer and metabolites from the tissue, the recirculation of both the tracer and its labeled metabolites, and the amount of tracer and metabolites remaining in the blood. The validity of all the underlying assumptions and the possible sources of error for each model when applied to the study of normal physiology and disease states must be clearly understood.

A final issue of great importance in the analysis of PET data is that of statistics. PET counts are statistical data by nature. Consequently, when comparing the data from several regions of interest to one another, one must use a correction for the potential error introduced by multiple comparisons. The selection of proper control subjects and regions of interest is also crucial to accurate data analysis.

Cerebral physiologic factors measured by positron emission tomography

Cerebral blood flow

CBF is the volume of blood delivered to a defined mass of tissue per unit time, generally in mL of blood per 100 g of brain per minute (mL/[100 g · min]). ^{15}O-labeled water is the most commonly used tracer for measurements of CBF and the method used in the author's laboratory [1]. The tracer kinetic models treat water as a freely diffusible tracer. Counts are nearly linearly proportional to CBF. Other methods are in common use as well, including ^{15}O-labeled butanol.

Cerebral blood volume

Cerebral blood volume (CBV) is the volume of blood within a given mass of tissue and is expressed as mL of blood per 100 g of brain tissue. Regional CBV measurements may serve as an indicator of the degree of cerebrovascular vasodilatation, as discussed in the text to follow. CBV can be measured by PET with either trace amounts of ^{15}O-labeled carbon monoxide or carbon dioxide [2]. Both carbon monoxide tracers label the red blood cells. Blood volume is calculated using a correction factor for the difference between peripheral vessel and cerebral vessel hematocrit.

Mean transit time

Mean transit time (MTT) is usually calculated as the ratio of CBV to CBF. By the central volume theorem, this ratio yields mean transit time, the hypothetical mean time for a particle to pass through the cerebral circulation. MTT is not measured directly with PET. Increased MTT is used as an indicator of autoregulatory vasodilatation. Some PET groups have advocated the use of the inverse of this ratio instead [3].

Oxygen extraction fraction

OEF is measured by an $O^{15}O$ inhalation scan and independent measurements of CBF and CBV [4]. The CBF accounts for the amount of oxygen delivered to the brain. The CBV corrects for oxygen in the blood that is not extracted. An alternative count-based method uses the ratio of the counts after an $O^{15}O$ inhalation scan to the counts from an $O^{15}O$ water scan, without CBV correction [5,6]. Other similar methods are also in common use.

Cerebral metabolic rate of oxygen

Cerberal metabolic rate of oxygen ($CMRO_2$) can be calculated from an equation using OEF, CBF, and arterial oxygen content (CaO_2) [4]. $CMRO_2$ is equal to the CBF multiplied by OEF and the CaO_2 (delivery of oxygen times the fraction extracted times the amount of available oxygen).

Glucose metabolism

Glucose metabolism (CMRGlu) is most frequently measured using the glucose analogue ^{18}F-FDG. CMRGlu measurements are limited in pathologic conditions such as ischemia, however, because the ratio of tissue uptake of glucose and its analogue, DG, varies with the severity of ischemia. CMRGlu can be measured directly with 1-^{11}C-D–glucose [7,8].

Molecular imaging studies

These studies in stroke patients have used several different labeled substances [9], including ^{11}C-labeled FK506 (tacrolimus) [10], copper-60, and a host of other labeled neurotransmitters [11].

Cerebral hemodynamics and metabolism

Whole brain mean CBF of the adult human brain is approximately 50 mL per 100 g per minute. Functional activation increases local or regional CBF, but global CBF remains unchanged. CBF for any brain region is determined by the ratio of cerebral perfusion pressure (CPP) and cerebral vascular resistance (CVR) in that region. CPP is the difference between the arterial pressure forcing blood into the cerebral circulation and intracranial pressure or the pressure in the venous system. The venous pressure is negligible under normal conditions, so the CPP is generally equal to the systemic (mean) arterial pressure (CPP = MAP). Several different pathologic processes result in reduced perfusion pressure secondary to venous disease. These include venous sinus thrombosis, dural arteriovenous fistulas, and possibly other conditions, such as jugular foraminal narrowing. The venous pressure also increases with increased intracranial pressure (CPP = MAP − ICP).

Under normal conditions, any change in regional CBF must be caused by a change in regional CVR. Vascular resistance is mediated by alterations in the diameter of small arteries or arterioles. In the resting brain with normal CPP, CBF is also closely matched to the metabolic rate of the tissue. Regions with higher metabolic rates have higher levels of CBF. For example, gray matter has a higher CBF than white matter. Although there is wide variation in levels of flow and metabolism, the ratio between the regional CBF (rCBF) and metabolism is nearly constant in all areas of the brain. Consequently, the maps of OEF and glucose extraction (not metabolism) from the blood show little regional variation [12]. One exception to this is seen in physiologic activation, where blood flow increases well beyond the metabolic needs of the tissue. This increase leads to a relative decrease of OEF and a reduction in local venous deoxyhemoglobin [13]. This phenomenon is the basis for the use of MR imaging to map brain function.

Responses to reductions in cerebral perfusion pressure

An arterial stenosis or occlusion may cause a reduction in perfusion pressure if collateral sources of flow are not adequate [14]. The mere presence of arterial stenosis or occlusion does not equate to hemodynamic impairment: as many as 50% of patients with complete carotid artery occlusion and prior ischemic symptoms have normally no evidence of reduced CPP [15]. The adequacy of collateral sources of flow largely determines whether an occlusive lesion will cause a reduction in perfusion pressure. When perfusion pressure falls owing to an arterial stenosis or occlusion and, in most cases, an inadequate circle of Willis, the brain and its vasculature can maintain the normal delivery of oxygen and glucose through two mechanisms, autoregulatory vasodilatation and increased OEF [16]. The presence of these mechanisms has been extensively studied, primarily in animal models employing acute reductions in perfusion pressure. The extent to which these models are applicable to humans with chronic regional reductions in perfusion pressure is not known.

Changes in perfusion pressure have little effect on CBF over a wide range of pressure, owing to vascular autoregulation. Increases in mean arterial pressure produce vasoconstriction of the pial arterioles, serving to increase vascular resistance and maintain CBF at a constant level [17]. Conversely, when the pressure falls, reflex vasodilatation will maintain CBF at near normal levels [18,19]. Two measurable parameters that indicate autoregulatory vasodilatation are MTT and CBV (Fig. 1). In addition, there is some slight reduction in CBF through the autoregulatory range, leading to a slight increase in oxygen extraction [16,20].

At some point, however, the capacity for autoregulatory vasodilatation may be exceeded. The threshold value for autoregulatory failure is variable between patients and can be shifted higher or lower by prior ischemic injury or long-standing hypertension. Beyond this point, CBF falls linearly as a function of pressure (see Fig. 1). Direct measurements of arteriovenous oxygen differences have demonstrated the brain's capacity to increase OEF and maintain normal $CMRO_2$ while the oxygen delivery diminishes owing to decreasing CBF [21]. The precise mechanism by which OEF increases is not completely understood. Oxygen passively diffuses from the blood to the tissue. Increases in the gradient between capillary and tissue partial pressures of oxygen and longer transit times that may allow for greater oxygen diffusion may be involved.

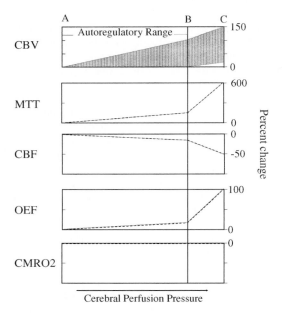

Fig. 1. Modified schematic of hemodynamic and metabolic responses to reductions in CPP after Derdeyn and colleagues [16]. The x-axis represents progressive reduction in perfusion pressure. The region between points A and B is the autoregulatory range. The region between points B and C is the region of autoregulatory failure where CBF falls passively as a function of pressure. Point C represents the exhaustion of compensatory mechanisms to maintain normal oxygen metabolism and the onset of true ischemia. CBV either remains unchanged or increases with autoregulatory vasodilatation, depending largely on the methods used to measure it. With autoregulatory failure, most investigations have found further increases in CBV. CBF falls slightly through the autoregulatory range. Once autoregulatory capacity is exceeded, CBF falls passively as a function of pressure down to 50% of baseline values. OEF increases slightly with the reductions in CBF through the autoregulatory range. After autoregulatory capacity is exceeded and flow falls as much as 50% of baseline, OEF may increase up to 100% from baseline. $CMRO_2$ remains unchanged throughout this range of CPP reduction owing to both autoregulatory vasodilatation and increased OEF.

Clinical positron emission tomography studies of chronic arterial occlusive disease (oligemia)

The identification of compensatory responses to reduced perfusion pressure, or hemodynamic impairment, as it is frequently called, may play an important role in medical decision making in a number of subacute or chronic arterial occlusive disorders. These conditions include atherosclerotic carotid occlusion, arterial dissection, moyamoya disease, subarachnoid hemorrhage-related vasospasm, and possibly asymptomatic atherosclerotic carotid stenosis. PET and other hemodynamic studies in these patient populations have been aimed primarily at determining whether the presence of these compensatory mechanisms is associated with future stroke risk (natural history studies) and whether particular medical or surgical interventions can improve cerebral hemodynamics (ie, using imaging as a secondary endpoint), or they have been pivotal intervention studies of efficacy based on hemodynamic criteria. In this section the author first reviews PET methods for identification of autoregulatory vasodilatation and increased OEF, then clinical studies in different patient populations.

Identification of compensatory responses to reduced perfusion pressure with positron emission tomography

As discussed earlier, the hemodynamic effect of an arterial stenosis or occlusion depends on the adequacy of collateral circulation as well as on the degree of stenosis. An occluded carotid artery, for example, often has no measurable effect on the distal CPP because the collateral flow through the circle of Willis is adequate. Many imaging techniques, such as arteriography, MR imaging, computed tomography angiography, and Doppler ultrasound, can identify the presence of these collaterals. These tools show us the highways for blood flow but not the traffic on them.

It is important to recognize that a single measurement of flow is meaningless when investigating the effects of an arterial lesion. Normal values of CBF

do not exclude the presence of autoregulatory vasodilatation, and reduced CBF may be present with normal perfusion pressure. This second situation may occur with prior stroke in the region of interest or in a remote area. Prior lacunar stroke in the basal ganglia may lead to profound reduction in metabolic demand of the overlying cortex and secondary reduction in flow. This phenomenon has been termed diaschisis (Fig. 2).

Three basic PET strategies for defining the degree of hemodynamic compromise caused by arterial occlusive disease have emerged, based on the known compensatory responses of the brain to reduction in CPP. Two approaches are used to identify autoregulatory vasodilatation, and the third identifies increased OEF. The first method relies on resting measurements of CBV and CBF. When CPP is reduced, autoregulatory vasodilatation will cause an increase in CBV (see Fig. 2). The CBV/CBF ratio (mean transit time) will increase. The second strategy employs paired measurements of rCBF at rest and during some form of vasodilatory stimulus, such as with acetazolamide or CO_2 inhalation. Reduction of the normal increase in CBF seen in response to these stimuli is taken as evidence of pre-existing autoregulatory vasodilatation, which would mute such an

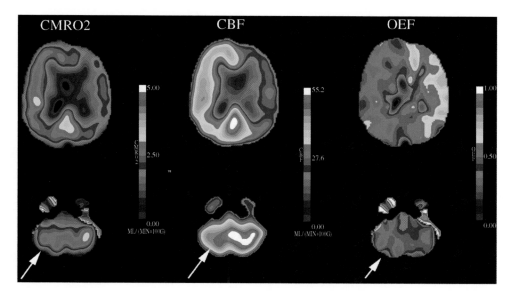

Fig. 2. Diaschisis. This patient has a high-grade stenosis of the left supraclinoid internal carotid artery and previous stroke in this territory. Consequently, the $CMRO_2$ image demonstrates reduced oxygen metabolism relative to the contralateral hemisphere. The reduced metabolic activity in the left frontal area has caused reduced metabolic activity in the structurally normal right cerebellar hemisphere. This phenomenon is known as diaschisis. The primary reduction in metabolism in the cerebellum leads to a reduction in CBF, and the OEF map remains symmetric. In contrast, the reduction in CBF is greater than the reduction in metabolism in the left cerebral hemisphere (*top row*), owing to flow reduction, not just metabolic reduction, and the OEF is increased (*top row*).

increase. The third approach involves direct measurements of OEF (Figs. 2 and 3).

Atherosclerotic carotid occlusion

The patient population that has been the focus of the most investigation has been that of atherosclerotic carotid artery occlusion. The presence of increased OEF as measured by PET has been established as a powerful and independent risk factor for future stroke in these patients [15]. Based on this information, a clinical trial of surgical revascularization is underway: the Carotid Occlusion Surgery Study [22]. The details of these natural history studies and the design and rationale of the current trial are described in this section.

Patients with complete atherosclerotic occlusion of the carotid artery are at high risk for future stroke [23]. A randomized trial of extracranial to intracranial arterial bypass (the EC/IC Bypass Trial) failed to show a benefit of surgical revascularization in more than 800 patients randomized to surgery or aspirin [24]. One possible reason for the failure of this study

to show a benefit was the lack of an effective tool to establish whether flow was normal or impaired. A procedure intended to improve flow is unlikely to provide any benefit if flow is normal. A benefit of bypass may have been missed for a subgroup at high risk owing to hemodynamic factors.

The St. Louis Carotid Occlusion Study was designed to determine whether such a subgroup existed [15]. This blinded, prospective study was designed to test the hypothesis that increased OEF in patients with symptomatic atherosclerotic carotid occlusion predicted future stroke risk. Eighty-one patients with complete carotid occlusion and ipsilateral ischemic symptoms were enrolled. At baseline, 17 clinical, epidemiologic, and laboratory stroke risk factors were recorded. PET measurements of oxygen extraction were obtained. Thirty-nine of the 81 patients had increased OEF. All 81 patients were followed for a mean duration of 3.1 years. Fifteen total and 13 ipsilateral ischemic strokes occurred during this period. Eleven of the 13 ipsilateral strokes occurred in the 39 patients with increased OEF. Multivariate analysis found only age and OEF as predictors of

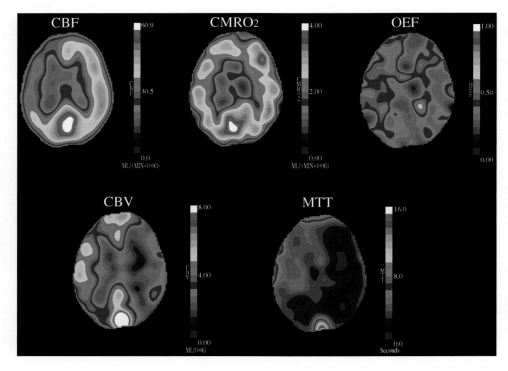

Fig. 3. PET images showing increased OEF (*top row*) and increased CBV (*bottom row*). This patient is a 58-year-old woman presenting with transient ischemic attacks in the hemisphere distal to an angiographically proven carotid occlusion. The PET examination was performed 35 days after the first event and 2 days after the most recent event. The images show reduced CBF (*top left*), normal CMRO$_2$ (*top middle*), and increased OEF in the hemisphere distal to the occluded carotid. CBV and MTT are elevated.

stroke risk. Log rank analysis demonstrated increased OEF to be a powerful predictor of subsequent stroke ($P = .004$). Similar results were found by Yamauchi and coworkers [25].

Prior studies with PET have shown that the superficial temporal artery to middle cerebral artery bypass procedure is capable of reversing the OEF abnormality [26,27]. Based on these facts, the Carotid Occlusion Surgery Study was funded by the National Institutes of Health and is under way. Patients with complete atherosclerotic carotid artery occlusion and recent (120 days) ipsilateral cerebral ischemic symptoms are eligible for enrollment. PET studies are obtained on enrollment. Patients with increased OEF are randomized to surgery or the best medical therapy.

Improvement in hemodynamics over time

In some patients with atherosclerotic carotid occlusion, hemodynamic impairment may improve over time, as collateral flow increases [28]. The author's team repeated PET measurements in 10 patients with complete atherosclerotic carotid artery occlusion with increased OEF by PET and no interval stroke 12 to 59 months after the initial examination. Quantitative regional measurements of CBF, CBV, $CMRO_2$, and OEF were obtained. Regional measurements of CMRGlu were also made on follow-up in five patients. As a group, the ratio of ipsilateral to contralateral OEF declined from a mean of 1.16 to 1.08 ($P = .022$). Greater reductions were seen with longer duration of follow-up ($P = .023$, $r = .707$). The CBF ratio improved from 0.81 to 0.85 ($P = .021$). No change in CBV or $CMRO_2$ was observed. CMRGlu was reduced in the ipsilateral hemisphere ($P=.001$ compared with normal), but the $CMRO_2$/CMRGlu ratio was normal.

This improvement in collateral sources of flow over time may be a factor that accounts for the reduction in stroke risk over time in all the major cerebral revascularization trials. The greatest risk for stroke in medically treated patients in the North American Symptomatic Carotid Stenosis Trial, the EC/IC Bypass Trial, the European Carotid Stenosis Trial, and the St. Louis Carotid Occlusion Study was in the first 2 years after stroke [24,29,30].

Moyamoya disease

Moyamoya disease is an obliterative vasculopathy of the anterior circulation at the circle of Willis. The cause is unknown. In North America, it most frequently affects women in their third and fourth decades. Ischemic symptoms of stroke or transient ischemic attacks are the most common presentation [31]. It is highly likely that hemodynamic mechanisms play a role in the pathogenesis of stroke in these patients. Hemodynamic assessment may be able to provide prognostic information regarding stroke risk in this patient population, analogous to the atherosclerotic carotid occlusion.

The author has studied eight patients with moyamoya disease with PET and found the degree of hemodynamic impairment to be variable. Pial collaterals from the posterior cerebral arteries are often capable of maintaining normal perfusion, despite the presence of severe stenosis or occlusion of the distal internal carotid artery. Interval improvement in OEF and CBF was found in one patient with increased OEF who underwent an indirect surgical revascularization procedure. This is an area for future study.

Acute ischemic stroke

If the perfusion pressure of the brain continues to fall beyond the capacity for increases in OEF to compensate, flow will become insufficient to meet the energy requirements of the brain [32]. Neurologic deficit may appear. This effect may be reversible if circulation is rapidly restored. Persistent or further declines in flow will lead to permanent tissue damage, depending on the duration and degree of ischemia. Below approximately 20 mL per 100 g per minute, normal brain electrical activity ceases and neurologic symptoms may appear. The energy supply becomes insufficient because of the inadequate supply of oxygen, preventing normal aerobic glycolysis. The high-energy phosphate stores of ATP and creatine phosphate (PCr) become depleted. Anaerobic metabolism of the small amount of glucose remaining in the intracellular stores or from the diminished blood flow leads to a lactic acidosis. Once CBF has fallen to 10 to 12 mL per 100 g per minute, the integrity of cell membranes is lost and intracellular K^+ leaks out of the cells while extracellular Ca^+ leaks in. Cell death ultimately follows unless reperfusion occurs quickly.

Once tissue damage has occurred, the normal mechanisms of cerebrovascular control may no longer operate [33]. Therefore, in some patients who have had transient ischemic attacks or mild ischemic strokes with subsequent recanalization, autoregulation or the normal cerebrovascular response to arterial carbon dioxide tension ($PaCO_2$) may be abnormal for up to several weeks [34]. Over time, flow will fall to match the metabolic needs of the tissue and autoregulatory capacity will be regained. Following reperfusion, the biochemical and ionic abnormalities resolve to a degree dependent on the severity of the initial ischemic insult. The acidosis of anaerobic glycolysis may be replaced by alkalosis.

Positron emission tomography studies in acute ischemic stroke

Human and animal PET studies have provided a detailed description of the time course of changes in CBF and metabolism that occur during and after transient and permanent interruption of normal blood flow. Pappata and colleagues [35] have shown in a baboon model of middle cerebral artery (MCA) occlusion that a zone of increased OEF first develops centrally and then moves progressively more peripherally over time. OEF reflects the mismatch between flow and metabolism. OEF was elevated in the MCA territory both at 1 hour and at 3 hours after occlusion. At 3 hours, the regional $CMRO_2$ ($rCMRO_2$) had fallen in the central or deep MCA territory, consistent with infarction. In peripheral, cortical regions, however, $CMRO_2$ was only moderately reduced, suggesting viability. These peripheral regions usually go on to infarction within hours even without further reduction in CBF. This gradual movement of reduced oxygen metabolism from central to peripheral has been termed the dynamic penumbra by Heiss and coworkers [36], who have described this phenomenon in cats as lasting up to 24 hours. Similar observations of potentially viable peri-infarct tissue that goes on to infarction have been made in humans.

A brief period of hyperperfusion often occurs immediately after the arterial occlusion ceases. This phenomenon is called luxury perfusion, where CBF becomes elevated in a region of infarction. A prolonged period of depressed CBF, below normal values, then follows. During this period of postischemic hypoperfusion, metabolism may recover or even rise above normal levels. Consequently, OEF may be increased. In one patient with persistently increased OEF 4 days after acute stroke, Wise and coworkers [37] raised the systemic blood pressure by means of angiotensin infusion. Flow to the infarcted region increased, OEF fell, but $CMRO_2$ remained unchanged and no neurologic improvement was observed. Later, CBF may rise above normal while metabolism falls. These changes are typically observed over a period of several days. CBF eventually returns to a level that

matches that of the reduced metabolic rate of the infarcted tissue.

PET studies performed in the setting of acute ischemia (<24 or 48 hours) have demonstrated regions of both decreased and increased blood flow [35,36]. The regions of decreased CBF are thought to be due to persisting ischemia or postischemic hypoperfusion. Regions with increased CBF are attributed to early postischemic hyperperfusion, caused by either clot lysis or collateral reperfusion. In acute ischemic stroke, focal reduction of CBF is accompanied by a reduction in $rCMRO_2$. The OEF is often elevated owing to a greater reduction in CBF than in $CMRO_2$ [33].

Marchal and colleagues [38] studied regional blood flow and oxygen metabolism in 18 patients with acute middle cerebral stroke between 5 and 18 hours after onset of symptoms and correlated their findings with neurologic outcome at 2 months. They could separate their patients into three groups based on the PET scan results. The first group had reduced blood flow and metabolism, suggesting irreversible damage. These patients had a poor outcome. The second group of patients demonstrated reduced flow and metabolism but to a lesser extent than the first group. This pattern was associated with a variable recovery of function. The third group showed increased perfusion and largely unchanged oxygen metabolism. This group had excellent return of function, suggesting that early spontaneous reperfusion and collaterals were able to maintain the minimum necessary flow during the period of occlusion.

Investigators have also used PET to measure central benzodiazapine receptor binding sites after acute ischemia. Sette and coworkers [39] measured ^{11}C-labeled flumazenil, an antagonist of central benzodiazepine receptors, ^{11}C-labeled PK 11195, a peripheral benzodiazepine receptor antagonist, and CBF, CBV, and OEF in a baboon model of stroke. They demonstrated a delayed (20–40 days to maximal binding) increase in the uptake of the peripheral antagonist, probably reflecting glial and macrophage reaction. More importantly, they noted a marked early and prolonged reduction in the uptake of the central receptor antagonist, ^{11}C-flumazenil, within the area of infarction that was unchanged after day 2 postinfarction. This reduction was time- and perfusion-independent.

Diaschisis

A common finding in PET studies of both acute and chronic stroke has been areas of reduced flow and metabolism at sites distant from the site of infarction. The remote reductions in flow and metabolism generally occur in areas linked by afferent or efferent pathways from the primary lesion. This phenomenon has been termed diaschisis [40]. The classic and most common example is seen in the contralateral cerebellar hemispheres after frontal infarction (see Fig. 3). Diaschisis has been observed in the visual cortex with local reduction in CMRGlu after infarction involving the optic radiations. Similar findings have been reported in other cortical sites, particularly those overlying subcortical infarctions. Decreased metabolism of the ipsilateral thalamus after cortical or subcortical infarction has been reported, as has the converse condition of decreased cortical metabolism after ipsilateral thalamic infarction.

References

[1] Raichle ME, Martin WRW, Herscovitch P, et al. Brain blood flow measured with intravenous $H_2^{15}O$. II. Implementation and validation. J Nucl Med 1983;24: 790–8.

[2] Martin WR, Powers WJ, Raichle ME. Cerebral blood volume measured with inhaled $C^{15}O$ and positron emission tomography. J Cereb Blood Flow Metab 1987;7:421–6.

[3] Sette G, Baron JC, Mazoyer B, et al. Local brain haemodynamics and oxygen metabolism in cerebrovascular disease. Brain 1989;113:931–51.

[4] Mintun MA, Raichle ME, Martin WRW, et al. Brain oxygen utilization measured with O-15 radiotracers and positron emission tomography. J Nucl Med 1984; 25:177–87.

[5] Jones T, Chesler DA, Ter-Pogossian MM. The continuous inhalation of oxygen-15 for assessing regional oxygen extraction in the brain of man. Br J Radiol 1976;49:339–43.

[6] Derdeyn CP, Videen TO, Simmons NR, et al. Count-based PET method for predicting ischemic stroke in patients with symptomatic carotid arterial occlusion. Radiology 1999;212:499–506.

[7] Baron JC, Frackowiak RSJ, Herholz K, et al. Use of PET methods for measurement of cerebral energy metabolism and hemodynamics in cerebrovascular disease. J Cereb Blood Flow Metab 1989;9:723–42.

[8] Powers WJ, Dagogo-Jack S, Markham J, et al. Cerebral transport and metabolism of 1-^{11}C-D-glucose during stepped hypoglycemia. Ann Neurol 1995;38: 599–609.

[9] Davies JR, Rudd JH, Weissberg PL. Molecular and metabolic imaging of atherosclerosis. J Nucl Med 2004;45:1898–907.

[10] Murakami Y, Takamatsu H, Noda A, et al. Pharmacokinetic animal PET study of FK506 as a potent neuroprotective agent. J Nucl Med 2004;45:1946–9.

[11] Abe K, Kashiwagi Y, Tokumura M, et al. Discrepancy between cell injury and benzodiazepine receptor binding after transient middle cerebral artery occlusion in rats. Synapse 2004;53:234–9.

[12] Baron JC, Rougemont D, Soussaline F, et al. Local interrelationships of cerebral oxygen consumption and glucose utilization in normal subjects and in ischemic stroke patients: a positron tomography study. J Cereb Blood Flow Metab 1984;4:140–9.

[13] Fox PT, Raichle ME. Focal physiological uncoupling of cerebral blood flow and oxidative metabolism during somatosensory stimulation in human subjects. Proc Natl Acad Sci USA 1986;83:1140–4.

[14] Powers WJ, Press GA, Grubb Jr RL, et al. The effect of hemodynamically significant carotid artery disease on the hemodynamic status of the cerebral circulation. Ann Intern Med 1987;106:27–35.

[15] Grubb Jr RL, Derdeyn CP, Fritsch SM, et al. The importance of hemodynamic factors in the prognosis of symptomatic carotid occlusion. JAMA 1998;280: 1055–60.

[16] Derdeyn CP, Videen TO, Yundt KD, et al. Variability of cerebral blood volume and oxygen extraction: stages of cerebral haemodynamic impairment revisited. Brain 2002;125:595–607.

[17] Forbes HS. The cerebral circulation. I. Observation and measurement of pial vessels. Arch Neurol Psychiatry 1928;19:751–61.

[18] Fog M. Cerebral circulation. The reaction of the pial arteries to a fall in blood pressure. Arch Neurol Psychiatry 1937;24:351–64.

[19] Rapela CE, Green HD. Autoregulation of canine cerebral blood flow. Circ Res 1964;15:I205–11.

[20] Schumann P, Touzani O, Young AR, et al. Evaluation of the ratio of cerebral blood flow to cerebral blood volume as an index of local cerebral perfusion pressure. Brain 1998;121:1369–79.

[21] McHenry Jr LC, Fazekas JF, Sullivan JF. Cerebral hemodynamics of syncope. Am J Med Sci 1961;80: 173–8.

[22] Grubb Jr RL, Powers WJ, Derdeyn CP, et al. The Carotid Occlusion Surgery Study. Neurosurg Focus 2003;14:1–9.

[23] Klijn CJM, Kappelle LJ, Tulleken CAF, et al. Symptomatic carotid artery occlusion: a reappraisal of hemodynamic factors. Stroke 1997;28:2084–93.

[24] The EC/IC Bypass Study Group. Failure of extracranial-intracranial arterial bypass to reduce the risk of ischemic stroke: results of an international randomized trial. N Engl J Med 1985;313:1191–200.

[25] Yamauchi H, Fukuyama H, Nagahama Y, et al. Significance of increased oxygen extraction fraction in five-year prognosis of major cerebral arterial occlusive disease. J Nucl Med 1999;40:1992–8.

[26] Powers WJ, Martin WR, Herscovitch P, et al. Extracranial-intracranial bypass surgery: hemodynamic and metabolic effects. Neurology 1984;34: 1168–74.

[27] Baron JC, Bousser MG, Rey A, et al. Reversal of focal

"misery perfusion syndrome" by extra–intracranial artery bypass in hemodynamic cerebral ischemia. A case study with O-15 positron emission tomography. Stroke 1981;12:454–9.

[28] Derdeyn CP, Videen TO, Fritsch SM, et al. Compensatory mechanisms for chronic cerebral hypoperfusion in patients with carotid occlusion. Stroke 1999;30:1019–24.

[29] North American Symptomatic Carotid Endarterectomy Trial (NASCET) Collaborators. Beneficial effect of carotid endarterectomy in symptomatic patients with high-grade carotid stenosis. N Engl J Med 1991;325:445–53.

[30] European Carotid Surgery Trialists' Collaborative Group. MRC European carotid surgery trial: interim results for symptomatic patients with severe (70–99%) or with mild (0–29%) carotid stenosis. Lancet 1991;337:1235–43.

[31] Chiu D, Shedden P, Bratina P, et al. Clinical features of moyamoya disease in the United States. Stroke 1998;29:1347–51.

[32] Marshall RS, Lazar RM, Mohr JP, et al. Higher cerebral function and hemispheric blood flow during awake carotid artery balloon test occlusions. J Neurol Neurosurg Psychiatry 1999;66:734–8.

[33] Powers WJ, Grubb Jr RL, Raichle ME. Physiological responses to focal cerebral ischemia in humans. Ann Neurol 1984;16:546–52.

[34] Powers WJ. Cerebral hemodynamics in ischemic cerebrovascular disease. Ann Neurol 1991;29:231–40.

[35] Pappata S, Fiorelli M, Rommel T, et al. PET study of changes in local brain hemodynamics and oxygen metabolism after middle cerebral artery occlusion in baboons. J Cereb Blood Flow Metab 1993;13:416–24.

[36] Heiss W-D, Graf R, Weinhard K, et al. Dynamic penumbra demonstrated by sequential multi-tracer PET after middle cerebral artery occlusion in cats. J Cereb Blood Flow Metab 1994;14:892–902.

[37] Wise RJS, Bernardi S, Frackowiak RSJ, et al. Serial observations on the pathophysiology of acute stroke. Brain 1983;106:197–222.

[38] Marchal G, Serrati C, Rioux P, et al. PET imaging of cerebral perfusion and oxygen consumption in acute ischemic stroke: relation to outcome. Lancet 1993;341:925–7.

[39] Sette G, Baron JC, Young AR, et al. In vivo mapping of brain benzodiazepine receptor changes by positron emission tomography after focal ischemia in the anesthetized baboon. Stroke 1993;24(12):2046–57.

[40] Feeney DM, Baron JC. Diaschisis. Stroke 1986;17:817–30.

ELSEVIER
SAUNDERS

Neuroimag Clin N Am 15 (2005) 351–365

NEUROIMAGING
CLINICS OF
NORTH AMERICA

Noninvasive Evaluation of Carotid Artery Stenosis: Indications, Strategies, and Accuracy

Javier M. Romero, MD[a,b,*], Robert H. Ackerman, MD, MPH[a,b,c],
Nayeli A. Dault, SB[a,b], Michael H. Lev, MD[a,b,d]

[a]Department of Radiology, Massachusetts General Hospital, Harvard Medical School, Boston, MA, USA
[b]Neurovascular Laboratory, Massachusetts General Hospital, Harvard Medical School, Boston, MA, USA
[c]Department of Neurology, Massachusetts General Hospital, Harvard Medical School, Boston, MA, USA
[d]Emergency Neuroradiology, Massachusetts General Hospital, Harvard Medical School, Boston, MA, USA

Motivation for noninvasive determination of degree of stenosis

Although there are many causes of anterior circulation stroke, emboli from carotid occlusive disease account for a significant percentage. A study of 189 consecutive stroke patients performed at Massachusetts General Hospital from 1998 to 1999 showed that almost 30% of ischemic strokes were due to extracranial carotid atherosclerotic disease (ie, "large vessel" stroke) [1]. Approximately 30% of cases were attributed to cardioembolic disease (ie, atrial fibrillation), and 20% were from small-vessel disease (ie, lacunar infarction), predominantly in patients who had hypertension and diabetes. The remaining 20% were attributable to other causes (up to 40% of these were due to aortic arch atherosclerotic disease, and almost 20% had no definite cause of stroke identified). Despite accounting for only a little over half of all strokes, infarcts caused by large-vessel disease or cardioembolic sources account for the

majority of stroke morbidity and mortality [1] and often result in paralysis, loss of language ability, or death. Although carotid dissection, an entity for which imaging plays a key role, is another significant source of anterior circulation stroke, a discussion of this topic is beyond the scope of this article.

Even before the North American Symptomatic Carotid Endarterectomy Trial (NASCET) demonstrated in 1991 strong evidence that, for symptomatic patients who have more than 70% stenosis, the reduction in ischemic stroke risk is greater for surgical than for medical treatment, imaging has played a pivotal role in defining which patients may benefit from carotid artery revascularization [2]. Carotid revascularization now includes carotid endarterectomy (CEA) and carotid angioplasty with stent placement as surgical options [3,4]. Other key roles for carotid imaging include following the progression of known stenosis and assessing potential restenosis after revascularization [5].

Indications for imaging

Noninvasive carotid imaging is performed on asymptomatic patients who have carotid bruits, patients who have experienced transient ischemic attacks (TIAs), and patients who have experienced ischemic stroke. Carotid bruits are easy to detect clinically but are neither sensitive nor specific for hemodynamically significant carotid atherosclerotic

Adapted from Ackerman RH, Romero JM, Lev MH. Ultrasonography of the extracranial carotid arteries. In: Latchaw, Kucharczyk, Mosely, editors. Imaging of the nervous system. Philadelphia: Elsevier; 2005. p. 421–38.

* Corresponding author. Department of Radiology, Massachusetts General Hospital, Harvard Medical School, Gray Building 254, 55 Fruit Street, Boston, MA 02114.

E-mail address: Javier_Romero@hms.harvard.edu (J.M. Romero).

disease. Approximately one third of patients who have bruits have no clinically relevant carotid disease. Conversely, one third of patients who have advanced stenoses have no detectable bruits. Moreover, asymptomatic patients who have carotid stenosis identified by bruit typically do not require revascularization, although they are often followed with serial ultrasound examinations to assess for disease progression [5].

All patients who have TIAs should be evaluated for carotid stenosis as soon as possible after their event and before significant irreversible ischemic damage occurs. There is an 11% overall stroke risk at 90 days for patients who have TIA. This risk exceeds 25% if there is a more than 70% ipsilateral carotid stenosis. All such patients should be evaluated for a potential cardiac source of emboli.

Although TIA has historically been defined as a focal neurologic deficit of vascular origin lasting less than 24 hours, stroke neurologists have long since informally discarded this definition in favor of a definition with a shorter time frame. A recent position article in the *New England Journal of Medicine* proposed a new formal definition for TIA: a focal neurologic deficit of vascular origin with symptoms lasting less than 1 hour and without evidence of acute infarction by imaging (when available) [6].

All patients who have carotid territory symptoms, especially if brain imaging studies show evidence of embolic or borderzone ischemic changes, should be referred for noninvasive evaluation to look for a carotid source.

Severity of carotid stenosis and indications for medical, surgical, or endovascular treatment

Because the efficacy of CEA in reducing ischemic events directly relates to severity of stenosis in symptomatic patients, it is important to appreciate how severity is determined and by which method. The degree of carotid stenosis can be expressed in terms of residual lumen area, residual lumen diameter in millimeters, or percent stenosis. Percent stenosis is the most common parameter used to determine severity of carotid stenosis and was the basis for quantifying severity of disease in the NASCET [2] and Asymptomatic Carotid Atherosclerosis Studies (ACAS) [7]. NASCET initially found that in symptomatic patients, asymptomatic patients with a stenosis of at least 70%, CEA was beneficial. A less dramatic benefit for endarterectomy was found in NASCET for symptomatic patients who had 50% to 69% stenosis and in ACAS for asymptomatic patients

who had more than 60% stenosis. The data indicate that in symptomatic patients who have more than 70% stenosis, fewer than eight CEAs are required to prevent one stroke. However, in asymptomatic patients, with the same disease severity, approximately 50 CEAs are required to prevent one stroke over 3 years [8]. No trial, including the European Carotid Surgery Trial (ECST) [9], demonstrated a clear surgical benefit for a stenosis of less than 50%. The asymptomatic carotid surgery trial (ACST) recently published results on 3120 patients that partially support the results obtained in ACAS. The ACST found an absolute reduction in 5-year stroke risk with surgery of 5.3%, compared with 5.1% in the ACAS trial. Major differences were related to morbidity and mortality. Subgroup analysis in the ACST led to the conclusion that surgical benefit was greater in men than in women. No benefit was demonstrated in asymptomatic women who had 50% to 69% stenosis [10]. Moreover, unlike the findings in the symptomatic trials, no direct relationship was found between severity of stenosis and absolute risk of stroke.

In the ECST, residual lumen diameter was compared with a hypothesized normal lumen at the same level as the stenosis. In the NASCET, the ACAS, and essentially all subsequent studies in North America, percent stenosis was measured by comparing lumen diameter at the point of maximum stenosis (m) with that of the normal internal carotid artery (ICA) distal to the bulb (d), such that percent stenosis $= (1 - m/d) \times 100$. In other words, for a given degree of stenosis in millimeters, the smaller the normal distal segment, the smaller the calculated percent stenosis (or the larger the residual lumen). The size of the normal ICA distal to a stenosis, therefore, becomes an important variable in the NASCET measurement (Table 1). Because the normal lumen of the distal ICA typically ranges from 5 to 8 mm, the same percent stenosis is not necessarily associated with the same residual lumen diameter or hemodynamic change in any two subjects. For example, when a distal ICA measures 5, 6, 7, and 8 mm, a 70% stenosis correlates with a 1.5, 1.8, 2.1, and 2.4 mm residual lumen diameter, respectively. Although the absolute differences in lumen diameter may be small, a 2.4 mm residual lumen diameter is 60% greater than a 1.5 mm measurement. If a percent stenosis value does not have a uniform quantitative anatomic substrate, it should not have the same hemodynamic or pathophysiologic relevance or the same relation to stroke risk in all patients.

Ackerman [11] has noted that when the residual lumen diameter is less than 1 mm, the carotid artery distal to the stenosis narrows ("slim" sign) due to a

Table 1
Effect of size of normal distal internal carotid on calculation of percent stenosis for a range of residual lumen diameters

Calculated stenosis (%)[a]	Diameter of normal distal internal carotid (mm)	Residual lumen diameter at stenosis (mm)
50	5	2.5
	6	3.0
	7	3.5
	8	4.0
60	5	2.0
	6	2.4
	7	2.8
	8	3.2
70	5	1.5
	6	1.8
	7	2.1
	8	2.4
80	5	1.0
	6	1.2
	7	1.4
	8	1.6
90	5	0.5
	6	0.6
	7	0.7
	8	0.8

[a] Depending on the size of the distal internal carotid a given percent stenosis will relate to a different severity of anatomic stenosis.

decrease in perfusion pressure. Whereas a fall in perfusion pressure in the intracranial resistance causes the vessels to dilate, a fall in perfusion pressure in the internal carotid artery causes the vessel to narrow. This narrowing can be appreciated on imaging studies and becomes of potential diagnostic significance. When an ICA distal to a stenosis is obviously smaller than the homologous segment of the contralateral normal vessel, this finding is essentially a pathognomonic sign that the residual lumen diameter of the stenosis is below 1 mm (Fig. 1). In conventional magnetic resonance angiography (MRA), signal dropout occurs at advanced stages of lumen narrowing, providing no landmarks for measurement of that segment. Although signal dropout may occur at a mode percent stenosis of 70%, its onset may be associated with a relatively broad range of values (eg, 40%–80%) (Fig. 2) [12,13]. Therefore, signal dropout cannot be used as a consistent criterion for severity of disease. The difference between a "string" sign and a "slim" sign should be noted here. Ojemann and Fisher [14] described the string sign as a narrowing of the extracranial ICA to the base of the skull as characteristic of a carotid dissection. A slim sign is a diffuse narrowing of the intra- and extra-

cranial ICA that is typically due to decreased perfusion pressure in the vessel.

Accuracy of ultrasound, magnetic resonance angiography, and computed tomographic angiography for stenosis assessment

The primary endpoint for carotid artery examination is the determination of luminal stenosis, although there is increasing interest in plaque morphology. Lumen diameter stenosis can be defined in terms of residual lumen in millimeters or percent stenosis. As a result of NASCET, percent stenosis has become the widely accepted parameter, categorized in broad ranges of severity (eg, 50%–69% and 70%–99%). We consider residual lumen diameter (RLD) to be a more scientifically sound reference unit than percent stenosis. RLD permits a more precise monitoring of disease progression. For example, a detection of a submillimeter decrement in RLD represents a smaller increment in stenosis than does a detection of a jump in percent stenosis from one broad category to another.

Numerous articles have explored the accuracy of carotid artery ultrasound, generally comparing the findings with percent stenosis determinations obtained by MRA, computed tomographic angiography (CTA), or transfemoral digital subtraction angiography (DSA). Methodologic differences between the studies make direct comparisons difficult for the following reasons: (1) The criteria for accuracy are not consistent. In some studies, "accuracy" is the identification of a stenosis greater than a single percent value, typically a threshold value between 50% and 70%. In other studies, "accuracy" represents correct placement of a stenosis percent value in one or more broad percent categories, such as 50% to 69% and 70% to 99%. (2) The percent ranges that define the categories may vary between centers. (3) The velocity values that are used to define percent stenosis categories are not always uniform. Some centers use older conventions, and others have created their own. (4) Some ultrasound devices may generate different velocity findings for a given degree of stenosis [15], which would affect the criteria developed by laboratories that have independently calibrated their own velocity data against their own angiographic findings. (5) The imaging standard against which ultrasound findings may be correlated is not uniform. Conventional angiography, MRA, or CTA may be used, each of which has its own source of error. (6) Different laboratories use different parameters for calculating results. These may include peak systolic velocity, end diastolic velocity, or ratios of ICA to common carotid

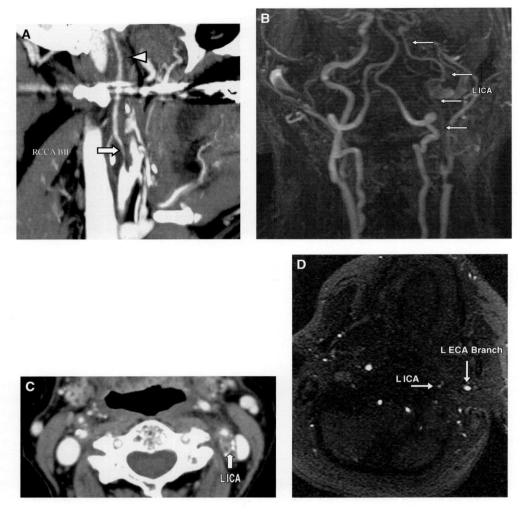

Fig. 1. Slim sign. (*A*) MIP from CT angiogram of the right internal carotid artery demonstrating a partially calcified hypo-dense atheromatous plaque in the proximal right ICA resulting in severe stenosis (*arrow*) and a distal slim sign extending into the skull base (*arrowhead*). (*B*) Elliptic centric contrast enhanced MRA of the head and neck shows significant narrowing of the distal left ICA (*arrows*) due to severe proximal stenosis. (*C*) Axial view from CT angiogram of the neck shows a severely narrowed left ICA lumen (*arrow*). (*D*) Axial 2D-TOF MRA of the neck demonstrating a significantly decreased flow-related enhancement of the left ICA with narrowing representing a slim sign (*arrow*). There is robust flow related enhancement in an ECA branch.

artery velocity values (peak systolic or end diastolic). (7) Different laboratories may use different strategies for deriving percent stenosis, which include not only the NASCET or ECST formulas but also formulas that use the common carotid artery diameter as the denominator [16]. These strategies may give varying results [16]. (8) The overall study designs may not be comparable because some may be methodologically deficient. Rothwell and colleagues [17], in addressing the problem of the quality of noninvasive carotid

artery studies, found that only 33% were prospective, only 45% studied a consecutive or random selection of patients, and only 38% reported on reproducibility. The sample sizes were often small. Additionally, tools, patients, and expertise vary between centers. It is difficult to know how to generalize the noninvasive findings from any single report.

Such apparent investigational bedlam may be what one might anticipate in a field in flux, where changing technology and insights continually pre-

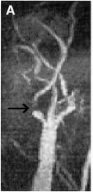 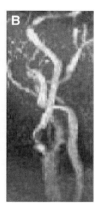

TE ~8.7ms   TE ~4.7 ms

Fig. 2. MRA signal drop out. (*A*) A 71-year-old symptomatic man. 2D-TOF MRA using an older 1.5-T GE signal
platform with the following specifications: SPGR-type
acquisition, a repetition time of 24 milliseconds, an echo
time (TE) of 8.6 milliseconds, flip angle of 60°, and a
number of excitations of 1. The typical axial images stack
consists of a set of contiguous 1.5-mm-thick axial images
that have a 24 × 18-cm field of view with a superior
saturation band. This image demonstrates signal dropout,
likely representing a severe focal stenosis. (*B*) The same
patient, imaged on a different scanner less than 48 hours
later, without change in clinical status. 2D-TOF MRA using
a 1.5-T GE LX platform. The only difference in imaging
parameters is a TE of 4.7 milliseconds. The previously noted
signal dropout is no longer appreciated, although the proximal ICA lumen is markedly narrowed.

sent new applications and new questions as clinicians
are consistently pressing for dependable guidelines.
Five recent articles [18–22] have examined the results of duplex ultrasound (DUS) findings relative to
DSA with those of at least one other noninvasive test
alone and in combination. Johnston and Goldstein
[18] looked retrospectively at the reports on all noninvasive studies in 569 consecutive patients undergoing
angiography at an academic and at a community-
based hospital over 3 years. CTA had to be dropped
from analysis because so few were done at that time.
For DUS studies, they found sensitivity, specificity, positive predictive values, and negative predictive
values of 87%, 46%, 73%, and 68%, respectively. For
MRA, the respective results were 75%, 88%, 84%,
and 80%. Respective concordant results using both
tests improved to 96%, 85%, 93%, and 92%. The
misclassification rate for ultrasound alone was 28%,
for MRA was 18%, and for both combined was 7.9%.
They concluded that surgical decisions based on one
test alone, particularly DUS, should be made with
caution and that concordant results lead to a lower
misclassification rate. With regard to CTA, one pro-

spective report (*n* = 40 patients) compared the efficacy of CTA alone with DSA and found that whereas
CTA was "excellent" in detecting 0% to 29%
or greater than 50% stenosis, it was not reliable
in distinguishing between 60% to 69% and 70% to
99% stenosis [23]. The sensitivity was 65% for 50%
to 69% stenosis and 73% for 70% to 99% stenosis.

A meta-analysis on studies done between 1994
and 2001 compared the findings of DUS or time-
of-flight MRA with DSA for the diagnosis of carotid
artery stenosis [19]. To be included in the review,
the absolute numbers of true positives, false negatives, true negatives, and false positives had to have
been available or derivable. The authors harvested
64 patient series on DUS and 21 on MRA. For the
diagnosis of 70% to 99% versus less than 70% stenosis, MR angiography had a pooled sensitivity/
specificity of 95%/90% and a DUS of 86%/87%. For
occlusion, the sensitivity/specificity for MRA was
98%/100% and for DUS was 96%/100%. The type of
MR scanner predicted the performance for diagnosing 70% to 90% stenosis. The authors concluded that
MRA has a better discriminatory power than DUS
in diagnosing 70% to 99% stenosis. A recent investigation provides the only available report that
directly compares DUS and contrast-enhanced
MRA (CE-MRA) with DSA [20]. For 35 high-grade
stenoses (70%–100%), sensitivities/specificities were
95%/79% for CE-MRA and 93%/82% for DUS.
Sensitivity/specificity was 95%/79% for CE-MRA
and 93%/82% for DUS. Combining the CE-MRA
and DUS data improved sensitivity/specificity to
100%/81%.

Few studies have compared DUS and CTA with
DSA, with or without MRA, and two of the most
current studies did not use the NASCET criteria for
determining the degree of stenosis. One report on
the results of 67 patients (34 with all four imaging
procedures) calculated percent stenosis by having the
common carotid normal diameter in the denominator
and evaluated accuracy as the ability to differentiate
a stenosis of 80% to 99% (an "operable lesion,"
according to their definition) from a lesion of less
than 80% stenosis or occlusion ("nonoperable lesions") [21]. In 80% of DUSs, CTA and MRA agreed
in the differentiation of operable from nonoperable
lesions. CTA tended to underestimate, MRA tended
to overestimate, and DUS tended to agree with DSA
findings. The most discrepancies occurred in patients
who had 75% to 80% stenosis on DSA. Interobserver
variability was best with DUS and worst with CTA
and MRA. A report that compared only DUS and
CTA with DSA included 30 patients who underwent all three imaging modalities [22]. The authors

calculated percent stenosis using ECST criteria and correlated CTA area and diameter measurements against ranges of percent stenoses derived from DUS. Correlation coefficients were 0.71 for measurement of CTA area versus DUS percent stenosis, 0.68 for DUS percent stenosis versus DSA diameter, and 0.61 for CTA diameter versus DSA diameter. These articles illustrate a number of the sources of potential difficulty that hinder the meaningful comparison of accuracy data from different investigations including variation in study design, sample sizes, and

the methods of calculating and interpreting critical stenosis (Table 3).

Whether carotid artery ultrasound studies or DUS in combination with MRA or CTA have made DSA redundant remains a source of controversy [24–27]. As many investigators have suggested, when the noninvasive tests are being used to help define indications for surgery or stent placement, we believe that at least two confirmatory noninvasive tests (ultrasound and MRA or CTA) are advisable. A conventional angiogram might be omitted if the results of

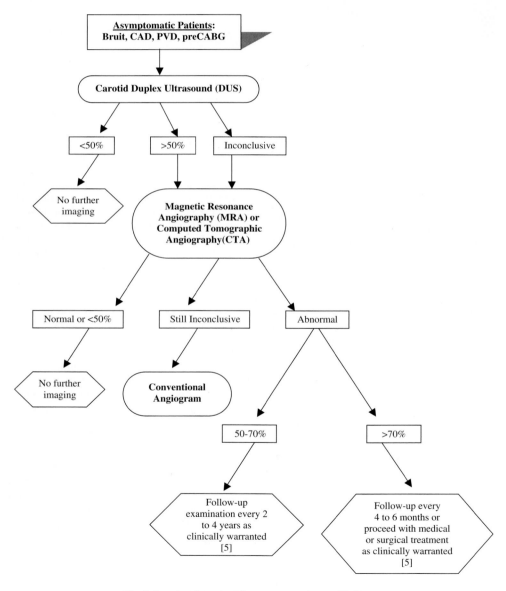

Fig. 3. Imaging flow chart for asymptomatic carotid disease.

both previous tests agree. In our experience, if the findings based on two noninvasive tests (any combination of ultrasound, MRA, or CTA) are contradictory or inconclusive, the probability is high that a conventional DSA rather than a third noninvasive test is required for a definitive answer (Fig. 3). In general, we recommend CTA as the second noninvasive test to confirm or clarify ultrasound findings, providing that clinically important MR imaging information (eg, diffusion/perfusion data) is not required. We have experience with CTA (going back to 1995) [28] and a dedicated reconstruction laboratory that optimizes vascular images. Not only does CTA show the details of the vascular lumen and the surrounding tissues, but it also demonstrates calcification. Although the latter can complicate interpretation of the status of the vascular lumen, one may participate in the reconstruction process by aiding in "peeling away" the calcium and carefully examining the source images to help overcome pitfall. The use of CTA to confirm ultrasound findings can be important before CEA and can provide a correlative anatomic baseline for nonsurgical candidates who are to be followed with ultrasound. This may be especially helpful when the initial ultrasound examination shows potential sources of error or produces uncertain results. When CTA or MRA are done as the first noninvasive examination and provide uncertain data about the severity of disease, an ultrasound examination may help resolve the discrepancy.

Sources of error

From the operator side, sources of error may arise due to inappropriate initial or poorly reproduced follow-up transducer placement and insonation angle. From the anatomic and physiologic aspects, possible errors may include incomplete tissue and rheologic sampling due to shadowing and hypoechoic disease and poorly differentiable resistance patterns in the internal and external carotid arteries (ICAs and ECAs, respectively). From the physics side, we have noted aliasing, which can confound determination of true peak velocities. Two other potential sources of error, occurring with very severe disease, are Doppler velocities falling off and subsequently undetectable Doppler flow. We discuss the effect of several anatomic configurations on carotid ultrasound findings, such as contralateral occlusion, stenosis, downstream or upstream pathology, and a high common carotid artery bifurcation.

The phenomenon of "velocities falling off" is one that is not widely recognized as a clinical problem [29]. Some laboratories believe that this phenomenon exists too transiently to be of concern (in essence, that when the vessel becomes tight enough for perfusion pressure to fall, the velocities rapidly drop out, basically to zero, such that the process itself is not frequently confronted in practice). Our experience is contrary to this and has indicated the phenomenon to be frequent enough that in formulating diagnostic impressions we are forced to raise the issue almost weekly. The process of velocities falling off results in a downward recapitulation of the velocity values into ranges associated with less severe stenoses and even normal carotids. In some cases, even if a repeat study is done within 2 to 4 months, one cannot always be sure from variations in the velocity data and waveform patterns whether or not the stenosis is moderately severe (with the values still in the rising phase) or if the stenosis is so critical that the velocities are declining as the vessel enters the preocclusive phase.

A resolution to the question of velocities falling off is not easy. We quickly move to CTA with tailored reformatting for the answer. The ultrasound clues that can provide some hints toward misleadingly low recorded velocities include a decrease in the resistance index, a dampening of the distal waveform, a pinpoint residual lumen on color flow images in longitudinal or transverse plane, and an abnormal ophthalmic artery flow direction on transcranial Doppler (TCD) study. TCD evidence of reversed ophthalmic artery flow occurs about the same time that frequencies begin to fall off and the ICA begins to narrow (ie, in association with a stenosis that narrows the residual lumen diameter to below 1 mm) (L. Marvel, R.H. Ackerman, unpublished observations). TCD monitoring of ophthalmic artery flow is a distinct process from periorbital Doppler ultrasonography. The latter examines other vascular and physiologic substrates [30] (Table 2).

Pseudo-occlusion of the cervical carotid is a related problem because it is the final phase of the process of velocities falling off. It remains uncertain whether any generally available ultrasonic technique, including power Doppler, can distinguish reliably between a hairline lumen and a complete occlusion, although ultrasonic contrast-enhancing agents may solve this problem (see below). CTA and MRA can also be more helpful in these situations, but they do not always provide correct information. DSA is the most definitive study. In a CTA study of 20 patients with suspected carotid artery occlusion and angiographic proof of diagnosis, readers achieved an accuracy of 85% to 95% in distinguishing a hairline lumen ($n = 7$) from total occlusion ($n = 13$) [31]. A potential diagnostic pitfall of this method is mistaking the ascending pharyngeal artery for a hairline ICA

Table 2
Hemodynamic correlates of degree of stenosis

Approximate stenosis		
%[a]	mm	Hemodynamic skin
50	3.0	Doppler frequency rises
60	2.4	Oculoplethysmosgraphy becomes abnormal
70	2.0	Supraorbital artery reverses (PDDU); CW = 10–12 kHz and PDF = 200–250 cm/s
75	1.8	ACA fills from opposite side (CA); TCD
80	1.2	Occipital artery reaches internal occipital protuberance before opercular vessels fill (CA)
85	0.9	Surpatrochlear arter reverses (PDDU); ECA branches over cranium fill before Sylvian vessels (CA); CW ≥ 20 mHz and PD ≥ 400 cm/s; retrograde opthalmic artery (TCD)
90	0.6	Doppler frequencies/velocities fall

Abbreviations: CA, conventional arteriography; CW, continuous-wave frequency; OPG, oculoplethysmography; PD, pulsed-wave Doppler velocity; PDDU, periorbital directional Doppler ultrasonography; TCD, transcranial Doppler.

[a] Based on original distal internal carotid artery lumen diameter of 6.0 mm.

lumen; examination of the contiguous axial CTA source images superiorly to the level of the petrous carotid canal at the skull base is essential to avoid this pitfall. A recent comparison of 3D gadolinium-enhanced MRA and DSA found that MRA missed two of nine pseudo-occlusions, which represented 28% of the pseudo-occlusion sample [32].

A unilateral occlusion or severe stenosis of the ICA may elevate contralateral Doppler velocities because of increased perfusion pressure in that system. If a stenosis is also present in the contralateral vessel, the velocities may be disproportionately increased to the degree of narrowing, suggesting a tighter lesion than actually exists. This represents a potential source of overestimating the severity of disease, but in our experience this compensatory elevation of velocities contralateral to an occlusion occurs in less than 50% of cases and depends on patterns of intracranial collateral flow (A.J. Walkey, R.H. Ackerman, unpublished observations). Other authors have found that ICA stenosis of 70% or more may artificially elevate the PSV in the contralateral ICA by a mean of 84 cm/s (ranging 10–159 cm/s) (Fig. 4) [33,34].

A number of downstream or upstream lesions can diffusely perturb the velocity waveform in one or both carotid systems. Severe proximal innominate or left common carotid artery stenosis can dampen the velocity waveform and slow the upstroke throughout the entire ipsilateral carotid system. Depending upon the size of the patient and how low down these lesions are located, these vessels may be seen with

Table 3
Accuracy of duplex ultrasound, magnetic resonance angiography, and CT angiography

First author, year [Ref.]	No. of patients	Modality	Sensitivity (%)[a]	Specificity (%)[a]	Criteria
Johnston, 2001 [18]	569	MRA	87	46	?
		DUS	75	88	
Anderson, 2000 [23]	40	CTA	73	92	Max stenosis of ICA/
		DUS	82	71	distal ICA diameter
Nederkoorn, 2003 [19]	85	MRA (non-CE)	95	90	NASCET
		DUS	93	82	
Borisch, 2003 [20][b]	35	MRA (CE)	95[b]	79[b]	NASCET
		DUS	93	82[b]	
Patel, 2002 [21][c]	67	CTA	65[c]	100[c]	NASCET
		MRA	100[c]	57[c]	
		DUS	85[c]	71[c]	

[a] 70%–99% stenosis.
[b] 70%–100% stenosis.
[c] 80%–99% stenosis.

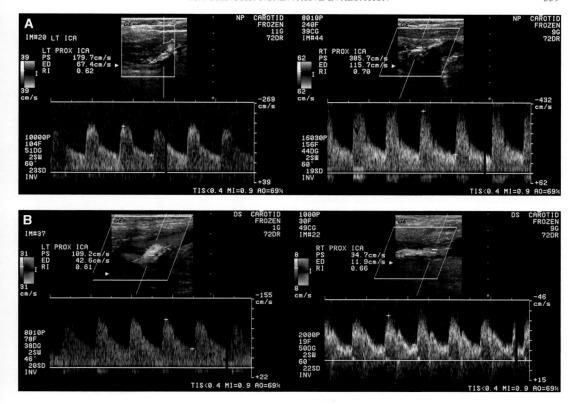

Fig. 4. Significant carotid stenosis and contralateral overestimation of stenosis. (*A*) Precarotid endarterectomy ultrasound demonstrates a severe lesion of the right ICA with a mild to moderate stenosis in the contralateral ICA. (*B*) Postcarotid endarterectomy shows a significant reduction of peak systolic velocities in the left internal carotid artery (70 cm/s) after carotid endarterectomy on the right side.

the 5 MHz duplex probe and reached with a 2 MHz TCD probe. In the case of an innominate lesion, the reduced ipsilateral radial artery pulse and brachial artery blood pressure provide confirmatory data. Severe aortic stenosis causes bilaterally dampened waveforms with slow upstrokes [34]. An intracranial AVM or fistula can produce an unexpectedly low resistance waveform with increased peak systolic velocity. The changes occur in the carotid system unilaterally or bilaterally, depending upon the lesion's size and location. Unilaterally increased carotid-system resistance can occur with a tandem ICA stenosis, distal ICA saddle embolus, supraclinoid carotid dissection, or tumor encasement (as by a meningioma). Bilaterally increased resistance can be found with bilateral carotid or intracranial vascular disease and with any intracranial pathology that raises CSF pressure.

The increased need to evaluate stent devices in carotid arteries has challenged our noninvasive techniques in the last years. Several sources of error and

artifact are attached to the metallic properties and unnatural stiffness of stent devices. DUS shows increased resistant indices (RIs) at the stent and possibly proximal to the stent due to decreased vessel distensibility. This change in RIs is due to increased stiffness of the stent device and to the compressed plaque under the stent placement (this is more frequently noted with older-generation and longer stent devices) (Fig. 5). Falsely elevated velocities may be present within the stent device, although these typically are not sufficient to alter the bottom line assessment or treatment [35].

MRA has limitations, most notably flow-related signal dropout in regions of turbulence or vortex flow. Although gadolinium may improve flow-related enhancement, turbulence and susceptibility effects from metallic stents continue to be a limiting factors in the assessment of carotid artery stenosis. Stent geometry, the relative orientation to the magnetic field, and alloy composition influence signal intensity alteration within the stent lumen (Fig. 6) [36].

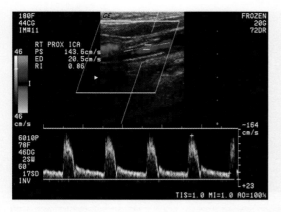

Fig. 5. Stent device in the right ICA. Ultrasound with pulsed-wave Doppler in the proximal stent demonstrates significantly elevated resistance indices (0.83) due to stent stiffness and length.

CTA also demonstrates significant limitations in determining the degree of stenosis due to the significant streak artifact produced by the stent, which obscures the evaluation of the residual lumen diameter. Extreme widening of the window settings and volume averaging may result in loss of intraluminal enhancement and overestimation of stenosis [37] (Fig. 7).

DUS demonstrates significant strengths in the evaluation of carotid stent devices due to its capacity

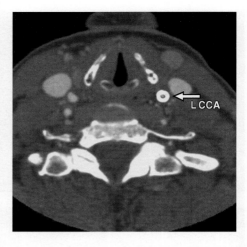

Fig. 7. CTA of left common carotid artery (CCA) stent. Axial images of the neck after contrast administration demonstrates a left CCA stent with significant difficulty for the assessment of the CCA residual lumen diameter. Widening of the window the stenosis seems to be significant; later DSA demonstrated only mild stenosis of this vessel.

to evaluate the residual lumen, vessel wall, and stent wall. Detection of carotid plaque echolucency has also been useful in the determination of stroke risk before carotid angioplasty [38].

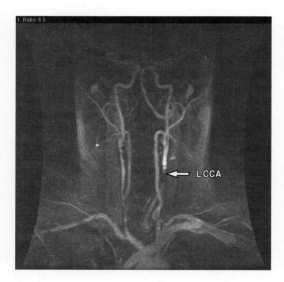

Fig. 6. Stent device in the distal left common carotid artery. Elliptic coronal MRA of the head and neck demonstrates loss of enhancement in the distal portion of the stent placement suggesting a severe stenosis; however, this patient had a subsequent U/S that confirmed patency of this vessel.

Assessment of plaque morphology using noninvasive techniques

In addition to degree of carotid artery stenosis, other potentially detectable pathologic features of the atheromatous plaque may further enhance the risk of stroke and warrant study. These include plaque ulceration, a thin fibrous cap, plaque rupture, and a large lipid core. In the late 1970s, intraplaque hemorrhage was invoked as a putative cause of ischemia on the basis that an expanding intraplaque hematoma could produce acute narrowing of the carotid artery lumen. Although intraplaque hemorrhage may be detected noninvasively with modern imaging techniques, the clinical rationale is wanting, as subsequent pathologic studies have suggested that intraplaque hemorrhage is not a marker of increased stroke risk but rather occurs almost equally in symptomatic and asymptomatic subjects [39,40].

Plaque ulceration has been postulated as playing a major role in the etiology of stroke from carotid atheromatous disease for many decades [41]. It is likely that the prevalence and number of ulcerations increase with the degree of stenosis [29] and that without concomitant ulceration a carotid artery stenosis might remain a benign process in patients who have good distal collateral flow [42]. No current routine imaging technique—including conventional arteriography [43], ultrasonography [44], CTA, and MRA [13]—is highly sensitive or specific for identifying ulceration. This means that the prevalence and hence the potential etiologic role of ulceration in patients with symptomatic carotid ischemic events remains unknown. The onset of ulceration in a previously stable plaque cannot be detected reliably; if it is identified, it cannot be confidently interpreted as evidence of increasing stroke risk. No general agreement exists as to the pathoanatomic changes that should be used to best characterize the degree of stroke risk represented by a persistent or newly evident ulceration [41]. Some ulcerations consist merely of intimal erosion, which can expose platelets to components of the atheromatous plaque, initiating aggregation of platelets, fibrin, and eventually red cells into a potentially embolic thrombus. Other ulcerations are "ugly" excavations that communicate with plaque contents, presumably due to recent or remote plaque rupture. A useful maxim may be that "small ulcers don't produce big strokes" (C.M. Fisher, personal communication). A number of processes can simulate the ugly ulcer on imaging studies, which is shown on conventional arteriography as a projection of contrast that apparently penetrates the inner border of the diseased vessel. This configuration can be simulated by a normal residual lumen between two atheromatous plaques, by an irregular plaque without intimal erosion, and by a reendothelialized ulcer. We call all such projections "outpouchings" to emphasize their indeterminate nature. On ultrasound, we have seen wall irregularities that resemble possible ulcers but that persist unchanged and asymptomatic for years (Fig. 8). The NASCET found a poor correlation between the arteriographic diagnosis of ulceration and the presence or absence of ulceration in the endarterectomy specimen [2]. Such reports underscore the difficulty in identifying a true ulcer that is biologically active. Benign, often large, irregularities in a stable atheromatous plaque, in our experience, may be over-read as ulcerations, whereas it is likely that relatively small plaque fissures that are part of the pathophysiologic stroke process may be missed routinely. Thus, incentive exists for finding ways to reliably detect, characterize, and follow ulcerations.

The aggregate of the thin fibrous cap, large lipid core, and ruptured plaque may be considered part of the "vulnerable plaque." Carotid plaque rupture can putatively occur when a thinning of the fibrous cap, accentuated by inflammation with the release of cytokines and proteinases, allows an expanding lipid core to discharge into the lumen [45]. This initiates intraluminal thrombosis. The concept of the "vulnerable plaque" has been imported from cardiology where characterization of the fibrous cap has become an imaging imperative. Major differences exist in the manifestations of the atherosclerotic process and in the pathophysiology of ischemic infarction in the coronary and carotid systems. Hence, the concept of the vulnerable plaque and the imaging requisites it mandates for the cardiologist may not be strictly applicable in the neurovascular setting. Some of the differences are listed here below.

1. Many myocardial infarctions in previously asymptomatic patients occur in patients whose coronary vessels have little or no underlying stenosis. The vessel accommodates the growing lipid core by expanding outward, rather than intruding into the lumen. However, as has been well demonstrated [2,9,46,47], the severity of carotid artery stenosis is a hallmark of relative risk for carotid-initiated stroke in symptomatic and asymptomatic patients. Moreover, carotid artery atheromatous disease intrudes into the lumen rather than causing outward expansion of the vessel wall.

2. Coronary atherosclerosis tends to be a diffuse disease in the involved artery, but carotid artery atheromatous disease is a focal process, most often occurring within 2 cm of the common carotid artery bifurcation.

3. Myocardial infarction due to coronary occlusion typically is a result of thrombosis, whereas strokes from carotid artery disease are typically caused by emboli. Therefore, for the coronary arteries, degree of stenosis may not be as reliable an index of ischemic risk as the characteristics of the fibrous plaque, but the reverse may be true for the carotid arteries. The neurovascular field could benefit from studying the possible role of a thinning fibrous cap in the pathophysiology of carotid territory stroke. Ultrasound and single-slice CTA [48] are not reliable tools for such investigations. Recent studies suggest that newer MR imaging techniques can accurately characterize an unstable cap [49,50]. The "vulnerable plaque" concept has the potential to offer further substratification of stroke risk beyond that of degree of stenosis.

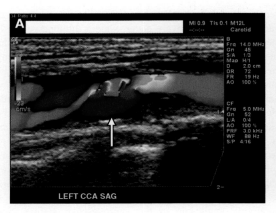
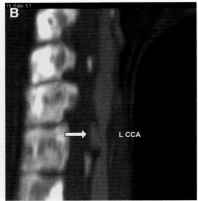

Fig. 8. Carotid outpouchings. Conventional transfemoral arteriographic images demonstrate in each patient a stenosis in the internal carotid artery bulb with a residual lumen diameter ≤ 1 mm (*arrowheads*). Proximal to each stenosis, one or more outpouchings are seen (*arrows*). (*A*) The upper outpouching is frequently called an ulcer but typically represents a remaining normal lumen between two atheromatous plaques. In this case, the outer wall has the configuration of the normal carotid bulb, of which the presumed full contour is simulated by the black dashes. The lower, smaller outpouching could represent an ulcer. (*B*) The outpouching (*arrow*) also probably represents carotid bulb, which in this case has become almost entirely encased by atheromatous plaque, except for the lower outer edge (*tip of arrow*), which could represent the lateral extent of the normal bulb. Outpouchings due to ulcers and to encroaching atheromatous changes are almost always proximal to the point of tightest stenosis.

Plaque echogenicity, as found with B-mode examination, is decreased in the region of the large lipid core, and this has been identified as a possible prognostic sign of enhanced stroke risk in patients who have carotid atherosclerosis [51]. Homogeneous, echolucent, lipid-rich plaques are putatively unstable and are likely to rupture into the lumen if the fibrous cap (Fig. 9) attenuates, whereas homogeneous echogenic plaques are said to be stable and fibrotic. Heterogeneous plaques fall in a spectrum between these two extremes. Two problems relate to using plaque echogenicity to infer stroke risk. First, studies of the intra- and interobserver reproducibility of subjective evaluation of echogenicity show poor correlations. These discrepancies are further degraded by differences in instrumentation and hardcopy storage techniques [52,53]. Second, when histologic studies have been done on plaques after scoring them for echogenicity, the B-mode characterizations have not always related well to the tissue findings from subsequent histologic studies. In a study in which plaques were graded as predominantly echolucent, heterogeneous, and predominantly echogenic, no significant difference was found in the fibrotic features between these classifications [52]. Recently, a method for normalizing B-mode gray-scale values was described that may overcome some of the problems involved in scoring plaque echogenicity [54].

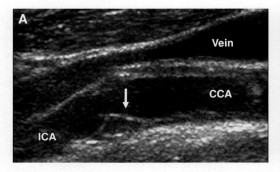
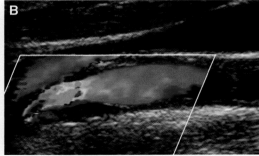

Fig. 9. Imaging plaque characteristics. (*A*) B-mode ultrasound image (9-MHz probe) demonstrates an intact fibrous cap (*arrow*) over an essentially homogeneous hypoechoic plaque, which produces no shadowing. The latter two features characterize a soft, echolucent plaque. (*B*) Color flow image of the same segment demonstrates a narrow lumen.

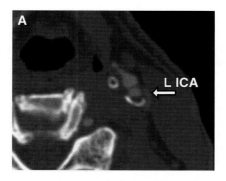

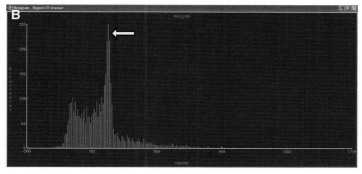

Fig. 10. (*A*) CTA plaque. (*B*) Histogram represented in Hounsfield units (*x* axis). The *y* axis represents number of pixels. Peak of calcific plaque in Hoursfield units (*arrow*).

Single-slice spiral CT has not been reliable for differentiating lipid core from fibrous cap [48]. High-resolution MR imaging may be more productive [55].

On the other hand, multiple studies have demonstrated that increased calcification may represent a more mature stage of carotid plaque and correspond to a surrogate marker for stable plaque [56,57]. Plaque calcification appears hyperechoic on B-mode ultrasound typically with signal loss (shadowing) distal to the lesion. On CT and x-ray, calcification of the plaque results in increased attenuation/density. A recent CT angiogram study evaluates the correlation of carotid calcification and the risk of stroke in the ipsilateral carotid territory. Nandalur and colleagues [58] demonstrated in a small group of patients (*n*=31) that calcified plaques were 21 times less likely to be symptomatic than noncalcified plaques (*P* = .030) (Fig. 10) [58].

High-resolution MR imaging has demonstrated strong correlation with pathologic specimens with impressive accuracy detecting lipid core, calcification, and necrotic cores [59,60]. Yaun and colleagues [61,62] suggest that MR findings of a thin fibrous capsule and an underlying lipid core are possible surrogates of unstable carotid atheromatous plaques. These findings need to be confirmed with larger studies.

Summary

The degree of internal carotid artery stenosis is an important risk factor for stroke. We have surveyed the major clinical trials related to stroke risk in symptomatic and asymptomatic patients with ICA stenosis; techniques for noninvasive screening of ICA stenosis including ultrasound, MRA, and CTA; and evolving algorithms for ICA evaluation. We also introduced the topic of "vulnerable plaque" as an additional stroke risk factor, a topic dealt with in more detail elsewhere in this issue.

References

[1] Gleason S, Furie KL, Lev MH, et al. Potential influence of acute CT on inpatient costs in patients with ischemic stroke. Acad Radiol 2001;8:955–64.

[2] Barnett HJM, and the North American Symptomatic

Carotid Endarterectomy Trial Collaborators. Beneficial effect of carotid endarterectomy in symptomatic patients with high-grade carotid stenosis. N Engl J Med 1991;325:445–53.

[3] Barnett HJM, Taylor DW, Eliasziw M, et al. Benefit of carotid endarterectomy in patients with symptomatic moderate or severe stenosis. The NASCET collaborators. N Engl J Med 1998;339:1415–25.

[4] Hobson Jr RW. Update on the Carotid Revascularization Endarterectomy versus Stent Trial (CREST) protocol. J Am Coll Surg 2002;194(Suppl):S9–14.

[5] Ackerman RH, Lev MH, Romero J. Ultrasonography of the extracranial carotid artery. In: Latchaw R, Kucharczyk W, editors. Neuroradiology. 2004. p. 421–38.

[6] Albers GW, Caplan LR, Easton JD, et al. Transient ischemic attack: proposal for a new definition. [editorial] N Engl J Med 2002;37:1713–6.

[7] Moore WS, Kempczinski RF, Nelson JJ, et al. Recurrent carotid stenosis: results of the asymptomatic carotid atherosclerosis study. Stroke 1998;29:2018–25.

[8] Biller J, Thies WH. When to operate in carotid artery disease. Am Fam Physician 2000;61:400–6.

[9] European Carotid Surgery Trialists' Collaborative Group. MCR European Carotid Surgery Trial: interim results for symptomatic patients with severe (70–99%) or with mild (0–29%) carotid stenosis. Lancet 1991; 337:1235–43.

[10] Halliday A, Mansfield A, Marro J, et al. Prevention of disabling and fatal strokes by successful carotid endarterectomy in patients without recent neurological symptoms: randomised controlled trial. MRC Asymptomatic Carotid Surgery Trial (ACST) Collaborative Group. Lancet 2004;363:1491–502 [erratum in Lancet 2004;364:416].

[11] Ackerman RH. Neurovascular non-invasive evaluation. In: Taveras JM, Ferrucci JT, editors. Radiology: diagnosis/ imaging/ intervention. Philadelphia: Lippincott; 1995.

[12] Enochs WS, Ackerman RH, Kaufman JA, et al. Gadolinium-enhanced MR angiography of the carotid arteries. J Neuroimaging 1998;8:185–90.

[13] Jackson MR, Chang AS, Robles HA, et al. Determination of 60% or greater carotid stenosis: a prospective comparison of magnetic resonance angiography and duplex ultrasound with conventional angiography. Ann Vasc Surg 1998;12:236–43.

[14] Ojemann RG, Fisher CM, Rich JC. Spontaneous dissecting aneurysm of the internal carotid artery. Stroke 1972;3:434–40.

[15] Kuntz KM, Polak JF, Whittemore AD, et al. Duplex ultrasound criteria for the identification of carotid stenosis should be laboratory specific. Stroke 1997; 28:597–602.

[16] Rothwell PM, Gibson RJ, Slattery J, et al. Equivalence of measurements of carotid stenosis: a comparison of three methods on 1001 angiograms. European Carotid Surgery Trialists' Collaborative Group. Stroke 1994; 25:2435–9.

[17] Rothwell PM, Pendlebury ST, Wardlaw J, et al. Critical appraisal of the design and reporting of studies of imaging and measurement of carotid stenosis. Stroke 2000;31:1444–50.

[18] Johnston DC, Goldstein LB. Clinical carotid endarterectomy decision making: noninvasive vascular imaging versus angiography. Neurology 2001;56: 1009–15.

[19] Nederkoorn PJ, Elgersma OE, van der Graaf Y, et al. Carotid artery stenosis: accuracy of contrast-enhanced MR angiography for diagnosis. Radiology 2003;228: 677–82.

[20] Borisch I, Horn M, Butz B, et al. Preoperative evaluation of carotid artery stenosis: comparison of contrast-enhanced MR angiography and duplex sonography with digital subtraction angiography. AJNR Am J Neuroradiol 2003;24:1117–22.

[21] Patel SG, Collie DA, Wardlaw JM, et al. Outcome, observer reliability, and patient preferences if CTA, MRA, or Doppler ultrasound were used, individually or together, instead of digital subtraction angiography before carotid endarterectomy. J Neurol Neurosurg Psychiatry 2002;73:21–8.

[22] Cinat ME, Casalme C, Wilson SE, et al. Computed tomography angiography validates duplex sonographic evaluation of carotid artery stenosis. Am Surg 2003; 69:842–7.

[23] Anderson GB, Ashforth R, Steinke DE, et al. CT angiography for the detection and characterization of carotid artery bifurcation disease. Stroke 2000;31: 2168–74.

[24] Moore WS. For severe carotid stenosis found on ultrasound, further arterial evaluation is unnecessary. Stroke 2003;34:1816–7.

[25] Rothwell PM. For severe carotid stenosis found on ultrasound, further arterial evaluation prior to carotid endarterectomy is unnecessary: the argument against. Stroke 2003;34:1817–9.

[26] Davis SM, Donnan GA. Is carotid angiography necessary? Editors disagree. Stroke 2003;34:1819.

[27] Derdeyn CP. Catheter angiography is still necessary for the measurement of carotid stenosis. AJNR Am J Neuroradiol 2003;24:1737–8.

[28] Lev MH, Ackerman RH, Chehade R, et al. The clinical utility of spiral computed tomographic angiography in the evaluation of carotid artery disease: review of our first 50 patients. Stroke 1996;27:179.

[29] Ackerman RH, Candia MR. Identifying clinically relevant carotid disease. Stroke 1994;25:1–3.

[30] Biller J, Thies WH. When to operate in carotid artery disease. Am Fam Physician 2000;61:400–6.

[31] Lev MH, Romero JM, Goodman DN, et al. Total occlusion versus hairline residual lumen of the internal carotid arteries: accuracy of single section helical CT angiography. AJNR Am J Neuroradiol 2003;24: 1123–9.

[32] Remonda L, Senn P, Barth A, et al. Contrast-enhanced 3D MR angiography of the carotid artery: comparison with conventional digital subtraction angiography. AJNR Am J Neuroradiol 2002;23:213–9.

[33] Henderson RD, Steinman DA, Eliasziw M, et al. Effect of contralateral carotid artery stenosis on carotid ultrasound velocity measurements. Stroke 2000;31: 2636–40.

[34] Romero JM, Lev MH, Chan S, et al. Sonography of neurovascular occlusive disease: interpretive pearls and pitfalls. Radiographics 2002;22:1165–76.

[35] Ringer AJ, German JW, Guterman LR, et al. Follow-up of stented carotid arteries by Doppler ultrasound. Neurosurgery 2002;51:639–43 [discussion: 64].

[36] Lenhart M, Volk M, Manke C, et al. Stent appearance at contrast-enhanced MR angiography: in vitro examination with 14 stents. Link J Radiol 2000;217: 173–8.

[37] Harada K, Nakahara I, Tanaka M, et al. Comparison of the findings of multislice CT and angiography after stenting for supraaortic arteries. No Shinkei Geka 2004;32:29–35.

[38] Biasi GM, Froio A, Diethrich EB, et al. Carotid plaque echolucency increases the risk of stroke in carotid stenting: the Imaging in Carotid Angioplasty and Risk of Stroke (ICAROS) study. Circulation 2004;110: 756–62.

[39] Fisher CM, Ojemann RG. A clinico-pathologic study of carotid endarterectomy plaques. Rev Neurol (Paris) 1986;142:573–89.

[40] Golledge J, Greenhalgh RM, Davies AH. The symptomatic carotid plaque. Stroke 2000;31:774–81.

[41] Wechsler LR. Ulceration and carotid artery disease. Stroke 1988;19:650–3.

[42] Eliasziw M, Streifler JY, Fox AJ, et al. Significance of plaque ulceration in symptomatic patients with high-grade carotid stenosis. North American Symptomatic Carotid Endarterectomy Trial. Stroke 1994; 25:304–8.

[43] Estol C, Claasen D, Hirsch W, et al. Correlative angiographic and pathologic findings in the diagnosis of ulcerated plaques in the carotid artery. Arch Neurol 1991;48:692–4.

[44] Sitzer M, Muller W, Rademacher J, et al. Color-flow Doppler-assisted duplex imaging fails to detect ulceration in high-grade internal carotid artery stenosis. J Vasc Surg 1996;23:461–5.

[45] Ogata J, Masuda J, Yutani C, et al. Rupture of atheromatous plaque as a cause of thrombotic occlusion of stenotic internal carotid artery. Stroke 1990;21: 1740–5.

[46] Feldmann E, Ackerman RH, Rosner B, et al. Progression of carotid disease and onset of ischemic symptoms: a study based on noninvasive/clinical correlations. Ann Neurol 1983;14:132.

[47] Chambers BR, Norris JW. Outcome in patients with asymptomatic neck bruits. N Engl J Med 1986;315: 860–5.

[48] Walker LJ, Ismail A, McMeekin W, et al. Computer tomography angiography for the evaluation of carotid atherosclerotic plaque: correlation with histopathology of endarterectomy specimens. Stroke 2002;33:977–81.

[49] Mitsumori LM, Hatsukami TS, Ferguson MS, et al. In vivo accuracy of multisequence MR imaging for identifying unstable fibrous caps in advanced human carotid plaques. J Magn Reson Imaging 2003;17: 410–20.

[50] Wasserman BA, Smith WI, Trout HH, et al. Carotid artery atherosclerosis: In vivo morphologic characterization with gadolinium-enhanced double-oblique MR imaging: initial results. Radiology 2002;223:566–73.

[51] Gronholdt ML, Nordestgaard BG, Schroeder TV, et al. Ultrasonic echolucent carotid plaques predict future strokes. Circulation 2001;104:68–73.

[52] Montauban van Swijndregt AD, Elbers HR, Moll FL, et al. Ultrasonographic characterization of carotid plaques. Ultrasound Med Biol 1998;24:489–93.

[53] Hartmann A, Mohr JP, Thompson JL, et al. Interrater reliability of plaque morphology classification in patients with severe carotid artery stenosis. Acta Neurol Scand 1999;99:61–4.

[54] Sabetai MM, Tegos TJ, Nicolaides AN, et al. Reproducibility of computer-quantified carotid plaque echogenicity: can we overcome the subjectivity? Stroke 2000;31:2189–96.

[55] Coombs BD, Rapp JH, Ursell PC, et al. Structure of plaque at carotid bifurcation: high resolution MRI with histological correlation. Stroke 2001;32:2516–21.

[56] O'Holleran LW, Kennelly MM, McClurken M, et al. Natural history of asymptomatic carotid plaque: five year follow-up study. Am J Surg 1987;154:659–62.

[57] Shaalan WE, Cheng H, Gewertz B, et al. Degree of carotid plaque calcification in relation to symptomatic outcome and plaque inflammation. J Vasc Surg 2004; 40:262–9.

[58] Nandalur KR, Baskurt E, Hagspiel KD, et al. Calcified carotid atherosclerotic plaque is associated less with ischemic symptoms than is noncalcified plaque on MDCT. AJR Am J Roentgenol 2005;184:295–8.

[59] Fayad ZA, Fuster V. Clinical imaging of the high-risk or vulnerable atherosclerotic plaque. Circ Res 2001; 89:305–16.

[60] Shinnar M, Fallon JT, Wehrli S, et al. The diagnostic accuracy of ex vivo MRI for human atherosclerotic plaque characterization. Arterioscler Thromb Vasc Biol 1999;19:2756–61.

[61] Yuan C, Mitsumori LM, Ferguson MS, et al. In vivo accuracy of multispectral magnetic resonance imaging for identifying lipid-rich necrotic cores and intraplaque hemorrhage in advanced human carotid plaques. Circulation 2001;104:2051–6.

[62] Hatsukami TS, Ross R, Polissar NL, et al. Visualization of fibrous cap thickness and rupture in human atherosclerotic carotid plaque in vivo with high-resolution magnetic resonance imaging. Circulation 2000;102:959–64.

NEUROIMAGING
CLINICS OF
NORTH AMERICA

ELSEVIER
SAUNDERS

Neuroimag Clin N Am 15 (2005) 367–381

Perfusion Imaging of Cerebrovascular Reserve

Clifford J. Eskey, MD, PhD[a],*, Pina C. Sanelli, MD[b]

[a]Division of Neuroradiology, Dartmouth Hitchcock Medical Center, Lebanon, NH, USA
[b]Division of Neuroradiology, New York Presbyterian Hospital, Weill Medical College of Cornell University, New York, NY, USA

Cerebral infarction results when nutrient supply is unable to meet minimum requirements needed to maintain cellular viability or when nutrient deprivation is sufficient to induce apoptosis. The conditions necessary to produce irreversible damage to the cerebral parenchyma have been studied extensively in experimental models and humans [1]. From these studies we know that cell death is a complex function of the duration of ischemia, the magnitude of ischemia, the nutrient and oxygen content of blood, and the specific cerebral structure involved. At the extreme represented by cessation of blood flow, we know that cell viability may be lost in as little as 20 minutes. For more mild but prolonged hypoperfusion, irreversible injury to gray matter will occur with a cerebral blood flow (CBF) below approximately 20 mL/100 mg/h. In between there is a wide spectrum of infarct-producing factor combinations.

In clinical practice, we group this spectrum into several distinct scenarios. These well-known entities include (1) acute ischemia resulting from sudden occlusion of a vessel by thromboembolism, (2) global hypoxic injury resulting from respiratory arrest, and (3) chronic borderline hypoperfusion due to the occlusion or stenosis of large arteries in the neck or circle of Willis.

This last scenario is the chief focus of efforts to measure cerebrovascular reactivity or reserve. Here, ischemia is the result of a combination of chronic and acute factors. There is long-standing and often slowly progressive narrowing of the large arteries (eg, internal carotid artery, middle cerebral artery). These stenoses act to decrease local perfusion pressure. The deficit is most marked at the regions farthest from the heart—the arterial border zones. These border zones are the regions at the margins of the territories supplied by the anterior, middle, and posterior cerebral arteries or between the cortical vessels and small penetrating arteries at the base of the brain. The baseline decrease in perfusion pressure makes these areas susceptible to fluctuations in systemic blood pressure, oxygen capacity, and local vascular resistance. When hypoperfusion is brief, transient neurologic deficits may occur. When perfusion pressure falls below critical levels for a sufficient time, infarction will result.

Cerebrovascular reactivity

The brains of mammals are protected from infarction to some extent by processes that maintain nutrient delivery to the brain in the face of blood pressure fluctuations. Chief among these systems is cerebrovascular reactivity [2]. The cerebral blood vessels themselves play a dynamic role in the control of local CBF. When perfusion pressure falls, vascular resistance decreases to maintain a constant blood flow. Of course, there is a point at which vascular resistance can no longer be decreased and therefore a perfusion pressure below which blood flow can no longer be maintained. This physiology of cerebrovascular reactivity can be described as a function of perfusion pressure [3] and is shown in Fig. 1.

In normal, healthy states, the local perfusion pressure is adequate to support a constant blood flow.

---
* Corresponding author. Division of Neuroradiology, Dartmouth Hitchcock Medical Center, 1 Medical Center Drive, Lebanon, NH 03756.

  E-mail address: clifford.j.eskey@hitchcock.org (C.J. Eskey).

neuroimaging.theclinics.com

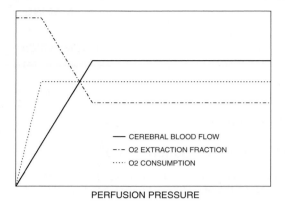

Fig. 1. Idealized depiction of cerebral autoregulation. CBF, oxygen extraction fraction, and oxygen consumption as a function of cerebral perfusion pressure.

In this condition (referred to as "stage I" by Powers [2]), blood flow to the brain may change in response to metabolic demand; however, there is little change in response to altered systemic pressure. The resistance in the cerebral circulation alters so as to maintain a constant blood flow (ie, cerebral autoregulation occurs). Because resistance to blood flow is largely mediated by changes in the diameter of small vessels, decreased perfusion pressure is accompanied by increased cerebral blood volume (CBV). In disease states produced by marked arterial stenosis, the local perfusion pressure distal to the stenosis may exceed the capacity of vascular reactivity to maintain blood flow. The vascular bed is maximally dilated, and decreases in perfusion pressure result in decreases in blood flow. With mild decreases in cerebral perfusion, cellular function is maintained by increased oxygen and nutrient extraction (referred to as "stage II"). As perfusion pressure falls further, oxygen extraction reaches a maximum, and any decreases in blood flow are accompanied by decreased oxygen consumption (referred to as "stage III"). When critical levels of oxygen and nutrient delivery cannot be met, cell viability is lost.

Therefore, in theory, determining where the cerebral tissue is functioning along the curve shown in Fig. 1 can assess the risk of infarction from hypoperfusion alone. Two principal approaches to making such a measurement exist. One is to make quantitative measurements of oxygen extraction, consumption, and blood flow. In clinical practice such measurements can be made using positron emission tomography (PET) with $^{15}O_2$ and $C^{15}O_2$ as radiopharmaceuticals. An area with impaired cerebrovascular reserve will show relatively decreased blood flow and increased fractional oxygen extrac-

tion. The second approach is to measure the response of local cerebral blood flow to a physiologic challenge. Such challenges include pharmacologic vasodilatation, elevated carbon dioxide levels, and decreased systemic pressure. The second approach is the focus of this article.

Perfusion measurement of cerebrovascular reactivity

Perfusion imaging, combined with a means of altering cerebral perfusion pressure or cerebrovascular resistance, can determine the state of cerebrovascular reserve and predict the risk of cerebral infarction. Perfusion measurements are becoming a standard part of cerebral imaging of stroke at tertiary care centers [4]. For acute stroke, perfusion imaging is used to determine the ischemic penumbra (ie, the area of tissue that is viable but at risk for infarction). However, for chronic impairment of cerebral perfusion, a single measure of CBF or blood volume is not sufficient.

The interpretation of any one-time perfusion measurement is made difficult by the physiologic variability of CBF. The blood flow that is "normal" or "adequate" varies from one person to another, varies from one region of the brain to another, varies between gray matter and white matter, and varies over time according to metabolic demands. Examine, for example, typical data for studies of the relationship between perfusion weighted imaging measures of CBF and extent of infarction [5]. The relationship between absolute CBF and progression to infarction varies widely both within and among subjects. This problem is particularly important when assessing chronic rather than acute hypoperfusion, because the degree of flow decrement is generally of the same order as that from the sources of variability already listed.

The difficulty of interpreting absolute perfusion measurements is compounded by the inaccuracies in the models used to derive CBF. Although this problem exists for all methods, the effect is perhaps greatest in those that depend on intravascular tracers. With these methods, a perfusion value is assigned from model-dependent calculations based on the dispersion of a tracer [6]. Regional perfusion, however, is only one of the factors that can affect this dispersion. Another important factor is intravascular dispersion arising from convection and diffusion during bulk flow in the large arteries between the heart and the capillaries. This intravascular dispersion may vary substantially and will depend on the degree of turbulence within the vessels and on the path length to the tissue of interest. Because this dispersion has effects on the tissue concentration versus time function that are similar to variation from capillary flow, variation in turbulence or path length will produce artifactual changes in the value obtained for tissue perfusion.

The measurement of cerebrovascular reserve (CVR) overcomes these limitations. Perfusion may be measured with any of several techniques; however, for CVR assessment, the measurement is made both before and after a physiologic or pharmacologic challenge. The baseline measurement serves as a control for the physiologic variations in flow described earlier and for a large portion of intravascular tracer dispersion. The change in flow on the post-challenge measurement then allows one to determine where the area in question lies on the graph in Fig. 1. As long as the inherent variability of the perfusion measure is substantially less than the magnitude of the effect

from the physiologic or pharmacologic challenge, reliable results will be obtained. For example, an area under stage II or III conditions will show stable or even decreased blood flow (see later discussion) after the administration of an appropriate cerebral vasodilator. A normal area will show an increase in blood flow (Fig. 2).

An important phenomenon affecting the results of CVR testing is that of "steal." In regions under stage II or III conditions, it is common to observe a decrease in blood flow after vasodilator administration [7,8]. This phenomenon is created by the interaction between regions of different CVR and the systemic effects of the agents used for physiologic or pharmacologic challenge. Areas without CVR impairment will vasodilate, lowering the perfusion pressure in the larger blood vessels supplying both normal and abnormal areas. This lower perfusion pressure results in a drop in blood flow in the regions that are already maximally dilated.

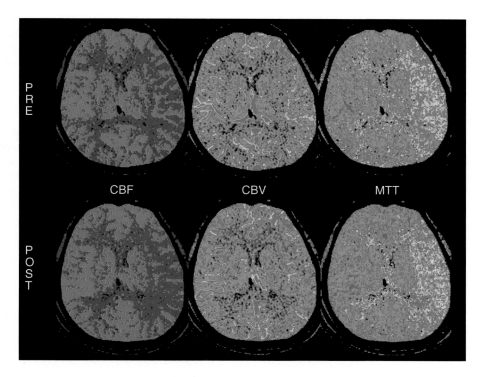

Fig. 2. Impaired cerebrovascular reserve. Patient with recent episodes of transient aphasia and severe stenosis of the left middle cerebral artery. Preacetazolamide CT perfusion (*top row*) shows markedly decreased CBF and prolonged mean transit time (MTT) in the left middle cerebral artery territory. The CBV is asymmetrically increased in this region, indicating compensatory vasodilatation. Postacetazolamide CT perfusion shows (*bottom row*) decreased CBF, slightly decreased CBV, and prolonged MTT in the left middle cerebral artery territory. The cerebral vasoreactivity has been exhausted, and there is shunting of blood flow away from the underperfused territory, representing "steal" phenomenon.

Methods of cerebrovascular reserve assessment

The list of methods used to assess CVR includes all of the major methods used to measure CBF in humans. Many of these methods are discussed at length in other portions of this monograph. The qualities that make any CBF measurement technique desirable—noninvasiveness, high spatial resolution, good signal-to-noise, availability—also apply here. However, some discussion is merited, because each one has particular advantages and disadvantages when applied to the assessment of CVR. Reproducibility is critical, because pre- and postchallenge studies must be compared. Absolute rather than relative flow assessment is important, because one needs to be able to recognize an absolute decrease in blood flow to identify the "steal" phenomenon. Sufficient spatial resolution is needed to separate the CVR of the different cerebral vascular territories, because the degree of impairment in each may be quite different. The necessary spatial resolution to separate gray and white matter structures is desirable, because the CVR responses of these tissues are different. Likewise, the capability to perform concurrent anatomic vascular and parenchymal imaging is desirable, because knowledge of the state of the large arteries is important for interpretation of CVR results.

Positron emission tomography

As mentioned earlier, PET is a fundamentally different method of assessing CVR from the perfusion methods that are the chief topic of this review. PET methods for making these measurements are varied, and each method has its own strengths and weaknesses [9], a topic beyond the scope of this article. In broad terms, rather than measure the vascular response to a pharmacologic or physiologic challenge, PET uses the juxtaposed measurement of CBF and oxygen use to determine whether perfusion pressure has fallen below levels where the oxygen demand of tissue can be met by changes in cerebrovascular resistance (Fig. 3). In the simple theoretic construct represented by Fig. 1, an increased oxygen extraction fraction (OEF) should correspond to the level where CVR is depleted when assessed by challenge tests. However, in practice, it has been shown that these two measures are strongly related but not the same [10,11]. Although OEF has been chosen by some as the measure of choice for CVR [12], it remains to be seen whether OEF or pharmacologic challenge of cerebrovascular reactivity provides a superior prediction of infarction risk.

In clinical practice, PET has disadvantages that currently limit its application. PET measurement of CVR requires isotopes, chiefly ^{15}O, with a very short half-life; it therefore requires an on-site cyclotron. The availability of this equipment is limited. PET studies of CVR are sufficiently cumbersome and expensive that they have been used more for clinical research than in routine clinical practice. The spatial resolution of PET has improved substantially, but the studies still require long acquisition times and are sensitive to patient motion.

Transcranial Doppler ultrasound

Transcranial Doppler ultrasound (TCD) has received extensive use in the assessment of cerebrovascular reserve [13]. TCD measures the velocity of flowing blood in the large arteries at the base of the brain and can be combined with any of the phar-

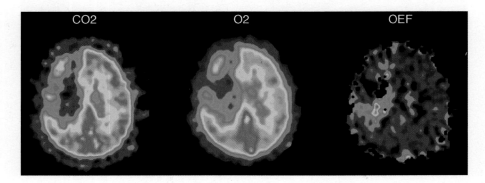

Fig. 3. PET measurement of oxygen extraction fraction (OEF). Patient with old right frontal infarct and recurrent transient worsening of his weakness. PET was performed using steady-state inhalation method where $C^{15}O_2$ is used to measure CBF and $^{15}O_2$ is used to measure oxygen consumption. OEF is decreased in the area of the old infarction but abnormally increased in a small area along the posterior margin of the infarct. (Courtesy of Steven B. Weiss, Boston, MA.)

macologic or physiologic challenges to blood flow that are described later. In theory, the velocities measured by TCD are proportional to the integrated blood flow in the territory supplied by that vessel. As long as the vessel diameter and velocity profile are stable, increased TCD velocities will reflect increases in blood flow. In practice, a correlation has been shown to exist between TCD measures of cerebrovascular reactivity and CBF-determined CVR [14–16]. TCD has qualities that make its use for CVR assessment particularly attractive—unlike any of the other methods discussed here, TCD is entirely noninvasive and free of ionizing radiation. It can be repeated quickly and as often as needed, and it is relatively inexpensive.

However, TCD has several shortcomings that limit the reliability of its CVR assessment. First, TCD only measures velocities in the large arteries at the base of the brain and does not allow one to map CVR within the brain. Regional areas of impaired CVR in a vessel's distribution may be missed when averaged with areas that are better perfused. Second, the correlation of TCD velocity changes and changes in CBF has been shown to be relatively weak, likely as a result of collateral circulation [17–19]. Third, the correlation between TCD velocities and quantitative flow measures is further impaired by changes in the diameter of the insonated vessel and in the velocity distribution [20]. Finally, because TCD results are operator-dependent and dependent on the presence of an adequately thin bone "window" to allow insonation, their reproducibility can be poor [21].

Single-photon emission CT

Single-photon emission CT (SPECT) has been used in conjunction with several radiopharmaceutical agents to measure CBF and test CVR [22]. These agents used include technetium-99m–hexamethyl-propyleneamine oxime (^{99m}Tc-HMPAO), ^{99m}Tc-ethylene cysteine dimer (^{99m}Tc-ECD), and N-isopropyl–[iodine-123]–iodoamphetamine (^{123}I-IMP). They are extracted by the brain in proportion to local CBF. They have a long half-life, measured in hours, permitting separate injection and imaging portions of the study and making possible the relatively long imaging times needed for high signal-to-noise images. The assessment of CVR with these agents has been performed with both qualitative and quantitative blood flow measurement. The qualitative methods are less invasive and more simply performed but only allow assessment of relative CBF (ie, comparison of the two hemispheres or comparison of cerebral hemispheres with cerebellum). Although the presence

of impaired CVR can be detected by these methods [23,24], the results have been mixed [25] and have compared unfavorably with quantitative methods of flow assessment [26,27]. These results are probably due in part to the fact that the qualitative assessment of CVR does not permit direct detection of the "steal" phenomenon. A degree of quantitation has been achieved with ^{123}I-IMP using a single arterial blood sample [27]. With this method, it has been shown that acetazolamide-induced CBF change measured with these agents correlates with quantitative CBF response [28].

SPECT performed with these agents has several disadvantages that have limited clinical use. The long half-life of the injected agents necessitates either a several-day delay between the pre- and postacetazolamide studies, the use of different radiopharmaceuticals, or the use of only a small tracer dose for the preacetazolamide study; each of these machinations introduces potential errors when the two studies are compared. Imaging time itself is long. The nominal spatial resolution of SPECT studies is inferior to that of the other imaging modalities, and coregistration with CT or MR imaging is needed when intrahemispheric variability in CVR is observed.

SPECT has also been performed with xenon-133 (^{133}Xe), a rapidly diffusible, inert radiotracer that is delivered by inhalation [29]. This method produces a quantitative CBF measurement [30,31]. Although it is free of some of the difficulties of the injectable SPECT agents, the imaging times are long, and the spatial resolution is even less than that achieved with the other agents. Furthermore, the substantial attenuation of the low-energy gamma particle emitted degrades the imaging of deep structures.

Xenon CT

Xenon CT also provides quantitative assessment of CBF and CVR [8]. An approximately 70:30 mixture of oxygen and nonradioactive xenon gas is delivered by inhalation for several minutes, and serial CT scans are acquired. Because the x-ray attenuation of xenon exceeds that of cerebral tissue, the accumulation of this tracer can be measured over time. Using the Kety-Schmidt model, CBF can be derived from the time course of xenon accumulation over 5 to 6 minutes. This method provides reliable CBF quantitation [26] combined with a high-resolution imaging method [32]. Although xenon inhalation at these concentrations is itself known to increase CBF after several minutes, the phenomenon has minimal effect with well-designed protocols [33]. The study can be performed before and after acetazolamide administration in the same session, because the xenon washes out of the brain rapidly.

These qualities make xenon CT well suited for CVR assessment, and this technique has received substantial clinical use and study [8]. It has been validated against the "gold standard" measures of blood flow [34] and correlates with PET-derived OEF [35].

However, few centers have developed the expertise necessary to perform these studies successfully. Although xenon CT is usually well tolerated at the concentrations used for these studies, feelings of inebriation, somnolence, or dysphoria may occur and interfere with the study [36]. The technique is sensitive to head motion, and it can be difficult to maintain immobility for the duration of combined pre- and postacetazolamide imaging.

Dynamic contrast bolus perfusion (CT and MR imaging)

Dynamic contrast bolus studies of cerebral perfusion with CT and MR have recently been used to study cerebrovascular reserve. The cerebral transit of an intravascular contrast agent is imaged and used to calculate CBV and CBF [37]. These techniques use CT or MR scanning to track the passage of an intravascular tracer through the cerebral circulation. The technology is now widely available, and the use of these techniques for acute stroke evaluation is increasing. The models used to derive absolute CBF from the data are less robust than those used for the freely diffusible tracers [34]. However, for CVR studies, the problem is mitigated, because the pre-acetazolamide study serves, in a sense, as a control for the postacetazolamide test (see introductory section). These techniques have some features that are attractive for CVR assessment. They can be performed rapidly, and pre- and postacetazolamide imaging can be performed in one session. The spatial resolution is high and the flow data easily mapped to the anatomic images. Anatomic vascular imaging (MR or CT angiography [MRA or CTA]) can be performed at the same time. Furthermore, these techniques are receiving increasing use in acute stroke assessment. The widespread availability of MR and multislice helical CT technology, the availability of commercial analysis software, the extensive experience with CT and MR contrast media, and the ease of use may make CT perfusion (CTP) and dynamic susceptibility contrast MR (DSC-MR) important techniques for CVR assessment.

The disadvantages of the two techniques differ. CTP requires repeated CT scanning of the region of interest and has a much higher radiation dose to the region of interest than any of the other techniques described here. The number of slices available with current CT scanners permits only limited coverage of the brain. The studies require the rapid intravenous bolus of iodinated contrast media with the associated risks of allergic reactions and extravascular contrast extravasation. DSC-MR lacks these risks but has the disadvantage of a more complex relationship between concentration and signal, making it more difficult to obtain reliable absolute quantitation [34].

CTP has received limited but promising use in CVR assessment. To date, published data consist of a case report in which impaired cerebrovascular reserve was demonstrated distal to an middle cerebral artery (MCA) stenosis and was improved after balloon angioplasty [38] and an anecdotal description of successful experience with the technique [39]. DSC-MR has received slightly more extensive study. Relative measures of CBF in normal subjects produced the expected response after acetazolamide [40]. Use of absolute CBF measurement by DSC-MR to assess CVR in normal adults and patients with acute or chronic cerebrovascular disease has produced expected responses [41,42].

Arterial spin-labeling MR perfusion

Arterial spin labeling (ASL) has also received preliminary study as a tool for CVR assessment. The effect of magnetic saturation or inversion of the protons in arterial blood on the MR signal is used to derive quantitative CBF measurements. This family of techniques has the advantage of requiring no exogenous contrast and no ionizing radiation and providing good spatial resolution and rapid repeatability. However, signal-to-noise is poor, and imaging times of 3 to 6 minutes have been needed to obtain satisfactory results for even single-slice imaging. Though water is a diffusible tracer, the arterial transit time and limited diffusibility of water have effects on CBF measurements with these techniques [43], a particularly important problem when studying patients with chronic cerebrovascular disease. Studies in humans are limited, but expected and reproducible CBF changes are seen when the technique is applied, in conjunction with acetazolamide or CO_2 manipulation, to healthy adults [43,44] and those with cerebrovascular disease [45]. A study of a small number of patients with chronic arterial stenosis showed that ASL perfusion imaging with acetazolamide challenge produced results comparable to those of ^{123}I-IMP SPECT [46].

Blood oxygenation level–dependent MR imaging

Blood oxygenation level–dependent (BOLD) imaging, used primarily for functional activation studies, has been applied to CVR assessment. BOLD imaging does not measure CBF directly; rather, it exploits the magnetic susceptibility differences between oxyhemoglobin and deoxyhemoglobin to provide a qualitative measure of regional oxygenation. The signal obtained from BOLD is dependent on several interdependent factors, including local CBF, CBV, oxygen delivery, oxygen consumption, hemoglobin level, and pH [47]. In healthy adults, BOLD signal has been shown also to change in response to carbon dioxide alteration or acetazolamide challenge [48–52], although there is substantial variability in response. The same maneuvers that increase regional CBF generally result in an elevated regional relative proportion of oxy-hemoglobin. However, the effects of these challenge maneuvers in the setting of chronic flow impairment are not well established. Complex interplay exists between the physiologic factors listed earlier, and BOLD signal will depend heavily on the degree and timing of these changes. Preliminary studies have tested BOLD imaging response to vasodilatory challenge in small numbers of patients with suspected CVR impairment [47,51,53,54]. Carbon dioxide BOLD response shows a moderate correlation ($R^2 = .49$) with SPECT imaging after acetazolamide challenge [47]. However, carbon dioxide–induced changes in hemispheric BOLD signal have not reliably matched the response on MCA flow velocity by TCD [54]. Larger studies and comparison with quantitative CBF or PET measures remain to be done.

Methods of physiologic challenge

For any of the methods of flow measurement, cerebrovascular reserve can only be measured through a challenge to perfusion pressure or cerebrovascular resistance. Such a challenge can take several forms. Although systemic hypotension could be used to test CVR, its use is limited; pharmacologically induced hypotension could result in permanent ischemic injury, particularly in the setting of already impaired CBF. Balloon test occlusion itself is a focal challenge to cerebral perfusion pressure; however, one is generally interested in whether current flow is adequate rather than in the effects of complete vessel occlusion. What is needed is a mild global challenge to cerebral perfusion that is unlikely to produce ische-

mia. The methods of physiologic challenge that meet these criteria and that have received substantial study for CVR assessment include acetazolamide infusion and carbon dioxide manipulation.

Acetazolamide

Acetazolamide is a carbonic anhydrase inhibitor that acts as a potent cerebral vasodilator. Administered intravenously, it slowly penetrates the blood–brain barrier, where it reversibly inhibits the carbonic anhydrase found throughout cerebral tissue. Carbonic anhydrase catalyzes the conversion of bicarbonate and hydrogen ion to water and carbon dioxide. Acetazolamide decreases the production of bicarbonate and results in a decrease in the extracellular pH in the brain [55–57]. This induced acidosis results in vasodilatation of the small arterioles [58–60].

Acetazolamide administration thus induces a considerable increase in CBF. Doses used in the assessment of CVR are in the 15–18 mg/kg range [61]; in many studies a standard total dose of 1 g has been used. Systemic blood pressure, heart rate, and respiratory rate are unaffected [62]. The effect on CBF may be seen within the first 5 minutes of administration, and steal phenomenon is most conspicuous at about 5 minutes [63]. Peak CBF augmentation occurs at approximately 10 minutes after bolus intravenous administration and diminishes little over the next 20 minutes. With these dose parameters, a 30% to 60% increase in CBF is achieved in normal subjects [8]. This response is little diminished in the healthy aged population [64]. The percentage increase in CBF after acetazolamide administration may be used to define CVR with Eq. 1:

$$CVR = \frac{CBF_{postacetozolamide} - CBF_{preacetozolamide}}{CBF_{preacetozolamide}} \times 100$$

$$(1)$$

Although a global, symmetric increase in blood flow by about 30% is accepted as normal, a variety of criteria have been used to define an abnormal response to acetazolamide. The definition has varied among the major studies in which it was used, including such criteria as a greater than 5% decrement in absolute CBF, a less than 10% increment in absolute CBF, an absolute change of less than 10 mL/100 g/min, and a value greater than two standard deviations below control values.

The bolus administration of acetazolamide over several minutes at these doses is generally well tolerated. The most commonly reported side effects of intravenous acetazolamide bolus include transient circumoral numbness, paresthesias, and headaches [62]. The theoretic concern of induced ischemia as a result of the "steal" phenomenon has not been borne out by clinical experience [8]. Drug interactions that may occur with the use of acetazolamide include (1) increased excretion of lithium and other drugs (eg, amphetamines, quinidine, procainamide, methenamine, phenobarbital, and salicylates) through alkalinization of urine, (2) increased cyclosporine trough concentrations, resulting in possible nephrotoxicity and neurotoxicity, (3) digitalis toxicity as a result of hypokalemia, (4) decreased primidone serum concentrations, and (5) salicylate-induced increases in acetazolamide effect with depression of the central nervous system and metabolic acidosis. Precautions must be taken for patients with hypersensitivity to acetazolamide, hypersensitivity to other sulfonamides, hepatic dysfunction, severe renal disease, adrenocortical insufficiency, decreased sodium or potassium levels, hyperchloremic acidosis, severe pulmonary obstruction, respiratory acidosis, and diabetes mellitus and with long-term use in glaucoma [65].

Carbon dioxide

Manipulation of systemic partial pressure CO_2 (PCO_2) has also been used to test cerebrovascular reactivity. Low-level hypercarbia results in a reproducible increase in CBF of $0.01-0.02$ mL/g/min for each 1 mm Hg rise in arterial carbon dioxide tension ($PaCO_2$). The effect is rapid and quickly reversible. It is mediated through a change in extracellular pH as well as nitric oxide and cyclic guanosine monophosphate and results from changes in vascular smooth muscle tone [66]. CO_2 manipulation has been performed with a number of schemes, including breath holding or hyperventilation, rebreathing, and inhalation of 3% to 5% CO_2. The effects of altered CO_2 tension on CBF have been quantified either as a fixed effect for particular CO_2 manipulation (similar to the quantification of acetazolamide effect) or as the slope of the CO_2–CBF relationship (Eq. 2) [10]:

$$CVR = \frac{CBF_{post-CO_2} - CBF_{pre-CO_2}}{CBF_{pre-CO_2}}$$
$$\times \frac{100}{Pa_{pre-CO2} - Pa_{post-CO2}} \quad (2)$$

In clinical practice, the magnitude of CBF changes is smaller than that achieved with acetazolamide. The average increase in CVR (percentage change in blood flow per mm Hg change in $PaCO_2$) is 1.1% to 2.9%. With 5% CO_2 inhalation, the CBF response is approximately half of the response to acetazolamide [67]. Furthermore, although CO_2 manipulation and acetazolamide in theory both produce vasodilatation and alter CBF in similar fashion, the correlation between CBF changes produced by the two has varied from poor [68] to moderate [15,67,69]. CO_2 manipulation also has the disadvantage of itself altering systemic blood pressure—mean blood pressure increase of about 10 mm Hg with 5% CO_2—an effect that may blunt the CBF response [68]. However, CO_2 manipulation is easily performed, generally well tolerated, and has no long-term side effects. The rapid response to CO_2 makes it particularly suitable for flow measurement techniques that allow continuous monitoring (eg, transcranial Doppler).

Clinical applications

Cerebral infarction risk assessment

CVR has been shown to be an important determinant of stroke risk in the setting of some types of advanced cerebrovascular disease. The clearest evidence of the prognostic ability of perfusion studies of CVR comes from patients with internal carotid or middle cerebral artery occlusions. In these patients the confounding effect of thromboembolic events is likely to be minimized. In one prospective study of symptomatic patients with internal carotid or middle cerebral artery occlusion, the risk of cerebral infarction in the territory of the affected vessel was greater (relative risk = 8.0) in subjects with evidence of diminished CVR by ^{133}Xe SPECT [70]. In this study, the annual risk of ipsilateral cerebral infarction in patients with diminished CVR was 23.7%. In a similar prospective study of symptomatic patients followed for 5 years with internal carotid or middle cerebral artery occlusion, the risk of cerebral infarction in the territory of the affected vessel was greater in subjects with evidence of diminished CVR by ^{133}Xe SPECT [31]. Most of the infarcts occurred within 8 months of entry into the study. Other studies of patients with internal carotid artery occlusion have shown a markedly higher incidence of cerebral infarction and transient ischemic attacks in those with diminished CVR by TCD [71,72]. The rate of infarction in all these studies is well above the 2% to 8% annual stroke incidence estimated for this population from other studies [73]. These studies corroborate those in which CVR has been assessed by PET measurement of OEF [74,75].

Even studies that include patients with severe stenosis have shown significantly increased incidence of cerebral infarction in those with diminished CVR [76–79]. Although one large study of this population failed to show any predictive value for CVR testing [25], this study used a qualitative SPECT measure of CVR [8].

Selection of patients for extracranial to intracranial bypass surgery

The logical extension of using CVR testing to assess infarction risk in the setting of occlusive cerebrovascular disease is using CVR testing to select patients for therapies that will diminish the risk of infarction from cerebral hypoperfusion. The primary surgical intervention for this problem has been extracranial to intracranial (EC-IC) bypass. In the past this procedure was considered for many patients with carotid stenosis in the neck or with severe stenosis or occlusion of the large intracranial arteries. However, a large, multicenter EC-IC bypass trial found no benefit from the procedure when all patients

with symptomatic stenosis or occlusion were included [80]. It is likely that this trial included many whose strokes were thromboembolic and many who never had impaired local perfusion pressure (Fig. 4). Thus, it has been hypothesized that a demonstrable benefit from the procedure will be shown if the patient population is more stringently defined [12]. Such a patient population would be composed of those with diminished cerebrovascular reserve and those in whom thromboembolic infarction is unlikely. Case series of such patients with impaired CVR who have undergone EC-IC bypass suggest a benefit from the procedure. Several case series have demonstrated full or partial reversal of impaired CVR after EC-IC bypass (Fig. 5) [7,81–84]. Studies have also shown reversal of CVR impairment by demonstrating reduced OEF in affected areas following EC-IC bypass procedures [2,85].

Outcome studies of internal carotid artery (ICA) or MCA occlusion have shown not only the reversal of impaired CVR but also clinical benefits. A case series of patients stratified for surgery on the basis of reduced CVR showed no infarcts in the patients with

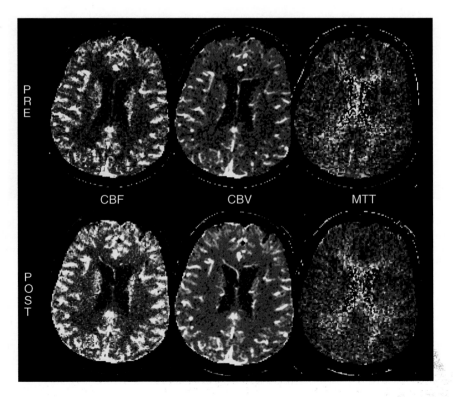

Fig. 4. Normal CVR response. Patient with severe right carotid artery stenosis. Preacetazolamide CTP demonstrates normal and symmetric CBF and mean transit time (MTT). CBV is slightly elevated in the right hemisphere, indicating compensatory vasodilatation. Post-acetazolamide CTP shows a normal response with symmetrically increased CBF and CBV.

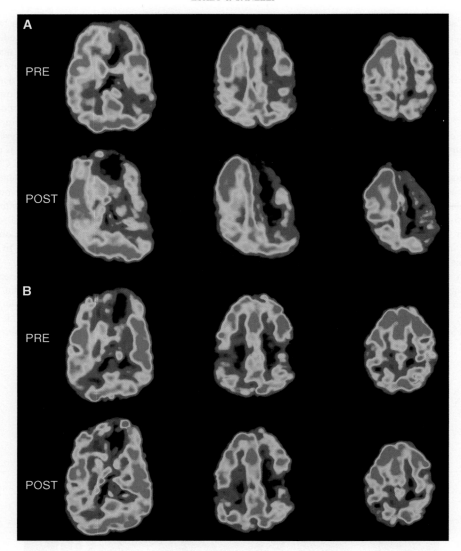

Fig. 5. Patient with left MCA occlusion and recurrent transient speech arrest. (*A*) Preoperative DSC-MR perfusion imaging (three selected levels) before and after acetazolamide administration shows a left frontoparietal region of baseline decreased CBF and a much larger area of decreased CBF after acetazolamide administration, consistent with markedly impaired cerebrovascular reserve. (*B*) Repeat CVR assessment after superficial temporal artery–MCA bypass shows substantial improvement in the CVR in most of the left frontal and parietal lobes.

normal CVR and no infarcts in those with diminished CVR who underwent superficial temporal artery to middle cerebral artery bypass; the small number of patients with impaired CVR who refused surgery suffered cerebral infarction [86]. A case series of 28 symptomatic patients with impaired CVR on [133]Xenon SPECT showed cessation of symptoms and no further infarcts after recovering from EC-IC bypass, although two suffered major perioperative infarcts [87]. EC-IC bypass can also result in im-proved cognitive function in patients with preopera-tively impaired CVR [88]. A large prospective, randomized trial of EC-IC bypass using PET CVR assessment to select patients for the procedure is under way [12].

Selection of patients for medical intervention

Although most studies of CVR testing have fo-cused on its role in guiding surgical treatment of cerebrovascular disease, CVR testing may play an important role in guiding medical therapy. In the setting of impaired CVR, primary consideration in medical management must be given to maintaining adequate cerebral perfusion pressure. Medical interventions in this setting include assurance of optimization of cardiac function, minimization of orthostatic changes in blood pressure (eg, with adequate hydration, support hose, and such medications such as midodrine or fludracortisone [89]), and limitation of antihypertensive medication. When CVR is normal, emphasis may be placed instead on minimizing hypertension and avoiding thromboembolism.

The relative merits of surgical and aggressive medical treatment for impaired CVR remain largely unstudied at this time. CVR may improve over time [70,90,91] without surgical revascularization. Temporizing with medical therapy for months to several years may allow the formation of sufficient collateral circulation to remove the risk of stroke from hypoperfusion. However, these same studies show that many patients fail to reverse their CVR deficits, and surgery may be the preferred option in many cases.

Moyamoya evaluation

Moyamoya deserves separate mention as a chronic cerebrovascular disease in which CVR testing appears to be useful. Multiple areas of proximal intracranial stenosis are present, and there is often extensive collateral development. Nonetheless, areas of impaired cerebrovascular reserve are common in this disease [92]. These areas are at great risk for infarction, particularly in children. Such revascularization procedures as superficial temporal artery–MCA bypass, encephaloduroarteriosynangiosis, and encephalomyoarteriosynangiosis are commonly performed, with cessation of ischemic events in many cases [93]. These results are reflected in studies of perioperative CVR measurement in which revascularization results in improved CVR [92,94–97]. The development of new vessels from the grafts occurs more reliably in areas of impaired CVR, independent of local CBF [98,99], suggesting that impaired CVR results in greater local angiogenic drive. CVR testing is likely to have an important role in selecting patients for revascularization and for the guidance of graft placement.

Assessing risk of hyperperfusion syndrome

Hyperperfusion syndrome is a rare but disastrous complication of carotid endarterectomy. Hyperperfusion, defined as increased CBF after surgery, results in cerebral edema and intracerebral hemorrhage [100,101]. The prognosis is poor, with mortality of 36% to 63%, and survivors have significant morbidity. CVR assessment offers promise as a means of predicting which patients are most at risk for this phenomenon. Postoperative hyperperfusion was only seen in patients following carotid endarterectomy with a reduced CVR (<10% CBF response to acetazolamide) [102]. If patients at risk for hyperperfusion syndrome can be identified preoperatively, strict control of blood pressure can be instituted in the early postoperative period [100,103].

Balloon test occlusion

Balloon test occlusion of the internal carotid artery is performed to assess the adequacy of collateral circulation before permanent carotid artery occlusion. Most patients who tolerate 20 to 30 minutes of carotid occlusion without developing neurologic deficits can safely undergo permanent occlusion. However, approximately 10% of people who pass the clinical evaluation suffer ipsilateral cerebral infarction after the permanent occlusion [104]. Several measures have been used to increase the sensitivity of balloon test occlusion, including pharmacologically induced hypotension, stump pressure measurements, and perfusion imaging; no consensus exists on the optimal protocol [105]. CVR testing has a strong theoretic advantage over mere CBF imaging for the same reasons that it provides superior evaluation in chronic cerebrovascular disease. CVR assessment by acetazolamide challenge has been performed during balloon test occlusion with promising initial results [104,106].

Summary

CVR reflects the capacity of the normal brain to maintain adequate blood flow in the face of decreased perfusion pressure. When this capacity is depleted, the brain approaches a state in which the risk of cerebral infarction is markedly increased. The imaging assessment of CVR provides valuable information beyond that given by the measurement of blood flow alone. Many means of assessing CVR exist, with the most widely used being perfusion imaging with acetazolamide challenge, PET, and TCD velocity reactivity to breath-hold–induced CO_2 elevation. Research to date has proved the value of CVR assessment in predicting the risk of cerebral infarction in the setting of occlusive cerebrovascular disease. Further research is needed to determine whether

CVR testing can be used to guide surgical and medical intervention.

References

[1] Baron JC. Perfusion thresholds in human cerebral ischemia: historical perspective and therapeutic implications. Cerebrovasc Dis 2001;11(Suppl 1):2–8.

[2] Powers WJ. Cerebral hemodynamics in ischemic cerebrovascular disease. Ann Neurol 1991;29:231–40.

[3] Ferrari M, Wilson DA, Hanley DF, et al. Effects of graded hypotension on cerebral blood flow, blood volume, and mean transit time in dogs. Am J Physiol 1992;262:H1908–14.

[4] Schaefer PW, Romero JM, Grant PE, et al. Perfusion magnetic resonance imaging of acute ischemic stroke. Semin Roentgenol 2002;37:230–6.

[5] Rohl L, Ostergaard L, Simonsen CZ, et al. Viability thresholds of ischemic penumbra of hyperacute stroke defined by perfusion-weighted MRI and apparent diffusion coefficient. Stroke 2001;32:1140–6.

[6] Bassingthwaighte JB, Goresky CA. Modeling in the analysis of solute and water exchange in the microvasculature. In: Renkin E, Michel C, editors. Handbook of physiology. Section 2: The cardiovascular system. Volume IV: The microcirculation. Bethesda (MD): American Physiology Society; 1984. p. 549–626.

[7] Vorstrup S, Brun B, Lassen NA. Evaluation of the cerebral vasodilatory capacity by the acetazolamide test before EC-IC bypass surgery in patients with occlusion of the internal carotid artery. Stroke 1986; 17:1291–8.

[8] Yonas H, Pindzola RR. Physiological determination of cerebrovascular reserves and its use in clinical management. Cerebrovasc Brain Metab Rev 1994; 6:325–40.

[9] Baron J, Frackowiak R, Kerholz K, et al. Use of PET methods for measurement of cerebral energy metabolism and hemodynamics in cerebrovascular disease. J Cereb Blood Flow Metab 1989;9:723–42.

[10] Kanno I, Uemura K, Higano S, et al. Oxygen extraction fraction at maximally vasodilated tissue in the ischemic brain estimated from the regional CO_2 responsiveness measured by positron emission tomography. J Cereb Blood Flow Metab 1988;8: 227–35.

[11] Nemoto EM, Yonas H, Kuwabara H, et al. Identification of hemodynamic compromise by cerebrovascular reserve and oxygen extraction fraction in occlusive vascular disease. J Cereb Blood Flow Metab 2004;24:1081–9.

[12] Adams HP, Powers WJ, Grubb RL, et al. Preview of a new trial of extracranial-to-intracranial arterial anastomosis: the carotid occlusion surgery study. Neurosurg Clin N Am 2001;12:612–24.

[13] Gur AY, Bornstein NM. TCD and the Diamox test for testing vasomotor reactivity: clinical significance. Neurol Neurochir Pol 2001;35(Suppl 3):51–6.

[14] Bishop CC, Powell S, Rutt D, et al. Transcranial Doppler measurement of middle cerebral artery blood flow velocity: a validation study. Stroke 1986;17: 913–5.

[15] Muller M, Voges M, Piepgras U, et al. Assessment of cerebral vasomotor reactivity by transcranial Doppler ultrasound and breath-holding: a comparison with acetazolamide as vasodilatory stimulus. Stroke 1995; 26:96–100.

[16] Dahl A, Lindegaard KF, Russell D, et al. A comparison of transcranial Doppler and cerebral blood flow studies to assess cerebral vasoreactivity. Stroke 1992;23:15–9.

[17] Demolis P, Tranh Dinh YR, Giudicelli J. Relationships between cerebral regional blood flow velocities and volumetric blood flows and their respective reactivities to acetazolamide. Stroke 1996;27:1835–9.

[18] Pindzola RR, Balzer JR, Nemoto EM, et al. Cerebrovascular reserve in patients with carotid occlusive disease assessed by stable xenon-enhanced CT cerebral blood flow and transcranial Doppler. Stroke 2001;32:1811–7.

[19] Brauer P, Kochs E, Werner C, et al. Correlation of transcranial Doppler sonography mean flow velocity with cerebral blood flow in patients with intracranial pathology. J Neurosurg Anesthesiol 1998;10:80–5.

[20] Lunt MJ, Jenkinson DF, Kerr D. Transcranial Doppler blood velocity measurement—the effect of changes in velocity profile. Ultrasound Med Biol 2000;26: 1145–51.

[21] Rohrberg M, Brodhyn R. Measurement of vasomotor reserve in the transcranial Doppler-CO_2 test using an ultrasound contrast agent (Levovist). Stroke 2001;32: 1298–303.

[22] Catafau AM. Brain SPECT in clinical practice. Part I: Perfusion. J Nucl Med 2001;42:259–71.

[23] Hirano T, Minematsu K, Hasegawa Y, et al. Acetazolamide reactivity on ^{123}I-IMP single photon emission computed tomography in patients with major cerebral artery occlusive disease: correlation with positron emission tomography parameters. J Cereb Blood Flow Metab 1994;14:763–70.

[24] Imaizumi M, Kitagawa K, Hashikawa K, et al. Detection of misery perfusion with split-dose ^{123}I-iodoamphetamine single-photon emission computed tomography in patients with carotid occlusive diseases. Stroke 2002;33:2217–23.

[25] Yokota C, Hasegawa Y, Minematsu K, et al. Effect of acetazolamide reactivity and long-term outcome in patients with major cerebral artery occlusive diseases. Stroke 1998;29:640–4.

[26] Yonas H, Pindzola RR, Meltzer CC, et al. Qualitative versus quantitative assessment of cerebrovascular reserves. Neurosurgery 1998;42:1005–12.

[27] Ogasawara K, Okuguchi T, Sasoh M, et al. Qualitative versus quantitative assessment of cerebrovascular reactivity to acetazolamide using iodine-123-N-isopropyl-

p-iodoamphetamine SPECT in patients with unilateral major cerebral artery occlusive disease. AJNR Am J Neuroradiol 2003;24:1090–5.

[28] Ogasawara K, Ito H, Sasoh M, et al. Quantitative measurement of regional cerebrovascular reactivity to acetazolamide using ^{123}I-N-isopropyl-p-iodoamphetamine autoradiography with SPECT: validation study using H$_2^{15}$O with PET. J Nucl Med 2003;44:520–5.

[29] Lassen NA, Henriksen L, Paulson OB. Regional cerebral blood flow in stroke by ^{133}Xe inhalation and emission tomography. Stroke 1981;12:284–7.

[30] Payne JK, Trivedi MH, Devous SR. Comparison of technetium-99m-HMPAO and xenon-133 measurements of regional cerebral blood flow by SPECT. J Nucl Med 1996;37:1735–40.

[31] Ogasawara K, Ogawa A, Terasaki K, et al. Use of cerebrovascular reactivity in patients with symptomatic major cerebral artery occlusion to predict 5-year outcome: comparison of xenon-133 and iodine-123-IMP single-photon emission computed tomography. J Cereb Blood Flow Metab 2002;22:1142–8.

[32] Yonas H, Darby JM, Marks EC, et al. CBF measured by Xe-CT: approach to analysis and normal values. J Cereb Blood Flow Metab 1991;11:716–25.

[33] Witt JP, Holl K, Heissler HE, et al. Stable xenon CT CBF: effects of blood flow alterations on CBF calculations during inhalation of 33% stable xenon. AJNR Am J Neuroradiol 1991;12:973–5.

[34] Latchaw RE, Yonas H, Hunter GJ, et al. Guidelines and recommendations for perfusion imaging in cerebral ischemia. Stroke 2003;34:1084–104.

[35] Nariai T, Suzuki R, Hirakawa K, et al. Vascular reserve in chronic cerebral ischemia measured by the acetazolamide challenge test: comparison with positron emission tomography. AJNR Am J Neuroradiol 1995;16:563–70.

[36] Holl K, Becker H, Haubitz B. Effect of xenon. Acta Neurol Scand Suppl 1996;166:38–41.

[37] Ostergaard L, Weisskoff RM, Chesler DA, et al. High resolution measurement of cerebral blood flow using intravascular tracer bolus passages. Part I: Mathematical approach and statistical analysis. Magn Reson Med 1996;36:715–25.

[38] Eastwood JD, Alexander MJ, Petrella JR, et al. Dynamic CT perfusion imaging with acetazolamide challenge for the preprocedural evaluation of a patient with symptomatic middle cerebral artery occlusive disease. AJNR Am J Neuroradiol 2002;23:285–7.

[39] Hoeffner EG, Case I, Jain R, et al. Cerebral perfusion CT: technique and clinical applications. Radiology 2004;231:632–44.

[40] Berthezene Y, Nighoghossian N, Meyer R, et al. Can cerebrovascular reactivity be assessed by dynamic susceptibility contrast-enhanced MRI? Neuroradiology 1998;40:1–5.

[41] Guckel FJ, Brix G, Schmiedek P, et al. Cerebrovascular reserve capacity in patients with occlusive cerebrovascular disease: assessment with dynamic susceptibility contrast-enhanced MR imaging and the acetazolamide stimulation test. Radiology 1996;201:405–12.

[42] Schreiber WG, Guckel F, Stritzke P, et al. Cerebral blood flow and cerebrovascular reserve capacity: estimation by dynamic magnetic resonance imaging. J Cereb Blood Flow Metab 1998;18:1143–56.

[43] Yen YF, Field AS, Martin EM, et al. Test-retest reproducibility of quantitative CBF measurements using FAIR perfusion MRI and acetazolamide challenge. Magn Reson Med 2002;47:921–8.

[44] Kastrup A, Li TQ, Glover GH, et al. Cerebral blood flow–related signal changes during breath-holding. AJNR Am J Neuroradiol 1999;20:1233–8.

[45] Detre JA, Samuels OB, Alsop DC, et al. Noninvasive magnetic resonance imaging evaluation of cerebral blood flow with acetazolamide challenge in patients with cerebrovascular stenosis. J Magn Reson Imaging 1999;10:870–5.

[46] Arbab AS, Aoki S, Toyama K, et al. Quantitative measurement of regional cerebral blood flow with flow-sensitive alternating inversion recovery imaging: comparison with [iodine 123]-iodoamphetamine single photon emission CT. AJNR Am J Neuroradiol 2002;23:381–8.

[47] Shiino A, Morita Y, Tsuji A, et al. Estimation of cerebral perfusion reserve by blood oxygenation level–dependent imaging: comparison with single-photon emission computed tomography. J Cereb Blood Flow Metab 2003;23:121–35.

[48] Rostrup E, Larsson HB, Toft PB, et al. Functional MRI of CO$_2$ induced increase in cerebral perfusion. NMR Biomed 1994;7:29–34.

[49] Kastrup A, Li TQ, Takahashi A, et al. Functional magnetic resonance imaging of regional cerebral blood oxygenation changes during breath holding. Stroke 1998;29:2641–5.

[50] Hedera P, Lai S, Lewin JS, et al. Assessment of cerebral blood flow reserve using functional magnetic resonance imaging. J Magn Reson Imaging 1996;6:718–25.

[51] Bruhn H, Kleinschmidt A, Boecker H, et al. The effect of acetazolamide on regional cerebral blood oxygenation at rest and under stimulation as assessed by MRI. J Cereb Blood Flow Metab 1994;14:742–8.

[52] Ohnishi T, Nakano S, Yano T, et al. Susceptibility-weighted MR for evaluation of vasodilatory capacity with acetazolamide challenge. AJNR Am J Neuroradiol 1996;17:631–7.

[53] Kleinschmidt A, Steinmetz H, Sitzer M, et al. Magnetic resonance imaging of regional cerebral blood oxygenation changes under acetazolamide in carotid occlusive disease. Stroke 1995;26:106–10.

[54] Lythgoe DJ, Williams SC, Cullinane M, et al. Mapping of cerebrovascular reactivity using BOLD magnetic resonance imaging. Magn Reson Imaging 1999;17:495–502.

[55] Heuser D, Astrup J, Lassen NA, et al. Brain carbonic acid acidosis after acetazolamide. Acta Physiol Scand 1995;93:385–90.

[56] Severinghaus JW, Cotev S. Carbonic acidosis and cerebral vasodilatation after Diamox. Scand J Clin Lab Invest Scand 1968;1(Suppl 102):E.

[57] Vorstrup S, Henriksen L, Paulson OB. Effect of acetazolamide on cerebral blood flow and cerebral metabolism rate for oxygen. J Clin Invest 1984;74: 1634–9.

[58] Gotoh F. Carbonic anhydrase inhibition and cerebral venous blood gases and ions in man. Arch Intern Med 1966;11:39–46.

[59] Kontos HA, Wei EP, Navari RM, et al. Responses of cerebral arteries and arterioles to acute hypotension and hypertension. Am J Physiol 1978;234:H371–83.

[60] Okazawa H, Yamauchi H, Sugimoto K, et al. Effects of acetazolamide on cerebral blood flow, blood volume, and oxygen metabolism: a positron emission tomography study with healthy volunteers. J Cereb Blood Flow Metab 2001;21:1472–9.

[61] Dahl A, Russell D, Rootwelt K, et al. Cerebral vasoreactivity assessed with transcranial Doppler and regional cerebral blood flow measurements: dose, serum concentration, and time course of the response to acetazolamide. Stroke 1995;26:2302–6.

[62] Sullivan HG, Kingsbury TB, Morgan ME, et al. The rCBF response to Diamox in normal subjects and cerebrovascular disease patients. J Neurosurg 1987; 67:525–34.

[63] Kuwabara Y, Ichiya Y, Sasaki M, et al. Time dependency of the acetazolamide effect on cerebral hemodynamics in patients with chronic occlusive cerebral arteries. Early steal phenomenon demonstrated by [^{15}O]H$_2$O positron emission tomography. Stroke 1995;26:1825–9.

[64] Petrella JR, DeCarli C, Dagli M, et al. Age-related vasodilatory response to acetazolamide challenge in healthy adults: a dynamic contrast-enhanced MR study. AJNR Am J Neuroradiol 1998;19:39–44.

[65] Lexi-Comp online. Available at: http://www.crlonline.com. Accessed February 10, 2005.

[66] Brian JE. Carbon dioxide and the cerebral circulation. Anesthesiology 1998;88:1365–86.

[67] Gambhir S, Inao S, Tadokoro M, et al. Comparison of vasodilatory effect of carbon dioxide inhalation and intravenous acetazolamide on brain vasculature using positron emission tomography. Neurol Res 1997;19: 139–44.

[68] Kazumata K, Tanaka N, Ishikawa T, et al. Dissociation of vasoreactivity to acetazolamide and hypercapnia. Comparative study in patients with chronic occlusive major cerebral artery disease. Stroke 1996; 27:2052–8.

[69] Ringelstein EB, Van Eyck S, Mertens I. Evaluation of cerebral vasomotor reactivity by various vasodilating stimuli: comparison of CO$_2$ to acetazolamide. J Cereb Blood Flow Metab 1992;12:162–8.

[70] Kuroda S, Houkin K, Kamiyama H, et al. Long-term prognosis of medically treated patients with internal carotid or middle cerebral artery occlusion: can acetazolamide test predict it? Stroke 2001;32:2110–6.

[71] Kleiser B, Widder B. Course of carotid artery occlusions with impaired cerebrovascular reactivity. Stroke 1992;23:171–4.

[72] Vernieri F, Pasqualetti P, Passarelli F, et al. Outcome of carotid artery occlusion is predicted by cerebrovascular reactivity. Stroke 1999;30:593–8.

[73] Settakis G, Molnar C, Kerenyi L, et al. Acetazolamide as a vasodilatory stimulus in cerebrovascular diseases and in conditions affecting the cerebral vasculature. Eur J Neurol 2003;10:609–20.

[74] Yamauchi H, Fukuyama H, Nagahama Y, et al. Significance of increased oxygen extraction fraction in five-year prognosis of major cerebral arterial occlusive diseases. J Nucl Med 1999;40:1992–8.

[75] Grubb Jr RL, Derdeyn CP, Fritsch SM, et al. Importance of hemodynamic factors in the prognosis of symptomatic carotid occlusion. JAMA 1998;280: 1055–60.

[76] Yonas H, Smith HA, Durham SR, et al. Increased stroke risk predicted by compromised cerebral blood flow reactivity. J Neurosurg 1993;79:483–9.

[77] Webster MW, Makaroun MS, Steed DL, et al. Compromised cerebral blood flow reactivity is a predictor of stroke in patients with symptomatic carotid artery occlusive disease. J Vasc Surg 1995;21: 338–44.

[78] Markus H, Cullinane M. Severely impaired cerebrovascular reactivity predicts stroke and TIA risk in patients with carotid artery stenosis and occlusion. Brain 2001;124:457–67.

[79] Gur AY, Bova I, Bornstein NM. Is impaired cerebral vasomotor reactivity a predictive factor of stroke in asymptomatic patients? Stroke 1996;27:2188–90.

[80] EC-IC Bypass Study Group. Failure of extracranial-intracranial arterial bypass to reduce the risk of ischemic stroke. Results of an international randomized trial. N Engl J Med 1985;313:1191–200.

[81] Batjer HH, Devous Sr MD, Purdy PD, et al. Improvement in regional cerebral blood flow and cerebral vasoreactivity after extracranial-intracranial arterial bypass. Neurosurgery 1988;22:913–9.

[82] Anderson DE, McLane MP, Reichman OH, et al. Improved cerebral blood flow and CO$_2$ reactivity after microvascular anastomosis in patients at high risk for recurrent stroke. Neurosurgery 1992;31:26–33.

[83] Yamashita T, Kashiwagi S, Nakano S, et al. The effect of EC-IC bypass surgery on resting cerebral blood flow and cerebrovascular reserve capacity studied with stable XE-CT and acetazolamide test. Neuroradiology 1991;33:217–22.

[84] Karnik R, Valentin A, Ammerer HP, et al. Evaluation of vasomotor reactivity by transcranial Doppler and acetazolamide test before and after extracranial-intracranial bypass in patients with internal carotid artery occlusion. Stroke 1992;23:812–7.

[85] Muraishi K, Kameyama M, Sato K, et al. Cerebral circulatory and metabolic changes following EC/IC bypass surgery in cerebral occlusive diseases. Neurol Res 1993;15:97–103.

[86] Kuroda S, Kamiyama H, Abe H, et al. Acetazolamide test in detecting reduced cerebral perfusion reserve and predicting long-term prognosis in patients with internal carotid artery occlusion. Neurosurgery 1993; 32:912–8.

[87] Schmiedek P, Piepgras A, Leinsinger G, et al. Improvement of cerebrovascular reserve capacity by EC-IC arterial bypass surgery in patients with ICA occlusion and hemodynamic cerebral ischemia. J Neurosurg 1994;81:236–44.

[88] Sasoh M, Ogasawara K, Kuroda K, et al. Effects of EC-IC bypass surgery on cognitive impairment in patients with hemodynamic cerebral ischemia. Surg Neurol 2003;59:455–60.

[89] Beers MH, Berkow R. The Merck manual of geriatrics. 3rd edition. Whitehouse Station (NJ): Merck Publishing Group; 2000.

[90] Hasegawa Y, Yamaguchi T, Tsuchiya T, et al. Sequential change of hemodynamic reserve in patients with major cerebral artery occlusion or severe stenosis. Neuroradiology 1992;34:15–21.

[91] Widder B, Kleiser B, Krapf H. Course of cerebrovascular reactivity in patients with carotid artery occlusions. Stroke 1994;25:1963–7.

[92] Kuwabara Y, Ichiya Y, Sasaki M, et al. Cerebral hemodynamics and metabolism in moyamoya disease—a positron emission tomography study. Clin Neurol Neurosurg 1997;99(Suppl 2):S74–8.

[93] Ishikawa T, Houkin K, Kamiyama H, et al. Effects of surgical revascularization on outcome of patients with pediatric moyamoya disease. Stroke 1997;28: 1170–3.

[94] Ikezaki K, Matsushima T, Kuwabara Y, et al. Cerebral circulation and oxygen metabolism in childhood moyamoya disease: a perioperative positron emission tomography study. J Neurosurg 1994;81:843–50.

[95] Kashiwagi S, Yamashita T, Katoh S, et al. Regression of moyamoya vessels and hemodynamic changes after successful revascularization in childhood moyamoya disease. Acta Neurol Scand Suppl 1996;166: 85–8.

[96] McAuley DJ, Poskitt K, Steinbok P. Predicting stroke risk in pediatric moyamoya disease with xenon-enhanced computed tomography. Neurosurgery 2004;55:327–32.

[97] Morimoto M, Iwama T, Hashimoto N, et al. Efficacy of direct revascularization in adult Moyamoya disease: haemodynamic evaluation by positron emission tomography. Acta Neurochir 1999;141:377–84.

[98] Nariai T, Suzuki R, Matsushima Y, et al. Surgically induced angiogenesis to compensate for hemodynamic cerebral ischemia. Stroke 1994;25:1014–21.

[99] Iwama T, Hashimoto N, Takagi Y, et al. Predictability of extracranial/intracranial bypass function: a retrospective study of patients with occlusive cerebrovascular disease. Neurosurgery 1997;40:53–9.

[100] Henderson RD, Phan TG, Piepgras DG, et al. Mechanism of intracerebral hemorrhage after carotid endarterectomy. J Neurosurg 2001;95:964–9.

[101] Piepgras DG, Morgan MK, Sundt TMJ, et al. Intracerebral hemorrhage after carotid endarterectomy. J Neurosurg 1988;68:532–6.

[102] Hosoda K, Kawaguchi T, Ishii K, et al. Prediction of hyperperfusion after carotid endarterectomy by brain SPECT analysis with semiquantitative statistical mapping method. Stroke 2003;34:1187–93.

[103] Reigel MM, Hollier LH, Sundt TM, et al. Cerebral hyperperfusion syndrome: a cause of neurologic dysfunction after carotid endarterectomy. J Vasc Surg 1987;5:628–34.

[104] Jain R, Hoeffner EG, Deveikis JP, et al. Carotid perfusion CT with balloon occlusion and acetazolamide challenge test: feasibility. Radiology 2004;231: 906–13.

[105] Morris P. Interventional and endovascular therapy of the nervous system. New York: Springer-Verlag; 2002.

[106] Okudaira Y, Arai H, Sato K. Cerebral blood flow alteration by acetazolamide during carotid balloon occlusion: parameters reflecting cerebral perfusion pressure in the acetazolamide test. Stroke 1996;27: 617–21.

ELSEVIER
SAUNDERS

Neuroimag Clin N Am 15 (2005) 383 – 395

NEUROIMAGING
CLINICS OF
NORTH AMERICA

Endovascular Treatment of Extracranial Carotid Artery Stenosis: Update on Carotid Angioplasty and Stenting

Sean P. Cullen, MD[a,b,*], Randall T. Higashida, MD[c]

[a]Cerebrovascular Center, Interventional Neuroradiology, Brigham and Women's Hospital, Boston, MA, USA
[b]Neurointerventional Radiology, Children's Hospital, Boston, MA, USA
[c]Division of Neurointerventional Radiology, University of California at San Francisco Medical Center, San Francisco, CA, USA

When it was first reported 25 years ago, endovascular treatment of carotid artery stenosis was an uncommon procedure consisting of simple balloon angioplasty, used mostly on patients who were believed to be poor surgical candidates or for surgically inaccessible lesions. Since then, the endovascular approach to carotid stenosis has undergone substantial modifications; it now consists typically of primary stenting (Fig. 1), with or without angioplasty, often using a distal embolic protection device (Fig. 2). The procedure is now widely performed, with more than 12,000 cases reported in the literature. In August 2004, the US Food and Drug Administration (FDA) approved the use of a stent and distal embolic protection device for the prevention of stroke in patients with carotid stenosis and recommended contingent approval for two additional devices [1]. In March 2005, the Centers for Medicare and Medicaid Services approved coverage of carotid artery stenting in selected high-risk patients, and reimbursement for the procedure by other insurers is expected. Several recently published randomized trials, including the Stenting and Angioplasty with Protection in Patients at High Risk for Endarterectomy (SAPPHIRE) and Carotid and Vertebral Artery Transluminal Angioplasty Study (CAVATAS) trials, have demonstrated that carotid artery stenting is as safe and effective in both high-risk and low-risk patients as carotid endarterectomy, which was previously the procedure of choice [2,3]. Other randomized clinical trials are currently in progress, including trials in North America (Carotid Revascularization Endarterectomy Versus Stent Trial [CREST]), Germany ([Stent-Protected Percutaneous Angioplasty of the Carotid vs. Endarterectomy] SPACE), and Great Britain (CAVATAS II). Indications exist that carotid artery stenting may continue to increase in frequency and become the standard treatment for patients with significant carotid stenosis at high risk for future stroke. A number of important issues remain to be clarified, however, including appropriate patient selection, standardization of training, and accrediting of operators.

The decision to treat carotid disease

Carotid stenosis is a common cause of stroke and has been estimated to be responsible for as many as 20%–25% of all ischemic events [4,5]. It is currently estimated that 175,000 to 200,000 cases of carotid endarterectomy are currently being performed on an annual basis in the United States alone. Distal embolization from a ruptured plaque, hemodynamic compromise from carotid occlusion or near-occlusion, or a combination of the two mechanisms is typically invoked as the explanation for stroke in the presence of ipsilateral carotid disease. Importantly, however, as many as 45% of strokes in patients with previously silent carotid disease are due to lacunes or cardioembolism [6].

* Corresponding author. Cerebrovascular Center, Interventional Neuroradiology, Brigham and Women's Hospital and Children's Hospital, 75 Francis Street, Boston, MA 02114.
  E-mail address: spcullen@gmail.com (S.P. Cullen).

1052-5149/05/$ – see front matter © 2005 Elsevier Inc. All rights reserved.
doi:10.1016/j.nic.2005.05.004

neuroimaging.theclinics.com

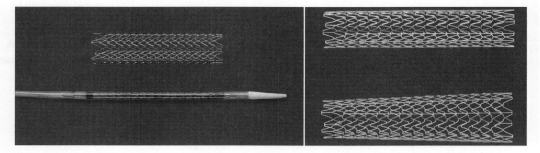

Fig. 1. US Food and Drug Administration–approved carotid artery self-expanding stent device: Acculink Carotid Stent System (Guidant Corporation, Indianapolis, Indiana). In delivery catheter (*bottom left*), in straight (*top right*), and tapered versions (*bottom right*). (Courtesy of Guidant Corporation; with permission.)

Appropriate management of carotid stenosis— whether this be no treatment, medical therapy, or open surgical or endovascular revascularization— depends on balancing future risk of stroke against the risk of the chosen therapy. Because the overall benefit of the treatment for an individual patient depends on weighing the actual outcome versus a speculative possible outcome without therapy, choice of treatment would be problematic even if the absolute risk of stroke and the absolute risk of therapy were known with certainty [7]. Reliably estimating future stroke risk and risk of therapy in an individual patient who has either previously silent carotid disease or prior symptoms is a complex task confounded by multiple factors. The natural history of atherosclerotic disease, as well as the risk profile of therapy, shows important differences among genders, races, and socioeconomic groups [5,8–10]. In addition, although risk stratification has commonly relied chiefly on estimation of percentage of stenosis—the main selection criterion

in the three major randomized clinical trials of carotid endarterectomy—mounting evidence gives importance to a number of factors besides the degree of narrowing. For example, the morphology of the atherosclerotic plaque, presence of ulceration or intraplaque hemorrhage, increased velocity, decreased volume of lumen in the diseased arterial segment, and the degree and severity of associated hemodynamic compromise distal to the lesion all probably affect the likelihood and severity of future ischemic events [11]. In the future, advanced neuroimaging techniques addressing these other features of carotid narrowing will likely be used increasingly to make appropriate treatment choices and may eventually be incorporated into future clinical studies. Finally, patients who undergo a successful revascularization procedure remain at risk for stroke from progression of atherosclerotic disease at other sites as well as stroke from other sources such as lacunar infarcts and cardioembolic causes. For these reasons, risk factor

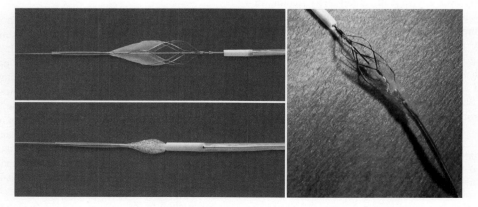

Fig. 2. US Food and Drug Administration–approved distal embolic protection system: Accunet Embolic Protection System (Guidant Corporation). Deployed (*top left*) and in retrieval position (*bottom left*). With debris (*right*). (Courtesy of Guidant Corporation; with permission.)

modification and medical therapy will always play crucial roles in stroke treatment and prevention.

Assessing the heterogeneous nature of carotid artery stenosis

Carotid disease that produces symptoms or that presents a significant risk of ischemic stroke is almost always due to atherosclerotic disease. Many other causes of carotid narrowing exist, however, and these must be considered when evaluating a patient with carotid narrowing, because natural history and treatment options will differ. Other processes that can result in carotid narrowing include fibromuscular dysplasia, dissection, Takayasu's arteritis, radiation-induced vasculopathy, and congenital variants [5]. Any approach to the treatment of carotid stenosis must address the nature of the stenosis, incorporate the natural history of that type of lesion into any risk

assessment, and identify the mechanisms by which it causes or may cause symptoms [5]. Currently, percentage stenosis is the most commonly used criterion for the assessment of carotid stenosis. Severity of stenosis, in general, has been shown to correlate with future stroke risk. For example, one study of nearly 700 patients with asymptomatic carotid narrowing identified by Doppler ultrasound and followed for an average of 41 months found a 1.3% per year stroke risk for patients with a stenosis of 75%; this increased to 10.5% per year for stenosis greater than 75% [12]. The North American Symptomatic Carotid Endarterectomy Trial (NASCET) found a 26% 2-year stroke rate for symptomatic patients with severe stenosis (70%–99%) despite best medical therapy. Five-year stroke rates on medical therapy were 22% and 19% for moderate stenosis (50%–69%) and mild stenosis (30%–49%), respectively [13].

Methods of measuring carotid stenosis are still somewhat controversial. The most common method

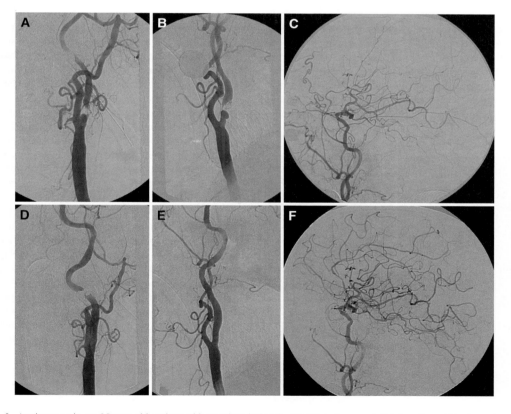

Fig. 3. Angiograms in an 85-year-old patient with transient ischemic attacks and severe left internal carotid artery stenosis, with cardiac disease. Anteroposterior (*A*) and lateral (*B*) left common carotid injection angiograms show severe proximal internal carotid stenosis. Lateral view of the head (common carotid injection) (*C*) shows preferential filling of the external carotid artery. Poststenting anteroposterior (*D*) and lateral (*E*) views of the left carotid show revascularization. Lateral view of the head (*F*) after stenting shows improved flow to the brain. There is extensive intracranial atherosclerosis.

of assessing stenosis is Doppler ultrasound. This method does produce two-dimensional images of the carotid artery and does depict extent of plaque, but percentage stenosis is usually inferred from the peak systolic velocity, not from the two-dimensional image. An excellent noninvasive screening modality, ultrasound can be operator dependent, and vascular laboratories employing this method should be carefully validated with more rigorous imaging techniques. Other pitfalls include erroneous measurements in the presence of tortuosity and artifactually low velocities in preocclusive lesions. Other noninvasive imaging techniques include MR angiography (MRA) and CT angiography (Figs. 3 and 4).

No strong published data validate the exclusive use of noninvasive imaging to assess carotid stenosis before endarterectomy or stenting. Many institutions, however, routinely use noninvasive imaging modalities and save diagnostic carotid angiography for instances where there are discrepant noninvasive findings. MRA and Doppler ultrasound tend to overestimate the degree of stenosis, and this method will tend to increase the volume of revascularization procedures performed at a given institution [11]. A pitfall of conventional time-of-flight MRA is that signal is derived from flow, which may lead to overestimating the degree of stenosis, although this is less of a problem when gadolinium-enhanced techniques are used. CT angiography has better anatomic

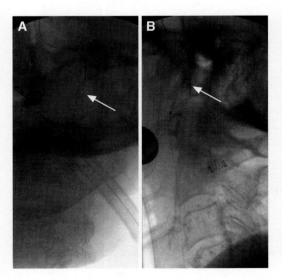

Fig. 4. FDA-approved protection device (Accunet). Anteroposterior (*A*) and lateral (*B*) views, unsubtracted, from the same case shown in Fig. 3 show the Accunet device deployed in the left internal carotid artery (*arrows*).

resolution than MR imaging, but evaluation of stenosis can be limited by beam hardening artifact in the presence of extensive calcification. The imaging method with the highest spatial resolution is digital subtraction angiography (DSA). A certain element of randomness or variability affects measurement of percentage stenosis even with DSA, depending on which segment of the vessel is measured and which segment is defined as normal for the NASCET criteria denominator.

Percentage stenosis, the major or only criterion used in the major carotid stroke trials, may be only one of a number of important markers of future stroke risk. As our understanding of atherosclerosis improves, it is likely that more sensitive and specific markers for stroke will be identified. Acute rupture of atherosclerotic plaques, not progressive gradual reduction in luminal caliber, is the main cause of vascular morbidity [14]. Atherosclerosis is a complex but specific molecular and cellular response of a given arterial segment that has been characterized as a predominantly inflammatory disease [15]. In keeping with the concept of segmental identity and vulnerability, plaque appears to accumulate at stereotypical sites in the carotid; this phenomenon may be due to the molecular identity of the vessel wall in these segments, although shear stress also appears to play an important role in atherogenesis [5]. If the process continues unabated, a complex atherosclerotic plaque appears that is composed of foam cells, smooth muscle cells, lymphocytes, monocytes, and a fibrous cap. Much of what is known about plaque morphology and behavior is derived from the study of the coronary arteries and may not be completely applicable to carotid occlusive disease. In most patients with myocardial infarction, erosion with uneven thinning or rupture of the fibrous cap where macrophages enter, accumulate, and are activated precipitates the event. Apoptosis may play an important role. Stable advanced lesions usually have smooth, uniformly dense fibrous caps. However, autopsy can identify active inflammation and plaque rupture at sites of nonocclusive and angiographically occult lesions, indicating that potentially dangerous lesions escape detection with many current imaging modalities [15].

Significant efforts are under way to improve the characterization of plaque morphology using noninvasive imaging methods like MR imaging [16]. Plaque ulceration can be readily identified using current noninvasive modalities and has been shown to be related to future stroke risk. One study examining the pathology of 44 endarterectomy specimens found that symptomatic patients were much more

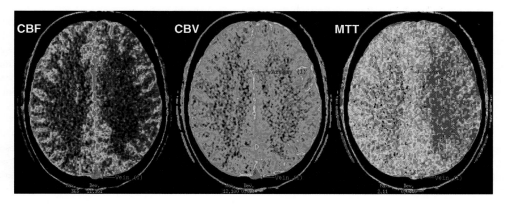

Fig. 5. CT perfusion images in a 39-year-old patient with an acute left carotid dissection. There is markedly prolonged mean transit time (MTT) and mildly elevated cerebral blood volume (CBV) in the left hemisphere. Cerebral blood flow (CBF) is mildly decreased.

likely to have plaque rupture (74%) than were asymptomatic patients (32%) for a similar degree of stenosis. Fibrous cap thinning and foam cell infiltration were also more commonly identified in the symptomatic patients [17]. In addition, in the medical treatment arm of NASCET, plaque ulceration increased the 2-year risk of ipsilateral stroke from 26.3% to 73.2% as the degree of stenosis progressed from 75% to 99% [13]. In patients without plaque ulceration, the 2-year stroke risk rate was 21.3% regardless of the degree of stenosis. One recent study found that plaque surface morphology as identified

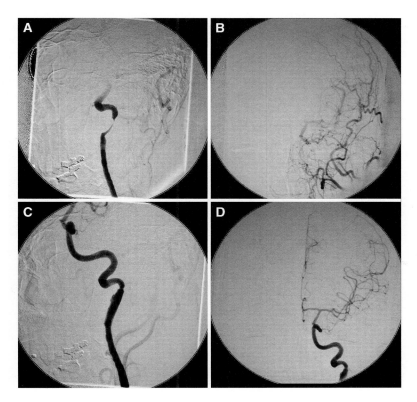

Fig. 6. Acute stenting of carotid dissection. Angiograms of same patient shown in Fig. 5 (all anteroposterior views) show the left internal carotid dissection (*A*) and paucity of intracranial flow (*B*). Excellent restoration of flow follows stent placement (*C,D*).

on carotid angiography correlated well with pathologic findings and was a highly sensitive marker for plaque instability [18]. Another study comparing microscopic plaque morphology in patients with and without stroke found that plaque ulceration and thrombosis were significantly more prevalent in symptomatic patients [19].

Hemodynamic factors

Whether a carotid stenosis will result in hemodynamic impairment (ie, a reduction in cerebral perfusion pressure) depends on the degree of narrowing but more importantly on the status of the collateral circulation, either via the circle of Willis or the presence of external-to-internal carotid anastomoses (Figs. 5 and 6). Not all patients with symptomatic carotid stenosis have hemodynamic impairment. Those who do, however, have a much higher risk of subsequent stroke [20–22]. It is likely that hemodynamic and embolic stroke mechanisms act synergistically. Hemodynamic impairment has been shown to be an independent risk factor for stroke in patients with carotid atherosclerotic disease [23]. In symptomatic patients, the presence of altered cerebral hemodynamics ipsilateral to a significant carotid stenosis would therefore provide further justification for revascularization therapy. More importantly, hemodynamic status may be an important variable to consider when evaluating asymptomatic patients with carotid

stenosis, although the prevalence of hemodynamic impairment in asymptomatic patients is low [20]. These patients form an important subgroup, however, because they are the most likely to benefit from a revascularization procedure over medical therapy. Some patients progress asymptomatically from carotid stenosis to occlusion, and many of these remain event free after their occlusion. These are patients with normal cerebral hemodynamics. This evidence suggests the existence of a small subset of patients with high-grade stenosis and minimal or no impairment of cerebral perfusion. These patients may be less likely to benefit from aggressive revascularization. However, subsequent contralateral disease places them at much higher risk, so, even in these cases, it is probably better to perform revascularization if this can be done with low risk.

This pattern may explain the lack of benefit identified in patients with near occlusion of the carotid artery, a group that previously was thought to be at extremely high risk for future stroke and was treated aggressively with urgent endarterectomy or stenting [24]. Many of these patients probably have abundant collaterals. Patients who progress to carotid occlusion without an ischemic event likely fall within this group. More studies clearly are needed to examine the relevance of baseline alterations in cerebral perfusion to future stroke risk in patients with carotid stenosis. At the authors' institution, carotid stenting is performed in a dedicated MR/x-ray imaging (XMR) suite (Fig. 7) [25]. This method

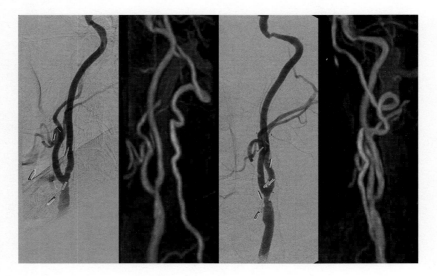

Fig. 7. Carotid revascularization in an XMR suite. Excellent correlation is seen between MR angiographic and digital subtraction angiograms.

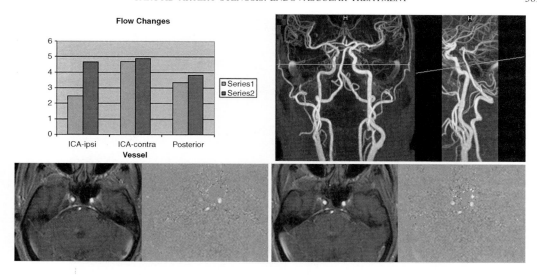

Fig. 8. Quantitative flow analysis may be performed, and data before (*bottom left*) and after (*bottom right*) stenting may be compared. ICA, intracranial hemorrhage. (*Modified from* Martin AJ, Saloner DA, Roberts TP, et al. Carotid stent delivery in an XMR suite: immediate assessment of the physiologic impact of extracranial revascularization. AJNR Am J Neuroradiol 2005;26:531–7; with permission.)

makes it possible to assess quantitative flow analysis in the treated and nontreated vessels, as well as to characterize diffusion and perfusion changes before and after revascularization (Figs. 8 and 9).

Carotid revascularization—surgery

DeBakey [26] performed the first true carotid endarterectomy in the United States on a patient with an occluded carotid artery in 1953. The procedure rapidly gained widespread acceptance, despite early reports of unacceptably high rates of perioperative stroke and death, and roughly 1 million carotid endarterectomies were performed worldwide between 1974 and 1985. Since then, a number of well-designed large randomized clinical trials have been performed, which have been well summarized elsewhere [27].

A few of the more important trials will briefly be reviewed here. The NASCET was begun in 1987, and its results were published in 1998 [13]. Conducted at 106 centers in the United States and Canada, NASCET analyzed 2885 patients with symptomatic carotid stenosis. This study found that patients with a symptomatic carotid stenosis of 70% or more benefited significantly from carotid endarterectomy over medical therapy alone, and that this benefit was durable for up to 5 years of follow-up. Surgery reduced the 2-year risk of ipsilateral stroke from 26% (medical group) to 9% (surgical

group), an absolute risk reduction of 17%. A 5.8% incidence of stroke and death (0.6%) was seen in the surgical group. When perioperative myocardial infarction is included, the complication rate increases to 6.7%. Benefit of surgery was twice as great for patients with very severe stenosis (90%–99%) compared with those with less severe stenosis (70%–79%).

Results of another large multicenter randomized trial, the European Carotid Surgery Trial (ECST), were in concordance with NASCET [28]. ECST calculated stenosis using an approximation of the normal carotid bulb diameter as the denominator rather than the distal normal diameter. Thus, in general, degree of stenosis was overestimated in ECST relative to NASCET. The authors enrolled 3024 patients with carotid stenosis who were symptomatic within 6 months. The risk of perioperative major stroke or death was reported to be 7%. The authors found a benefit for the surgical group when the stenosis was greater than 80%, with Kaplan-Meier estimate for major stroke or death equaling 26.5% at 3 years for the control group and 14.9% for the surgical group. This result was an absolute risk reduction of 11.6% at 3 years.

A significant percentage of patients with carotid stenosis are asymptomatic. These patients may present with a bruit, or an incidental carotid narrowing may be identified on noninvasive imaging performed for some other reason. The first two trials evaluating potential benefit for carotid endarterectomy in

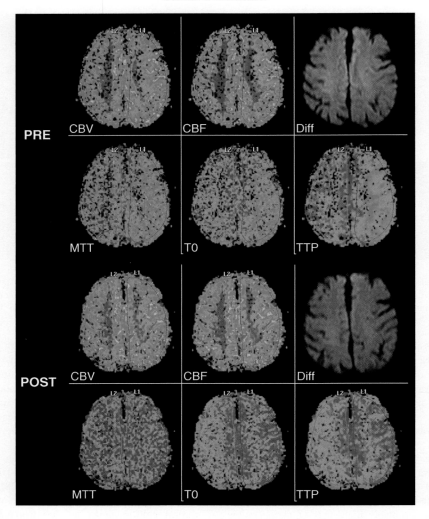

Fig. 9. Changes in MR perfusion and diffusion may be tracked before (*top*) and after (*bottom*) revascularization. CBF, cerebral blood flow; CBV, cerebral blood volume; MTT, mean transit time. (*Modified from* Martin AJ, Saloner DA, Roberts TP, et al. Carotid stent delivery in an XMR suite: immediate assessment of the physiologic impact of extracranial revascularization. AJNR Am J Neuroradiol 2005;26:531–7; with permission). Diff, diffusion; T0, contrast arrival time; TTP, time to peak.

asymptomatic patients were not conclusive. The CASANOVA trial did not demonstrate a significant difference in outcome between surgical and non-surgical arms, although the design of the trial permitted a large percentage of patients in the nonsurgical cohort ultimately to undergo endarterec-tomy [29]. The Veterans Affairs Cooperative Study also failed to show a significant difference between endarterectomy and medical therapy, although the authors speculated that a modest benefit might not have been detected because of the small sample size (444 males were enrolled with stenosis ≥50%) [30]. The Asymptomatic Carotid Atherosclerosis Study

study enrolled 1662 patients at 39 centers and had a median follow up of 2.7 years [31]. An absolute risk reduction favoring endarterectomy of 5.9% was found, with a 5-year risk of ipsilateral stroke or death with a carotid stenosis of 60% or more for 5.1% for the surgical arm and 11% for the medical arm. The 30-day perioperative stroke and death rate was very low (2.3%), with more than half of these complications attributed to diagnostic cerebral an-giography. Interestingly, no significant benefit of endarterectomy was found for females in this study, nor was there a correlation demonstrated between degree of stenosis and benefit of surgery.

In summary, a clear and statistically significant benefit appears to derive from performing endarterectomy over medical therapy on patients who are symptomatic with stenosis of 70% or greater, with less of a benefit for patients with symptomatic stenoses of 50%–69% and asymptomatic stenoses of 60% or greater. The benefit appears to be reduced for women. Periprocedural complication rates must be kept extremely low, or the benefit is negated. It should be noted that patients in many of the trials were highly selected, and outcomes can be significantly worse in a nonselected patient population [8].

Carotid revascularization—angioplasty and stenting

Endovascular treatment of carotid stenosis offers a number of inherent advantages over open surgical therapy. In most cases, the procedure can be performed under local anesthesia and conscious sedation, allowing continuous monitoring of the patient's neurologic status. No cervical incision or dissection is necessary, eliminating the risk of cranial nerve palsy, neck hematoma, and infection. Recovery time is generally shorter, with one hospital night stay routine. Although many investigators have assumed that the cost is reduced for the endovascular approach, one recent study found no significant difference in cost [32].

Reports of carotid angioplasty were first published in 1980 [33,34]. Early case series reported high technical success and low morbidity and mortality that compared favorably with ECST and NASCET [27]. Restenosis after angioplasty alone is a concern, with studies reporting rates of 0%–16% (versus 10% for carotid endarterectomy), although many patients with restenosis remain asymptomatic [27]. Other disadvantages of angioplasty alone in the treatment of carotid stenosis include the risk of dissection, elastic recoil of the artery, and distal embolization of particulate material. For these reasons, the experience with endovascular stenting combined with angioplasty in nonneuroradiologic applications has been rapidly assimilated into the endovascular approach to carotid stenosis. Stenting decreases the incidence of dissection, vessel recoil, and distal embolization, and endovascular carotid revascularization is currently most commonly performed using stents. A large number of carotid stent case series and registries have been published, with mortality ranging from 0.6% to 4.5% and major stroke rates from 0% to 4.5% [27].

The SAPPHIRE trial is a large, recently published randomized trial directly comparing endarterectomy to stenting [2]. This study, which was industry supported, enrolled 334 patients at 29 centers in the United States and compared carotid artery stenting with the use of a protection device to endarterectomy in patients who had either a symptomatic stenosis of 50% or greater or an asymptomatic stenosis of 80% or greater. Of the 413 patients who were not randomized, all but seven underwent stenting. Randomized patients were required to have at least one comorbid condition that potentially increased the risk of surgery. These included significant cardiac or pulmonary disease, contralateral carotid occlusion, and age of at least 80 years. The surgical group did not undergo angiography and thus was not exposed to this risk. The primary end point—major cardiovascular event at 1 year (death, stroke, or myocardial infarction)—occurred in 20 patients in the stenting arm and 32 patients in the surgical arm (12.2% versus 20.1%). This was an absolute difference of 7.9% with a 95% confidence interval. Conditions for noninferiority of stenting were met and highly significant ($P = .004$); conditions for superiority showed near-statistical significance ($P = .053$) in favor of stenting. Based on these data, the authors concluded that, among patients with severe carotid artery stenosis and coexisting high-risk medical or surgical conditions, stenting is at least as good as endarterectomy. Similarly, a smaller randomized trial in a community hospital that enrolled 85 patients, randomized them to endarterectomy or stenting, and followed them for 4 years found the techniques to be roughly equivalent in efficacy and to have similar rates of complications [35].

A number of other trials are under way, comparing carotid stenting and endarterectomy. One of the larger trials, CREST, will compare endarterectomy and stenting in both symptomatic and asymptomatic patients at 80 centers in North America. The study has a planned enrollment of 2500 patients.

The CAVATAS trial randomized over 500 patients with carotid stenosis to surgery or endovascular therapy and found no difference in the major risks or benefits of carotid angioplasty or stenting versus surgery, although confidence intervals were wide [3]. Minor complications were less commonly seen with the endovascular approach. Major outcome events at 30 days (disabling stroke or death) were high in both groups: 6.4% and 5.9% for endovascular stenting and surgery, respectively. The endovascular techniques were early in their development, with only 26% of patients receiving stents and the remainder treated with angioplasty alone. This factor probably explains the high rate of recurrent stenosis seen (10.5%) [36]. The International Carotid Stenting Study, also known as "CAVATAS-2," is a prospective randomized trial under way at 27 centers in Canada, Europe, and Australia that has enrolled over 400 patients and will compare carotid stenting to endarterectomy in symptomatic patients suitable for either treatment. A number of other trials and device-related registries of carotid stenting are in progress, including the Boston Scientific EPI-A Carotid Stenting Trial for High Risk Surgical Patients (BEACH) and the Carotid Artery Revascularization Using the Boston Scientific FilterWire and the EndoTex NexStent (CABERNET) trials. A listing of relevant carotid stents and stroke-related trials is available at www.stroketrials.org.

Carotid stenting: technique

Patients are routinely placed on double antiplatelet therapy, beginning at least 3 days before the procedure. A standard regimen includes aspirin 325 mg/d and a secondary platelet inhibitor, such as clopidogrel 75 mg/d. In most cases, the procedure can be performed with minimal sedation. In some patients, only local anesthesia is used for femoral artery puncture. An external cardiac pacer is placed, and intravenous atropine (0.5 mg) or glycopyrolate (0.2–0.4 mg) is on hand for the uncommon occurrence of bradycardia during angioplasty near the carotid sinus. A complete diagnostic angiogram is performed, including imaging of the origin of the vertebral arteries and intracranial circulation to identify other potentially significant atherosclerotic lesions.

A Simmons-type catheter is often used to decrease the chances of inadvertently crossing a significant stenosis with a guidewire. The optimal working projection is reached for the carotid lesion. (This is often an ipsilateral oblique projection with some cranial or caudal angulation, to avoid the external branches or metallic dental work.) Measurements are made, estimating percentage stenosis according to NASCET methods. Once the decision is made to proceed with the stenting, the patient is given heparin, with a target activated clotting time of between 250 and 300 seconds. This measure is accomplished with a weight-based bolus, and the patient is then placed on a continuous heparin infusion. A suture groin closure device is used before sizing up the groin sheath. An 8F guiding catheter or a 6F guide sheath is placed in the distal common carotid artery. If the lesion is severely narrowed, predilatation may be performed. If a distal embolic protection device is to be used, this is

navigated distal to the stenosis and deployed. A small noncompliant balloon is then placed across the lesion. This balloon is gently inflated until the waist of the lesion disappears. There is no need aggressively to predilate the lesion. The appropriately sized stent for the lesion diameter and length is chosen, then placed across the stenosis. An angiogram may be performed to confirm adequate stent placement, because the configuration of the vessel, and thus the location of the stenosis relative to other landmarks, may have changed after introduction of the stent introducer system. The stent is then deployed and the introducer device withdrawn, leaving the protection device in place.

If the poststenting angiogram shows significant residual stenosis, a poststent angioplasty may be performed. The balloon is sized to the normal vessel diameter. It is generally believed that this maneuver, poststent angioplasty, is the most likely to dislodge embolic particles, which may be sheared off the vessel wall against the stent. After the poststent angiogram of the treated vessel, a biplane angiogram of the intracranial circulation should always be performed, looking for branch occlusions. The sheath is then removed and suture-closure of the arteriotomy completed. The authors typically allow the heparin to wear off without reversal with protamine. Care is taken not to let the patient become hypertensive in the immediate postprocedure period, to ward against hyperperfusion syndrome. Preprocedure assessment of hypoperfusion is helpful in this context. The patient is admitted overnight to a neurointensive care unit and may be transferred to a step-down floor the following day, with home discharge routine on the second day post-procedure. Aspirin 325 mg/d is continued indefinitely, and clopidogrel 75 mg/d is taken for at least 6 weeks, when a follow-up ultrasound is typically performed to ensure stent patency. Angiographic follow-up on asymptomatic patients is not routinely needed.

Table 1
Adverse events of endovascular versus surgical revascularization of carotid artery stenosis

Adverse events	Endovascular	Surgery	P value
CAVATAS (at 30 d)	N = 251	N = 253	
Death	3%	4%	NS
Stroke	7%	8%	NS
Myocardial infarction	0%	1%	NS
SAPPHIRE (at 1 y)	N = 167	N = 167	
Death	7.4%	13.5%	0.08
Stroke	6.2%	7.9%	0.60
Myocardial infarction	5%	12%	0.07

Box 1. Eligibility criteria of SAPPHIRE trial comparing carotid angioplasty and stenting to carotid endarterectomy in high-risk patients

General inclusion criteria

- Unilateral or bilateral atherosclerotic or restenosed lesions in native carotid arteries
- Symptoms, plus stenosis of more than 50%
- No symptoms, plus stenosis of more than 80%

Criteria for high risk (at least one required)

- Clinically significant cardiac disease
- Severe pulmonary disease
- Contralateral carotid occlusion
- Contralateral laryngeal-nerve palsy
- Previous radical neck surgery or radiation therapy to the neck
- Recurrent stenosis after endarterectomy
- Age >80 y

Data from Yadav JS, Wholey MH, Kuntz RE, et al. Protected carotid-artery stenting versus endarterectomy in high-risk patients. N Engl J Med 2004;351: 1493–501.

Training, competency, and standards

Formal training in performing carotid angiography and carotid angioplasty and stenting has until recently been a component of few fellowship programs in the United States. Because carotid angioplasty and stenting carries the risk of significant complication, including stroke, concern about standardization of operator training has been expressed [1]. It is currently recommended that operators (1) have a minimum of 6 months of formal cognitive neuroscience training in an Accreditation Council for Graduate Medical Education–approved program in neuroradiology, neurosurgery, neurology, or vascular neurology, (2) have performed a minimum of 100 diagnostic cerebral/carotid angiograms before postgraduate training in carotid stenting procedures, and (3) have performed either 25 noncarotid stenting procedures plus a hands-on course plus four super-

vised carotid stenting procedures or 10 supervised carotid stenting procedures. Although these recommendations have met with criticism from some practitioners, they are significantly less stringent than those adopted by the American College of Cardiology regarding the performance of coronary interventions [1].

Reimbursement

In March 2005, the Centers for Medicare and Medicaid Services (CMS) clarified the National Coverage Policy for Carotid Stenting. CMS will cover patients at high risk for carotid endarterectomy who have symptomatic carotid artery stenosis of at least 70%. Coverage is available for high-risk symptomatic patients with a stenosis of 50% to 70% and for high-risk asymptomatic patients with a stenosis of 80% or greater who are participating in a clinical trial. Coverage is limited to procedures performed using FDA-approved carotid artery stenting systems and embolic protection devices.

Summary

An expanding range of treatment options is now available for patients with carotid artery occlusive disease, including endovascular angioplasty and

Box 2. Reimbursement criteria for carotid angioplasty and stenting for Centers for Medicare and Medicaid Services

1. Patients at high risk for endarterectomy with symptomatic carotid artery stenosis >70%
2. Patients at high risk for endarterectomy with symptomatic carotid artery stenosis of between 50% and 70%, as part of an approved clinical trial
3. Patients at high risk for endarterectomy with asymptomatic carotid artery stenosis >80%, as part of an approved clinical trial
4. Must be performed using FDA-approved carotid artery stenting systems and embolic protection devices
5. Must be performed at approved medical centers

> **Box 3. Definition of high risk for endarterectomy according to Centers for Medicare and Medicaid Services**
>
> - Congestive heart failure class III/IV
> - Left ventricular ejection fraction < 30%
> - Unstable angina
> - Contralateral carotid occlusion
> - Recent myocardial infarction
> - Previous carotid endarterectomy with recurrent stenosis
> - Prior radiation treatment to the neck

stenting. Treatment decisions will continue to rely on the best assessment of future risk of stroke weighed against the risk of therapy. In the future, advanced neuroimaging techniques will be used to refine this risk assessment, which until now has chiefly been made by measuring percentage stenosis and determining whether the patient is symptomatic. Plaque morphology, presence of ulceration, and extent and severity of hemodynamic compromise will likely become additional important factors that can revise risk estimates (Table 1 and Box 1).

Large, well-designed randomized prospective trials have shown that carotid endarterectomy provides a significant and durable benefit to selected patients with significant carotid narrowing. Many trials are currently under way comparing endovascular stenting and surgery. Two recently published trials suggest that endovascular stenting is at least as good as carotid endarterectomy in terms of safety and efficacy. In the future, carotid stenting may become the standard procedure for patients with significant carotid occlusive disease and a high estimated risk of future stroke (Boxes 2 and 3).

References

[1] Sacks D, Connors III JJ. Carotid stent placement, stroke prevention, and training. Radiology 2005;234: 49–52.

[2] Yadav JS, Wholey MH, Kuntz RE, et al. Protected carotid-artery stenting versus endarterectomy in high-risk patients. N Engl J Med 2004;351:1493–501.

[3] CAVATAS Investigators. Endovascular versus surgical treatment in patients with carotid stenosis in the Carotid and Vertebral Artery Transluminal Angioplasty study (CAVATAS): a randomized trial. Lancet 2001; 357:1729–37.

[4] Dyken M. Stroke risk factors in prevention of stroke. In: Norris JW, Hachinski VC, editors. Prevention of stroke. New York: Springer-Verlag; 1991. p. 83–102.

[5] Berenstein A, Lasjaunias P, Ter Brugge KG. Occlusive vascular disease. In: Surgical neuroangiography 2.1: clinical and endovascular treatment aspects in adults. 2nd edition. Berlin: Springer Verlag; 2004. p. 3–117.

[6] Inzitari D, Eliasziw M, Gates P, et al. The causes and risk of stroke in patients with asymptomatic internal-carotid-artery stenosis. N Engl J Med 2000;342: 1693–700.

[7] Rothwell PM, Mehta Z, Howard SC, et al. From subgroups to individuals: general priniciples and the example of carotid endarterectomy. Lancet 2005;365: 256–65.

[8] Wennberg DE, Lucas FL, Birkmeyer JD, et al. Variation in carotid endarterectomy mortality in the Medicare population. JAMA 1998;279:1278–81.

[9] Alamowitch S, Eliasziw M, Barnett HJ for the North American Symptomatic Carotid Endarterectomy Trial (NASCET) and the ASA and Carotid Endarterectomy (ACE) Trial Groups. The risk and benefit of endarterectomy in women with symptomatic internal carotid artery disease. Stroke 2005;36:27–31.

[10] Rothwell PM, Eliasziw M, Gutnikov SA, et al. Sex difference in the effect of time from symptoms to surgery on benefit from carotid endarterectomy for transient ischemic attack and nondisabling stroke. Stroke 2004;35:2855–61.

[11] Derdeyn CP. Catheter angiography is still necessary for the measurement of carotid stenosis. AJNR Am J Neuroradiol 2003;24:1737–8.

[12] Norris JW, Zhu CZ, Bornstein NM, et al. Vascular risks of asymptomatic carotid stenosis. Stroke 1991;22: 1485–90.

[13] Barnet HJ, Taylor DW, Eliasziw M, et al for the North American Symptomatic Carotid Endarterectomy Trial Collaborators. Benefit of carotid endarterectomy in patients with symptomatic moderate or severe stenosis. N Engl J Med 1998;339:1415–25.

[14] O'Rourke F, Dean N, Akhtar N, et al. Current and future concepts in stroke prevention. CMAJ 2004;170: 1123–33.

[15] Ross R. Atherosclerosis—an inflammatory disease. N Engl J Med 1999;340:115–26.

[16] Wasserman BA. Clinical carotid atherosclerosis. Neuroimaging Clin N Am 2002;3:403–19.

[17] Carr S, Rarb A, Pearce WH, et al. Atherosclerotic plaque rupture in symptomatic carotid artery stenosis. J Vasc Surg 1996;23:755–65.

[18] Lovett JK, Gallagher PJ, Hands LJ, et al. Histological correlates of carotid surface morphology on lumen contrast imaging. Circulation 2004;110:2190–7.

[19] Fisher M, Paganini-Hill A, Martin A, et al. Carotid plaque pathology. Thrombosis, ulceration and stroke pathogenesis. Stroke 2005;36:253–7.

[20] Powers WJ, Derdeyn CP, Fritsch SM, et al. Benign prognosis of never-symptomatic carotid occlusion. Neurology 2000;54:878–82.

[21] Derdeyn CP. Cerebral hemodynamics in carotid occlusive disease. AJNR Am J Neuroradiol 2003;24:1497–8.

[22] Grubb Jr RL, Derdeyn CP, Fritsch SM, et al. Importance of hemodynamic factors in the prognosis of symptomatic carotid occlusion. JAMA 1998;280:1055–60.

[23] Derdeyn CP, Grubb RL, Powers WJ. Cerebral hemodynamic impairment. Methods of measurement and association with stroke risk. Neurology 1999;53:251–9.

[24] Rothwell PM, Gutnikov SA, Warlow CP for the European Carotid Surgery Trialists' Collaboration. Re-analysis of the final results of the European Carotid Surgery Trial. Stroke 2003;34:514–23.

[25] Martin AJ, Saloner DA, Roberts TP, et al. Carotid stent delivery in an XMR suite: immediate assessment of the physiologic impact of extracranial revascularization. AJNR Am J Neuroradiol 2005;26:531–7.

[26] DeBakey ME. Carotid endarterectomy revisited. J Endovasc Surg 1996;3:4.

[27] Higashida RT, Meyers PM, Phatouros CC, et al for the Technology Assessment Committees of the American Society of Interventional and Therapeutic Neuroradiology and the Society of Interventional Radiology. Reporting standards for carotid artery angioplasty and stent placement. Stroke 2004;35:e112–33.

[28] European Carotid Surgery Trialists' Collaborative Group. Randomised trial of endarterectomy for recently symptomatic carotid stenosis: final results of the MRC European Carotid Surgery Trial (ECST). Lancet 1998;351:1379–87.

[29] The CASANOVA Study Group. Carotid surgery versus medical therapy in asymptomatic carotid stenosis. Stroke 1991;22:1229–35.

[30] Hobson RW, Weiss DG, Fields WS, et al. Efficacy of carotid endarterectomy for asymptomatic carotid stenosis. The Veterans Affairs Cooperative Study Group. N Engl J Med 1993;328:221–7.

[31] Executive Committee for the Asymptomatic Carotid Atherosclerosis Study. Endarterectomy for asymptomatic carotid artery stenosis. JAMA 1995;273:1421–8.

[32] Ecker RD, Brown Jr RD, Nichols DA, et al. Cost of treating high-risk symptomatic carotid artery stenosis: stent insertion and angioplasty compared with endarterectomy. J Neurosurg 2004;101:904–7.

[33] Mullan S, Duda EE, Patronas NJ. Some examples of balloon technology in neurosurgery. J Neurosurg 1980;52:321–9.

[34] Kerber CW, Cromwell LD, Loehden OL. Catheter dilatation of proximal carotid stenosis during distal bifurcation endarterectomy. AJNR Am J Neuroradiol 1980;1:348–9.

[35] Brooks WH, McClure RR, Jones MR, et al. Carotid angioplasty and stenting versus carotid endarterectomy for treatment of asymptomatic carotid stenosis: a randomized trial in a community hospital. Neurosurgery 2004;54:318–24.

[36] McCabe DJ, Pereira AC, Clifton A, et al on behalf of the CAVATAS Investigators. Restenosis after carotid angioplasty, stenting or endarterectomy in the Carotid and Vertebral Artery Transluminal Angioplasty Study (CAVATAS). Stroke 2005;36:281–6.

ELSEVIER
SAUNDERS

Neuroimag Clin N Am 15 (2005) 397 – 407

NEUROIMAGING
CLINICS OF
NORTH AMERICA

Unenhanced CT and Acute Stroke Physiology

Thomas Kucinski, MD*

Department of Neuroradiology, University Medical Center Hamburg-Eppendorf, Hamburg, Germany

The invention [1,2] and implementation [3] of CT has altered current practice in many fields of clinical medicine. Imaging intracranial pathology in the emergency setting remains the most beneficial application of CT, with acute stroke representing an important indication. CT is fast, available, and easily obtained in severely ill patients who are dependent on support and monitoring devices. In industrially developed countries, CT scanners are used in every hospital with community-based emergency service 24 hours a day, 7 days a week.

Ischemic stroke occurs most frequently in the middle cerebral artery (MCA) territory [4–6], resulting in the largest burden of mortality and permanent disability [7]. Occlusion of the MCA stem or its branches is usually caused by emboli arising from the heart or upstream atherosclerotic lesions. The most severe strokes of the anterior circulation are associated with occlusion of the internal carotid artery, particularly if the intracranial segment, including the anterior cerebral artery (ACA)-MCA bifurcation (the so called "carotid T occlusion") is involved [8,9].

The result of an arterial occlusion is a well-delineated, hypodense region on unenhanced CT corresponding to the territory of the affected vessel (Fig. 1A). Hypodensity (or reduced tissue attenuation) results from tissue water increase within the ischemic territory [10–13] and is a continuously evolving process that peaks during the first 3 to 10 days post ictus. Fig. 1B through 1D show progressive demarcation of early cerebral infarcts resulting in a clearly delineated, territorial hypodensity

(Fig. 1A). Water increase alters the volume of brain tissue, which can lead to critical edema. Other early ischemic signs (EIS) include sulcal effacement and dense vessel.

In some cases, several days to weeks after the initial ischemic insult, hypodensity is followed by near iso-density compared with the surrounding viable tissue—the so-called "fogging effect" [14]—which is caused by macrophage invasion, proliferation of capillaries, and sometimes extravasation of blood cells through damaged vessel walls. With fogging, the acute edema phase of stroke has resolved, but the tissue cavitation phase has not occurred. After weeks, a final characteristic hypodense defect is usually recognizable, consisting of glial scarring of necrotic tissue and cerebrospinal fluid cavity [15]. Hemorrhagic transformation is seldom seen within the first 24 hours but occurs in more than 40% of all territorial infarctions in the subacute stage [16,17].

Hounsfield units

CT measures physical tissue density and is dependent on the same principles of x-ray attenuation, as is plain film radiography. In contrast to plain radiography, a CT image is generated by computer algorithms reconstructing the density values (Hounsfield units [HU]) of the imaged structure from the projected photon counts at different detector angles [18]. HU are defined as $HU = 1000 \times ([u_v - u_{H2O}]/u_{H2O})$, where u_{H2O} is the linear x-ray attenuation of water, and u_v is the linear x-ray attenuation of the voxel being measured. According to this arbitrary definition, the zero point of the HU scale represents the density of pure water, and not that of air, which is approximately -1000 HU.

---

* Department of Neuroradiology, University Medical Center Hamburg-Eppendorf, Martinistrasse 52, 20246, Hamburg, Germany.

E-mail address: kucinski@uke.uni-hamburg.de

neuroimaging.theclinics.com

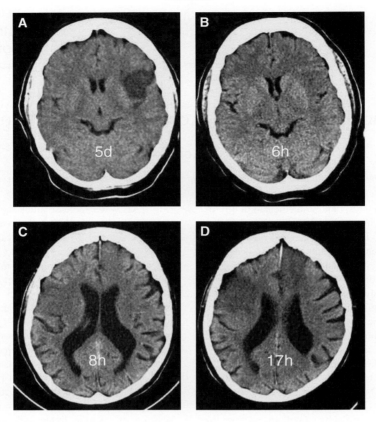

Fig. 1. Development of a clearly delineated cerebral infarction. (*A*) CT obtained 5 days after sudden onset of right-sided hemiparesis and aphasia. The hypodense lesion matches the territory of a frontal MCA branch and is well demarcated relative to the surrounding unaffected tissue. (*B*) At initial presentation 6 hours after onset, the hypodensity in this region is subtle but present. Another patient, imaged at 8 and 17 hours after onset of left hemiparesis, shows simultaneous right MCA and left ACA infarctions. The evolution of more hypodensity over time can be monitored in the sequence (*B*) to (*D*) and finally (*A*).

Because the HU scale ranges from about -1000 for air to 3000 for metal and because the human eye can discern approximately only 128 shades of gray, the roughly 10 HU density difference between gray matter (~40 HU) and white matter (~30 HU) is typically visible only with the use of narrow "window width" image display settings, with the "center level" centered between the two at 35 HU [19]. Gray matter/white matter conspicuity can be improved by increasing the image signal-to-noise ratio through raising the scan acquisition mAs (milliampere per second) setting, which provides increased photon flux and decreases quantum mottle. Although increasing tube current, and thus photon counts at the detector, is the most efficient method to decrease image noise, it exposes the patient to higher radiation, which should be accounted for in developing scan protocols, and is an increasingly important and recognized issue with the advent of faster and more powerful multi-slice CT systems [20]. For a given image acquisition, interactive adjustment of window width and center level settings has been shown to increase EIS detection for CT images reviewed on picture archiving and communicating system workstations [19].

Early hypodensity

Until the early 1990s, it was widely assumed that unenhanced CT was normal within the first 6 hours of ischemic stroke onset, despite reports on early hypodensities dating from the 1980s [21–24]. These subtle hypodense changes, referred to as "early ischemic signs" strictly within the first 6 hours after symptom onset, are increasingly recognized [25] as more acute stroke patients receive local [26,27] and systemic thrombolysis [28,29].

EIS are more easily detected if the reviewer follows a disciplined procedure for image review and is aware of typical stroke patterns. For example, with proximal MCA occlusion effecting the deep M1 region perforators, the margins of the lentiform nucleus vanish [23,24,30] due to isodensity (caused by edema) relative to the surrounding inner and outer capsule (Fig. 2A).

This phenomenon of obscuration also occurs typically in the insular cortex—the so-called "loss of insular ribbon" sign [31]. Normally, insular gray matter on either side of the Sylvian fissure lies in close proximity, and the cortex is visible as a thin but clearly hyperdense band adjacent to the external capsule (Fig. 2C). With infarction, the lobar cortical ribbon fades (Fig. 3A), accompanied by the effacement of adjacent cerebral sulci [32–34]. Rarely, swelling can occur early, without significant hypodensity, possibly due to collateral vascular supply increasing cerebral blood volume (vasodilatation),

before the occurrence of blood-brain barrier breakdown and hence the development of edema (Fig. 3C).

The prevalence of early hypodensity within the first 6 hours of acute stroke onset has been estimated to be approximately 44% but may reach 80% in certain patient populations, such as those selected by arteriographic findings or with appropriate soft copy image review using narrow "window width" and "center level settings" [19,35,36]. The application of a fixed image review strategy, such as that advocated by the Alberta Stroke Project Early CT Score (ASPECTS), can further facilitate detection of ischemic hypodensities and quantification of EIS [37–39].

Dense vessel

In the clinical setting of acute stroke, an MCA vessel segment of higher density than other parts of the same vessel, the contralateral MCA, or the basi-

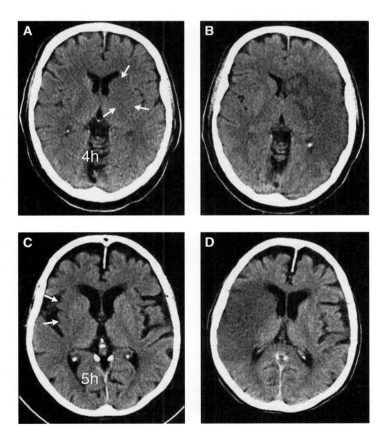

Fig. 2. EIS. Obscuration of the lentiform nucleus (*A, arrows*) and insular ribbon (*C, arrows*). In both patients, 24-hour follow-up scans show significantly larger infarctions than predicted by EIS on CT. EIS within 6 hours of symptom onset have limited gray matter conspicuity and minimal, if any, white matter conspicuity (*B* and *D*).

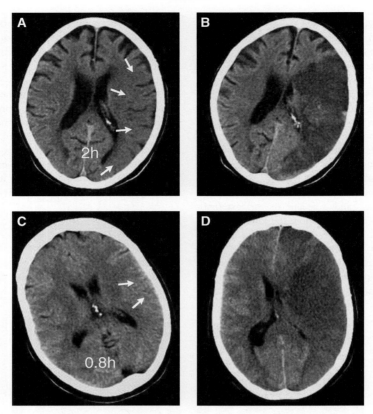

Fig. 3. Cortical hypodensity of more than one third of the MCA territory (*A*, *arrows*). Follow-up scan shows completed infarction with space occupying edema 3 days later (*B*). In cases with severe cerebral blood flow reduction, the early ischemic edema (EIE) may be more severe and the cortical EIS more pronounced (compare (*A*) with Fig. 2A and C). (*C*) A 60-year-old patient studied ultra-early after onset of hemiplegia showed only sulcal effacement (*arrows*) on CT. She had a carotid "T" occlusion (CTO) and died soon after from herniation due to space-occupying edema despite systemic thrombolysis (*D*). Cerebral blood volume increase related to dilated leptomeningeal collateral channels might contribute to early tissue volume increase.

lar artery has been designated as the hyperdense MCA sign (HMCAS) [40,41]. The higher-density results from the intravascular blood clot, which typically has HU values of 60 to 90 HU, whereas in vivo, unclotted blood (without extruded plasma) typically has soft-tissue HU values ranging from 30 to 60 HU range (Fig. 4A).

Dense vessel typically consists of "red" thrombus, a loose network of predominantly red blood cells with some fibrin, in distinction to "white" thrombus, which consists of cellular debris, fibrin, and platelets but only few red cells [42]. This feature may help to predict the likelihood of recanalization because it has been postulated that the more compact, fibrin-rich white clot may hinder thrombolysis due to its more retracted state associated with reduced clot permeability, whereas red clot permits more deep penetration of thrombolytic agents [42].

Even though HMCAS is frequently associated with a more severe clinical course [43,44], it is not an unequivocal sign of MCA occlusion, nor does it predict tissue fate, and, although it is highly specific, it is a relatively insensitive indicator of occlusive thrombus: Sensitivity has been estimated to range between 5% and 50%, depending on the population under study [33,45]. The negative predictive value of HMCAS is therefore low [46,47], and false-positive mimics caused by high hematocrit or vessel wall calcifications are not infrequent and must be differentiated from "true" HMCAS [48].

Clinical Implications of early ischemic signs

Because EIS on CT are believed to occur with irreversible ischemic change, they represent tissue

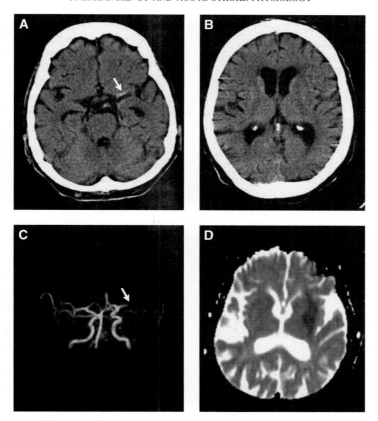

Fig. 4. HMCAS depicting acute clot in the MCA, indicating an M1 occlusion (*A*). A different patient with a corresponding occlusion confirmed by MRA (*C*) showed minimal hypodensity of the left lentiform nucleus 2 hours after symptom onset (*B*). On a subsequent ADC map (*D*), the low-signal ischemic lesion is well established.

with very high probability of final infarction. Patients who have extended EIS (hypodensity larger than one third of the MCA territory or ASPECTS ≤ 7) have a small chance of good clinical outcome after stroke [25,49–51].

CT remains an accepted imaging modality for the assessment of hemorrhagic risk after thrombolysis, based largely on the results of the ECASS trials [34,52]. It has been suggested that patients who have a greater than one third MCA territory hypodensity on admission CT should be excluded from thrombolysis due to the high risk of hemorrhage. Within 3 hours of stroke onset, however, decisions based on EIS were problematic; the earlier the patient was scanned, the more unreliable was the delectability of the EIS [35,53–55]. Under these circumstances, EIS may not be predictive of hemorrhage [55].

Thrombolysis treatment benefit declines with time post ictus, due in large part to infarct progression [29]. The ideal time window, for IV lysis especially, is a point of much controversy, although it seems

clear from the literature that less than 90 minutes is optimal. For these reasons, a more detailed understanding of the pathophysiology of acute stroke and the early ischemic edema (EIE) is desirable.

Early ischemic signs and stroke physiology

In this section, animal studies and clinical observations are integrated to provide an overview of the proposed evolution of EIE. Within minutes after cerebral artery occlusion, cerebral blood flow (CBF) drops in the downstream territory, with more severe changes in the center compared with the periphery [56,57]. The outer zones typically remain better perfused by collateral blood flow, originating from leptomeningeal anastomoses of distal arterial segments at the pial brain surface [58,59]. Theoretically, the regions of depressed CBF can be quantified to distinguish three zones: (1) a central "core" (with irreversible damage), (2) a "salvageable penumbra" with

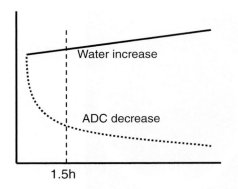

Fig. 5. Diagrammatic time course of brain tissue. Water increase (EIE) (*solid line*). Diffusion restriction (ADC decrease, *discontinuous line*) in acute stroke. (*From* Kucinski T, Vaterlein O, Glauche V, et al. Correlation of apparent diffusion coefficient and computed tomography density in acute ischemic stroke. Stroke 2002;33:1786–91; with permission.)

morphologically intact but stunned neurons (which may recover with early robust recanalization), and (3) an "oligemic penumbra" (low flow but without risk of cell death) [60]. The prognostic values of the reported thresholds for tissue fate in acute stroke, however, are routinely low due to the typically unknown time-to-recanalization and to the instability of collateral circulation.

ATP depletion in the infarct core results in cell membrane depolarization due to termination of ion-

pump function; cell swelling ("cytotoxic" edema) follows within minutes [61,62]. Simultaneously, an exponential reduction of the apparent diffusion coefficient (ADC) of water can be observed by diffusion MR imaging [63], with a rapid initial drop and a more gradual decrease after the first few hours [64–66]. Ischemic edema (net water increase) occurs with a delay of 15 to 30 minutes after stroke onset [67–69] but is typically not detectable as CT hypodensity until at least 45 minutes [8]. CT density is inversely correlated with water content [70] and thus may provide a tool to monitor EIE. In contrast to the time course of ADC, CT density declines linearly in the initial hours after stroke [65] (Fig. 5). Cell swelling (as measured by ADC decrease) and net water content (as measured by CT hypodensity) can be correlated in terms of their severity but not their time course, suggesting a certain independency [71]. However, a third common factor determining the severity of ADC reduction and the time course of EIE development is the degree of CBF reduction [72].

The metabolic impairment of Na/K-ATPase after acute vascular occlusion has been shown to correlate with an increase of net water content [73], which occurs roughly 30 minutes after the initial CBF drop [67,69]. Cell swelling is not inexorably linked to net water increase. Changes in cell volume due to extracellular to intracellular water shift are unlikely to be correlated with net water increase because the vasogenic edema attributable to disruption of the blood-

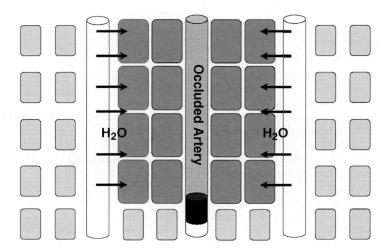

Fig. 6. Diagram of pathophysiology of the development of EIE. Cerebral blood flow is severely decreased in the ischemic core (*dark gray, swollen cells*) immediately surrounding the occluded supplying artery. Metabolic impairment due to oxygen depletion with associated energy failure results in a loss of Na/K-ATPase function, and osmotic cell swelling ensues. Narrowing of the extracellular space and changes in ion concentrations give rise to osmotic water migration through the blood-brain barrier, increasing the net water content.

brain barrier appears hours to days later [74,75]. What, then, might be a reason for the early water increase? A potential explanation involves an increase in osmolarity of the extracellular space due to shrinkage related to changes in cation concentration, which may result in passive water movement from the intravascular space (Fig. 6) into ischemic brain interstitium [76–78]. A very early increase in blood-brain barrier permeability may support this process [79,80]. EIE correlates with changes in cell volume and thus ADC [65], both of which are driven by CBF decrease [72]. As with ADC, a CBF threshold for the development of the EIE has been postulated [81], but the earliest changes in brain water content may be unobservable in humans due to the insensitivity of our current methods.

The differing time courses of the CT versus ADC signal changes after stroke contribute to the marked difference in lesion conspicuity between these techniques. Typically, in the time that it takes for ADC to drop about 20%, EIE results in only a 0.1% decrease in HU on CT. Stated another way, our results indicate a roughly 1.5 HU decrease for every 1% increase in tissue water [65]. This corresponds well with recent animal experiments [70] but is less than was initially suspected [82]. Such small changes explain the relative insensitivity of CT within the first 3 hours of stroke onset.

CT and MR imaging can be used to assess vessel status (using CTA and MRA) (Figs. 4C and 7D). DWI has a higher sensitivity for ischemia detection than does CT, especially for small lacunar or brain-

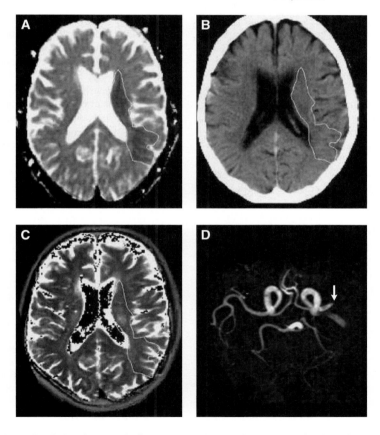

Fig. 7. T2-weighted MR signal elevation as an indicator of water increase in severely ischemic regions. A 73-year-old patient studied 2 hours (CT) (*B*) and 2.5 hours (MR imaging) (*A*, *C*) after onset of hemiparesis. MRA (*D*) shows MCA-trunk occlusion (*arrow*). ADC (*A*), CT (*B*), and quantitative T2 (*C*) data sets have been normalized into a common 3D space for direct transfer of regions of interest between the modalities. In regions corresponding to that of the ADC reduction, a decrease of only 1.2 HU was present on the CT scan, and an increase of only 5 milliseconds signal intensity units was present on the quantitative T2 maps. No conspicuous early changes on the CT or T2-weighted MR images would have been discernible without knowledge of the ADC findings, except perhaps for slightly hyperintense regions lateral to the left ventricle and at the temporal-parietal area on the T2 map.

stem infarctions [83–87]. Examples of the improved visualization of ischemic regions by ADC maps are given in Figs. 4 and 7.

EIS hypodensities on CT are typically smaller and less conspicuous than are corresponding ADC lesions [65]. This has been confirmed in an analysis by Somford and colleagues [88]. Somford and colleagues also demonstrated that more severe ADC decreases were present in regions with EIS on CT. These observations could be important because the severity of the ADC decrease, and thus that of the EIS, corresponds with more frequent hemorrhagic events after thrombolysis [89–91] and with the development of malignant MCA infarctions [92]. The concept that more severe hemorrhages are associated with hypodensities of $\geq 1/3$ the MCA territory owes much to ECASS I [34,52].

Theoretically, some of the CT hypodensity observed with very early stroke might be attributable not to edema but to marked reduction in local cerebral blood volume (CBV) in the setting of complete vascular occlusion [93]. This makes some sense because the in vivo density of blood is higher than that of normal brain tissue [94]; however, this mechanism for early hypodensity is thought to be unlikely for the following reasons: (1) CT hypodensity evolves slowly over time, rather than immediately after occlusive stroke onset. (2) CBV reduction would not account for the observed increase in quantitative T2 signal intensity, even in the setting of reduced blood flow. In severely ischemic tissue (Fig. 7), the increase in T2 relaxation time correlates strongly with the time course of the edematous CT HU changes [72,95]). (3) Our group's preliminary observations indicate that, on quantitative T2* images, the centers of even severely ischemic regions do not seem to be hemoglobin deficient.

Summary

Early ischemic edema develops only in regions with an initially severe reduction in blood flow. The presence of ischemic hypodensity on admission-unenhanced CT typically indicates irreversible infarction [25,36,96], and, in the 3 to 6 hour time range for the ECASS trials, the size of that hypodensity is an important risk factor for symptomatic hemorrhage after thrombolysis [34,52]. In NINDS patients, however, in the 0 to 3 hour range, there was a lack of prognostic significance for EIS $\geq 1/3$ the MCA territory [55]. In the angiographically controlled PROACT II study [27,50], there was no relevance of EIS for predicting symptomatic hemorrhage [97].

Regardless of their implications for forecasting clinical outcome, EIS remain the simplest, most available, and most specific indicators of definite brain infarction, and hence their recognition is important for acute stroke evaluation. Rapid, accurate quantification of EIS on unenhanced CT remains a major challenge for neuroradiologists and stroke physicians. Standardization of the "one third rule", with a more detailed checklist of suspected EIS locations as accomplished with ASPECTS [38], may help readers detect these sites of early, irreversible edema.

If clearly marginated hypodensity is present in suspected early stroke victims, the time window from onset must be carefully checked because an HU decrease of more than 4 to 6 HU may not be apparent within the first 6 hours of onset. After hemorrhage, the visualization of EIE on CT or MR imaging is the next and most important task in current acute stroke imaging. Other important variables, such as site and degree of occlusion and core/penumbra mismatch, can be accomplished with multimodal CT [98] or MR imaging [99,100]; these data may prove to be critical as the next generation of acute stroke treatments becomes available. The insights regarding acute stroke physiology provided by studying the CT evolution of early ischemic signs continue to be valuable for informed interpretation of all stroke images.

References

[1] Hounsfield GN. Computerized transverse axial scanning (tomography): 1. Description of system. Br J Radiol 1973;46:1016–22.

[2] Cormack AM. Reconstruction of densities from their projections, with applications in radiological physics. Phys Med Biol 1973;18:195–207.

[3] Ambrose JA. The usefulness of computerized transverse axial scanning in problems arising from cerebral haemorrhage, infarction or oedema. Br J Radiol 1973; 46:736.

[4] Ringelstein EB, Zeumer H, Schneider R. Contribution of computer tomography of the brain to differential typology and differential therapy of ischemic cerebral infarct. Fortschr Neurol Psychiatr 1985;53: 315–36.

[5] Lee BI, Nam HS, Heo JH, et al. Yonsei Stroke Registry: analysis of 1,000 patients with acute cerebral infarctions. Cerebrovasc Dis 2001;12:145–51.

[6] de Freitas G, Bogousslavsky J. Classification of stroke. In: Hennerici M, editor. Imaging in stroke. London, Chicago: Remedica; 2003. p. 1–17.

[7] Paciaroni M, Arnold P, Van Melle G, et al. Severe disability at hospital discharge in ischemic stroke survivors. Eur Neurol 2000;43:30–4.

[8] Kucinski T, Koch C, Grzyska U, et al. The predictive

value of early CT and angiography for fatal hemispheric swelling in acute stroke. AJNR Am J Neuroradiol 1998;19:839–46.

[9] Arnold M, Nedeltchev K, Mattle HP, et al. Intra-arterial thrombolysis in 24 consecutive patients with internal carotid artery T occlusions. J Neurol Neurosurg Psychiatry 2003;74:739–42.

[10] Alcala H, Gado M, Torack RM. The effect of size, histologic elements, and water content on the visualization of cerebral infarcts. Arch Neurol 1978; 35:1–7.

[11] O'Brien MD. Ischemic cerebral edema: a review. Stroke 1979;10:623–8.

[12] Rieth KG, Fujiwara K, Di Chiro G, et al. Serial measurements of CT attenuation and specific gravity in experimental cerebral edema. Radiology 1980;135: 343–8.

[13] Torack RM. Computed tomography and stroke edema: case report with an analysis of water in acute infarction. Comput Radiol 1982;6:35–41.

[14] Becker H, Desch H, Hacker H, et al. CT fogging effect with ischemic cerebral infarcts. Neuroradiology 1979;18:185–92.

[15] Constant P, Renou AM, Caille JM, et al. Cerebral ischemia with CT. Comput Tomogr 1977;1:235–48.

[16] Hornig CR, Bauer T, Simon C, et al. Hemorrhagic transformation in cardioembolic cerebral infarction. Stroke 1993;24:465–8.

[17] Jaillard A, Cornu C, Durieux A, et al. Hemorrhagic transformation in acute ischemic stroke: the MAST-E study. Stroke 1999;30:1326–32.

[18] Cormack AM, Doyle BJ. Algorithms for two-dimensional reconstruction. Phys Med Biol 1977; 22:994–7.

[19] Lev MH, Farkas J, Gemmete JJ, et al. Acute stroke: improved nonenhanced CT detection—benefits of soft-copy interpretation by using variable window width and center level settings. Radiology 1999;213: 150–5.

[20] Berrington de Gonzalez A, Darby S. Risk of cancer from diagnostic X-rays: estimates for the UK and 14 other countries. Lancet 2004;363:345–51.

[21] Inoue Y, Takemoto K, Miyamoto T, et al. Sequential computed tomography scans in acute cerebral infarction. Radiology 1980;135:655–62.

[22] Kuroiwa T, Seida M, Tomida S, et al. Discrepancies among CT, histological, and blood-brain barrier findings in early cerebral ischemia. J Neurosurg 1986; 65:517–24.

[23] Tomura N, Uemura K, Inugami A, et al. Early CT finding in cerebral infarction: obscuration of the lentiform nucleus. Radiology 1988;168:463–7.

[24] Bozzao L, Bastianello S, Fantozzi LM, et al. Correlation of angiographic and sequential CT findings in patients with evolving cerebral infarction. AJNR Am J Neuroradiol 1989;10:1215–22.

[25] von Kummer R, Bourquain H, Bastianello S, et al. Early prediction of irreversible brain damage after ischemic stroke at CT. Radiology 2001;219:95–100.

[26] Zeumer H, Ringelstein EB, Hassel M, et al. Local fibrinolysis therapy in subtotal stenosis of the median cerebral artery. Dtsch Med Wochenschr 1983;108: 1103–5.

[27] Furlan A, Higashida R, Wechsler L, et al. Intra-arterial prourokinase for acute ischemic stroke. The PROACT II study: a randomized controlled trial. Prolyse in acute cerebral thromboembolism. JAMA 1999;282:2003–11.

[28] The National Institute of Neurological Disorders and Stroke rt-PA Stroke Study Group. Tissue plasminogen activator for acute ischemic stroke. N Engl J Med 1995;333:1581–7.

[29] Hacke W, Donnan G, Fieschi C, et al. Association of outcome with early stroke treatment: pooled analysis of ATLANTIS, ECASS, and NINDS rt-PA stroke trials. Lancet 2004;363:768–74.

[30] Okada Y, Sadoshima S, Nakane H, et al. Early computed tomographic findings for thrombolytic therapy in patients with acute brain embolism. Stroke 1992; 23:20–3.

[31] Truwit CL, Barkovich AJ, Gean-Marton A, et al. Loss of the insular ribbon: another early CT sign of acute middle cerebral artery infarction. Radiology 1990;176:801–6.

[32] von Kummer R, Nolte PN, Schnittger H, et al. Detectability of cerebral hemisphere ischaemic infarcts by CT within 6 h of stroke. Neuroradiology 1996; 38:31–3.

[33] von Kummer R, Holle R, Grzyska U, et al. Interobserver agreement in assessing early CT signs of middle cerebral artery infarction. AJNR Am J Neuroradiol 1996;17:1743–8.

[34] von Kummer R, Allen KL, Holle R, et al. Acute stroke: usefulness of early CT findings before thrombolytic therapy. Radiology 1997;205:327–33.

[35] Roberts HC, Dillon WP, Furlan AJ, et al. Computed tomographic findings in patients undergoing intra-arterial thrombolysis for acute ischemic stroke due to middle cerebral artery occlusion: results from the PROACT II trial. Stroke 2002;33:1557–65.

[36] Kucinski T, Koch C, Eckert B, et al. Collateral circulation is an independent radiological predictor of outcome after thrombolysis in acute ischaemic stroke. Neuroradiology 2003;45:11–8.

[37] Barber PA, Demchuk AM, Zhang J, et al. Validity and reliability of a quantitative computed tomography score in predicting outcome of hyperacute stroke before thrombolytic therapy. ASPECTS Study Group. Alberta Stroke Programme Early CT Score. Lancet 2000;355:1670–4 [erratum: Lancet 2000;355:2170].

[38] Pexman JH, Barber PA, Hill MD, et al. Use of the Alberta Stroke Program Early CT Score (ASPECTS) for assessing CT scans in patients with acute stroke. AJNR Am J Neuroradiol 2001;22:1534–42.

[39] Coutts SB, Demchuk AM, Barber PA, et al. Interobserver variation of ASPECTS in real time. Stroke 2004;35:e103–5.

[40] Tomsick TA, Brott TG, Olinger CP, et al. Hyperdense

middle cerebral artery: incidence and quantitative significance. Neuroradiology 1989;31:312–5.

[41] Bastianello S, Pierallini A, Colonnese C, et al. Hyperdense middle cerebral artery CT sign: comparison with angiography in the acute phase of ischemic supratentorial infarction. Neuroradiology 1991;33:207–11.

[42] Kirchhof K, Welzel T, Mecke C, et al. Differentiation of white, mixed, and red thrombi: value of CT in estimation of the prognosis of thrombolysis phantom study. Radiology 2003;228:126–30.

[43] Tomsick T, Brott T, Barsan W, et al. Prognostic value of the hyperdense middle cerebral artery sign and stroke scale score before ultraearly thrombolytic therapy. AJNR Am J Neuroradiol 1996;17:79–85.

[44] Manelfe C, Larrue V, von Kummer R, et al. Association of hyperdense middle cerebral artery sign with clinical outcome in patients treated with tissue plasminogen activator. Stroke 1999;30:769–72.

[45] Leys D, Pruvo JP, Godefroy O, et al. Prevalence and significance of hyperdense middle cerebral artery in acute stroke. Stroke 1992;23:317–24.

[46] Tomsick T, Brott T, Barsan W, et al. Thrombus localization with emergency cerebral CT. AJNR Am J Neuroradiol 1992;13:257–63.

[47] Barber PA, Demchuk AM, Hill MD, et al. The probability of middle cerebral artery MRA flow signal abnormality with quantified CT ischaemic change: targets for future therapeutic studies. J Neurol Neurosurg Psychiatry 2004;75:1426–30.

[48] Rauch RA, Bazan CD, Larsson EM, et al. Hyperdense middle cerebral arteries identified on CT as a false sign of vascular occlusion. AJNR Am J Neuroradiol 1993;14:669–73.

[49] Hill MD, Rowley HA, Adler F, et al. Selection of acute ischemic stroke patients for intra-arterial thrombolysis with pro-urokinase by using ASPECTS. Stroke 2003;34:1925–31.

[50] Wechsler LR, Roberts R, Furlan AJ, et al. Factors influencing outcome and treatment effect in PROACT II. Stroke 2003;34:1224–9.

[51] Coutts SB, Lev MH, Eliasziw M, et al. ASPECTS on CTA source images versus unenhanced CT: added value in predicting final infarct extent and clinical outcome. Stroke 2004;35:2472–6.

[52] Hacke W, Kaste M, Fieschi C, et al. Intravenous thrombolysis with recombinant tissue plasminogen activator for acute hemispheric stroke. The European Cooperative Acute Stroke Study (ECASS). JAMA 1995;274:1017–25.

[53] Grotta JC, Chiu D, Lu M, et al. Agreement and variability in the interpretation of early CT changes in stroke patients qualifying for intravenous rtPA therapy. Stroke 1999;30:1528–33.

[54] Kalafut MA, Schriger DL, Saver JL, et al. Detection of early CT signs of >1/3 middle cerebral artery infarctions: interrater reliability and sensitivity of CT interpretation by physicians involved in acute stroke care. Stroke 2000;31:1667–71.

[55] Patel SC, Levine SR, Tilley BC, et al. Lack of clinical significance of early ischemic changes on computed tomography in acute stroke. JAMA 2001;286:2830–8.

[56] Fiehler J, Knab R, Reichenbach JR, et al. Apparent diffusion coefficient decreases and magnetic resonance imaging perfusion parameters are associated in ischemic tissue of acute stroke patients. J Cereb Blood Flow Metab 2001;21:577–84.

[57] Kucinski T, Naumann D, Knab R, et al. Tissue at risk is overestimated in perfusion-weighted imaging: MRI in acute stroke patients without vessel recanalization. AJNR Am J Neuroradiol 2005;26:815–9.

[58] Weidner W, Hanafeewmarkham CH. Intracranial collateral circulation via leptomeningeal and rete mirabile anastomoses. Neurology 1965;15:39–48.

[59] Liebeskind DS. Collateral circulation. Stroke 2003;34:2279–84.

[60] Baron JC. Perfusion thresholds in human cerebral ischemia: historical perspective and therapeutic implications. Cerebrovasc Dis 2001;11(Suppl 1):2–8.

[61] Busza AL, Allen KL, King MD, et al. Diffusion-weighted imaging studies of cerebral ischemia in gerbils: potential relevance to energy failure. Stroke 1992;23:1602–12.

[62] Hossmann KA, Fischer M, Bockhorst K, et al. NMR imaging of the apparent diffusion coefficient (ADC) for the evaluation of metabolic suppression and recovery after prolonged cerebral ischemia. J Cereb Blood Flow Metab 1994;14:723–31.

[63] Pierpaoli C, Alger JR, Righini A, et al. High temporal resolution diffusion MRI of global cerebral ischemia and reperfusion. J Cereb Blood Flow Metab 1996;16:892–905.

[64] van der Toorn A, Dijkhuizen RM, Tulleken CA, et al. Diffusion of metabolites in normal and ischemic rat brain measured by localized 1H MRS. Magn Reson Med 1996;36:914–22.

[65] Kucinski T, Vaterlein O, Glauche V, et al. Correlation of apparent diffusion coefficient and computed tomography density in acute ischemic stroke. Stroke 2002;33:1786–91.

[66] Fiehler J, Kucinski T, Knudsen K, et al. Are there time-dependent differences in diffusion and perfusion within the first 6 hours after stroke onset? Stroke 2004;35:2099–104.

[67] Kato H, Kogure K, Ohtomo H, et al. Characterization of experimental ischemic brain edema utilizing proton nuclear magnetic resonance imaging. J Cereb Blood Flow Metab 1986;6:212–21.

[68] Mellergard P, Bengtsson F, Smith ML, et al. Time course of early brain edema following reversible forebrain ischemia in rats. Stroke 1989;20:1565–70.

[69] Gerriets T, Stolz E, Walberer M, et al. Middle cerebral artery occlusion during MR-imaging: investigation of the hyperacute phase of stroke using a new in-bore occlusion model in rats. Brain Res Brain Res Protoc 2004;12:137–43.

[70] Dzialowski I, Weber J, Doerfler A, et al. Brain tissue

water uptake after middle cerebral artery occlusion assessed with CT. J Neuroimaging 2004;14:42–8.

[71] Matsuoka Y, Hossmann KA. Cortical impedance and extracellular volume changes following middle cerebral artery occlusion in cats. J Cereb Blood Flow Metab 1982;2:466–74.

[72] Kucinski T, Majumder A, Knab R, et al. Cerebral perfusion impairment correlates with the decrease of CT density in acute ischaemic stroke. Neuroradiology 2004;46:716–22.

[73] Yang GY, Chen SF, Kinouchi H, et al. Edema, cation content, and ATPase activity after middle cerebral artery occlusion in rats. Stroke 1992;23:1331–6.

[74] Gotoh O, Asano T, Koide T, et al. Ischemic brain edema following occlusion of the middle cerebral artery in the rat. I: the time courses of the brain water, sodium and potassium contents and blood-brain barrier permeability to 125I-albumin. Stroke 1985;16:101–9.

[75] Go KG. The normal and pathological physiology of brain water. Adv Tech Stand Neurosurg 1997;23: 47–142.

[76] Young W, Rappaport ZH, Chalif DJ, et al. Regional brain sodium, potassium, and water changes in the rat middle cerebral artery occlusion model of ischemia. Stroke 1987;18:751–9.

[77] Hatashita S, Hoff JT, Salamat SM. Ischemic brain edema and the osmotic gradient between blood and brain. J Cereb Blood Flow Metab 1988;8:552–9.

[78] Odland RM, Sutton RL. Hyperosmosis of cerebral injury. Neurol Res 1999;21:500–8.

[79] Sampaolo S, Nakagawa Y, Iannotti F, et al. Blood-brain barrier permeability to micromolecules and edema formation in the early phase of incomplete continuous ischemia. Acta Neuropathol (Berl) 1991; 82:107–11.

[80] Betz AL, Keep RF, Beer ME, et al. Blood-brain barrier permeability and brain concentration of sodium, potassium, and chloride during focal ischemia. J Cereb Blood Flow Metab 1994;14:29–37.

[81] Murr R, Berger S, Schurer L, et al. Relationship of cerebral blood flow disturbances with brain oedema formation. Acta Neurochir Suppl (Wien) 1993;59: 11–7.

[82] Unger E, Littlefield J, Gado M. Water content and water structure in CT and MR signal changes: possible influence in detection of early stroke. AJNR Am J Neuroradiol 1988;9:687–91.

[83] Urbach H, Flacke S, Keller E, et al. Detectability and detection rate of acute cerebral hemisphere infarcts on CT and diffusion-weighted MRI. Neuroradiology 2000;42:722–7.

[84] Lansberg MG, Albers GW, Beaulieu C, et al. Comparison of diffusion-weighted MRI and CT in acute stroke. Neurology 2000;54:1557–61.

[85] Fiebach J, Jansen O, Schellinger P, et al. Comparison of CT with diffusion-weighted MRI in patients with hyperacute stroke. Neuroradiology 2001;43:628–32.

[86] Barber PA, Darby DG, Desmond PM, et al. Identification of major ischemic change: diffusion-weighted imaging versus computed tomography. Stroke 1999; 30:2059–65.

[87] Saur D, Kucinski T, Grzyska U, et al. Sensitivity and interrater agreement of CT and diffusion-weighted MR imaging in hyperacute stroke. AJNR Am J Neuroradiol 2003;24:878–85.

[88] Somford DM, Marks MP, Thijs VN, et al. Association of early CT abnormalities, infarct size, and apparent diffusion coefficient reduction in acute ischemic stroke. AJNR Am J Neuroradiol 2004;25:933–8.

[89] Tong DC, Adami A, Moseley ME, et al. Prediction of hemorrhagic transformation following acute stroke: role of diffusion- and perfusion-weighted magnetic resonance imaging. Arch Neurol 2001;58:587–93.

[90] Oppenheim C, Samson Y, Dormont D, et al. DWI prediction of symptomatic hemorrhagic transformation in acute MCA infarct. J Neuroradiol 2002;29: 6–13.

[91] Fiehler J, Remmele C, Kucinski T, et al. Reperfusion after severe local perfusion deficit precedes hemorrhagic transformation: an MRI study in acute stroke patients. Cerebrovasc Dis 2005;19:117–24.

[92] Thomalla GJ, Kucinski T, Schoder V, et al. Prediction of malignant middle cerebral artery infarction by early perfusion- and diffusion-weighted magnetic resonance imaging. Stroke 2003;34:1892–9.

[93] Zimmerman RD. Stroke wars: episode IV CT strikes back. AJNR Am J Neuroradiol 2004;25:1304–9.

[94] Hubener KH, Schmitt WG. Computer tomographic densitometry of human blood: the effect of absorption by parenchymatous organs and effusions. ROFO Fortschr Geb Rontgenstr Nuklearmed 1979;130:185–8.

[95] Kucinski T, Vaterlein O, Fiehler J, et al. Correlation of apparent diffusion coefficient and computed tomography density in acute ischemic stroke: response. Stroke 2003;34:E17–8.

[96] von Kummer R, Meyding Lamade U, Forsting M, et al. Sensitivity and prognostic value of early CT in occlusion of the middle cerebral artery trunk. AJNR Am J Neuroradiol 1994;15:9–15 [discussion: 16–8].

[97] Kase CS, Furlan AJ, Wechsler LR, et al. Cerebral hemorrhage after intra-arterial thrombolysis for ischemic stroke: the PROACT II trial. Neurology 2001;57: 1603–10.

[98] Lev MH, Segal AZ, Farkas J, et al. Utility of perfusion-weighted CT imaging in acute middle cerebral artery stroke treated with intra-arterial thrombolysis: prediction of final infarct volume and clinical outcome. Stroke 2001;32:2021–8.

[99] Sorensen AG, Buonanno FS, Gonzalez RG, et al. Hyperacute stroke: evaluation with combined multi-section diffusion-weighted and hemodynamically weighted echo-planar MR imaging. Radiology 1996; 199:391–401.

[100] Eastwood JD, Lev MH, Wintermark M, et al. Correlation of early dynamic CT perfusion imaging with whole-brain MR diffusion and perfusion imaging in acute hemispheric stroke. AJNR Am J Neuroradiol 2003;24:1869–75.

NEUROIMAGING
CLINICS OF
NORTH AMERICA

ELSEVIER
SAUNDERS

Neuroimag Clin N Am 15 (2005) 409–419

Alberta Stroke Program Early CT Score in Acute Stroke Triage

Andrew M. Demchuk, MD, Shelagh B. Coutts, MD*

Department of Clinical Neurosciences, Foothills Medical Centre, University of Calgary, Calgary, AB, Canada

CT is currently the imaging modality of choice for evaluation of patients with acute stroke. Most acute stroke patients present to community hospitals without available MR imaging facilities [1].

CT was the only imaging tool in the pivotal National Institute of Neurological Disorders and Stroke (NINDS) Recombinant Tissue Plasminogen Activator (rt-PA) Stroke Study, which demonstrated efficacy of rt-PA for treatment of acute ischemic stroke within 3 hours of symptom onset [2]. In that trial, CT was used as a screening tool to exclude intracranial hemorrhage (ICH) before rt-PA administration. Among multiple baseline clinical factors, only early time to treatment predicted an improved outcome [3,4]. No other clinical or imaging factors were associated with a treatment-modifying effect.

The extent of early ischemic change (EIC) on the baseline CT did not influence patient eligibility in the NINDS study. Initial review of baseline CT scans in this trial was based on EIC definitions of edema and mass effect. Edema consisted of focal or diffuse regions of hypodensity that, on visual inspection, were less dense (darker) than white matter but denser (whiter) than cerebrospinal fluid (CSF). Mass effect consisted of effacement of the cerebral sulci, Sylvian fissures and/or basal cisterns, or ventricular system. A total of 5.2% of cases had evidence of such findings.

When these findings were present, there was a higher risk of symptomatic ICH, but no treatment-modifying effect was demonstrated.

Early ischemic change on unenhanced CT and the one-third middle cerebral artery rule

EIC on CT before the administration of acute stroke therapies may predict functional outcome and the risk of ICH [5–7]. The European Cooperative Acute Stroke Study (ECASS-1) [8] identified a trend toward increased mortality with rt-PA treatment for patients with EIC of one third or greater of the middle cerebral artery (MCA) territory in patients treated up to 6 hours after symptom onset. Despite no clear statistical interaction, this led to an assumption that patients should not receive thrombolysis if CT demonstrates early changes of a recent greater than one-third MCA territory infarction with features of sulcal effacement, mass effect, or edema. In fact, this study demonstrated that rt-PA was associated with an increased risk for fatal brain hemorrhage in the greater than one-third MCA territory EIC group as well as in the normal CT scan group (without EIC) [9]. The importance of the greater than one-third MCA territory rule could not be confirmed in the ECASS-2 trial, however, where no association with increased mortality was seen with rt-PA [10]. To this day, the guidelines for stroke thrombolytic therapy do not stipulate that greater than one-third MCA territory EIC involvement is a contraindication to rt-PA [11].

Despite the inconsistent data in a population predominantly 3 to 6 hours from symptom onset, the

* Corresponding author. Department of Clinical Neurosciences, Foothills Medical Center, University of Calgary, 1403 29th Street NW, Calgary, AB, Canada T2N 2T9.

E-mail address: shelagh.coutts@calgaryhealthregion.ca (S.B. Coutts).

one-third MCA territory rule did appear in the approval language and package insert for the US Food and Drug Administration (FDA) approval of rt-PA for stroke in the less than 3-hour window [12]. To address this issue, a more detailed re-review of EIC using definitions of (1) loss of gray/white matter distinction, (2) hypodensity or hypoattenuation, and (3) compression of CSF spaces was subsequently applied to the NINDS rt-PA Stroke Study scans. Using these EIC definitions in the NINDS rt-PA Stroke Study [13] resulted in a higher prevalence of EIC (31%). EIC was significantly associated with baseline National Institutes of Health Stroke Scale (NIHSS) score and time from stroke onset to baseline CT scan, but no EIC treatment interaction was demonstrated. EIC did not seem to be important for response to rt-PA therapy. When the one-third MCA rule was applied using these EIC definitions, no treatment-modifying interaction was demonstrated.

Further difficulty with the one-third MCA rule is the poor interrater reliability by multiple groups [14–16]. Methods to improve the one-third MCA rule have resulted in better reliability but have not been tested among less experienced readers [7].

Given the controversies regarding EIC definitions and importance, and the difficulties with reliability of the one-third MCA rule, we developed the Alberta Stroke Program Early CT Score (ASPECTS) [17]. This was devised to provide a simple systematic approach to assessing EIC in brain regions supplied by the MCA.

Early ischemic change on unenhanced CT and the Alberta Stroke Program Early CT Score

The ASPECTS is a scoring system that divides the MCA territory into 10 regions of interest. The ASPECTS is therefore a topographic scoring system, which applies a quantitative approach. Areas of the MCA territory are weighted based on functional importance (localization weighted) rather than extent, with equal weighting given to smaller structures, such as the internal capsule, basal ganglia, and caudate, as is given to larger structures, such as the posterior temporal (M3) and inferior frontal (M1) lobes.

As opposed to the greater than one-third MCA territory rule, physicians are not asked to estimate ischemic volumes from two-dimensional images. Rather, the ASPECTS is determined from evaluation of two standardized regions of the MCA territory: (1) the basal ganglia level, where the thalamus, basal ganglia, and caudate are visible, and (2) the supraganglionic level, which includes the corona radiata and centrum semiovale (Fig. 1). The boundary of these two levels is the caudate head. All cuts with basal ganglionic or supraganglionic structures visible are required to determine if an area is involved. If 5-mm axial cuts are used, the abnormality should be visible on at least two consecutive cuts to ensure that it is truly abnormal rather than a volume-averaging effect.

To compute the ASPECTS, a single point is subtracted from 10 for any evidence of EIC (eg, focal

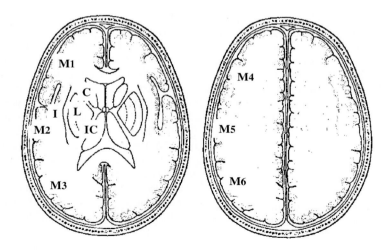

Fig. 1. The Alberta Stroke Program Early CT Score system (see text). (*From* Barber PA, Demchuk AM, Zhang J, et al for the ASPECTS Study Group. Validity and reliability of a quantitative computed tomography score in predicting outcome in hyperacute stroke before thrombolytic therapy. Lancet 2000;355:1671; with permission.)

swelling, parenchymal hypoattenuation) for each of the 10 ASPECTS-defined regions (M1–M6, I = insula, IC = internal capsule, L = lenticular, and C = caudate; see Fig. 1). A score of 10 therefore reflects the highest possible score and a normal CT scan, without evidence of EIC in the MCA territory. Conversely, a score of 0 indicates diffuse ischemic involvement throughout all 10 ASPECTS-defined regions of the MCA territory.

Parenchymal hypoattenuation is defined as abnormally decreased density of brain tissue relative to attenuation of other parts of the same structure or of the contralateral hemisphere. Focal brain swelling or mass effect is defined as any focal narrowing of the CSF space as a result of compression by adjacent structures, such as effacement of cortical sulci or ventricular compression.

Alberta Stroke Program Early CT Score and outcome prediction

Using this scoring system, we have achieved good agreement among CT observers ($\kappa = 0.71 - 0.89$ when the affected hemisphere was known). By systematically quantifying early CT findings with the ASPECTS, we were able to predict functional out-

come and the risk of symptomatic hemorrhage in rt-PA–treated stroke patients [17]. Improved EIC detection was demonstrated in this study compared with the one-third MCA territory rule.

This relation to functional outcome has been subsequently confirmed in the Canadian Activase for Strokes Effectiveness Study of rt-PA treated patients in a Canadian rt-PA registry. The ASPECTS was a strong predictor of outcome in rt-PA–treated patients, with lower scores implying a lower probability of an independent functional outcome (odds ratio [OR] = 0.81 and 95% confidence interval [CI]: 0.75–0.87, per 1-point decrement in the ASPECTS; Fig. 2) [18].

Detailed methodology of the ASPECTS has subsequently been published, which clarifies how each region is scored and highlights differences and challenges in interpretation among ASPECTS readers [19]. When assessed in real-time clinical practice, ASPECTS values correlate closely with expert interpretation [20]. EIC on noncontrast CT (NCCT) with the ASPECTS also correlates well with diffusion-weighted imaging (DWI) abnormalities and DWI ASPECTS values [21]. With training, a systematic approach, and careful scrutiny, the information available with a CT scan can sometimes be as clinically valuable as that obtained from a MR-DWI imaging scan.

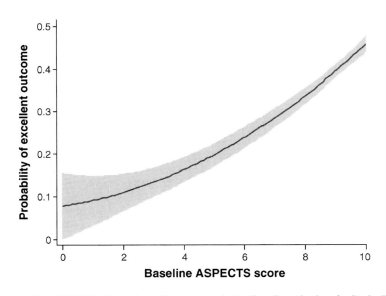

Fig. 2. Relation between the ASPECTS value and excellent outcome in the Canadian Alteplase for Stroke Effectiveness Study (see text). (*From* Hill MD, Buchan AM for the Canadian Alteplase for Stroke Effectiveness Study (CASES) Investigators. Thrombolysis for acute ischemic stroke: results of the Canadian Alteplase for Stroke Effectiveness Study. Can Med Assoc J 2005;172:1309; with permission.)

The ASPECTS represents the first system for EIC detection that may be clinically useful for treatment decision making. When the Prourokinase Acute Cerebral Infarct Trial–II (PROACT-II) scans were re-evaluated for EIC using the ASPECTS, a clear treatment interaction was identified. PROACT-II patients represented a fairly homogeneous cohort of patients with proximal MCA occlusion. Half received intra-arterial therapy a mean of 5.3 hours after symptom onset. Specifically, this reanalysis demonstrated that patients treated with intra-arterial pro-urokinase did better than controls only when they had a baseline ASPECTS greater than 7. The magnitude of the benefit for these patients was large, with a number needed to treat (NNT) of 3 to yield functional independence at 90 days, compared with an NNT of 16 to 100 when patients were treated with pro-urokinase and had evidence of significant EIC (ASPECTS $\leq$ 7) [22]. We think that this finding of a treatment effect in a predominant 3- to 6-hour time window is important because it sheds light onto what an ideal target population for intra-arterial therapy would be in the greater than 3-hour time window for patients with MCA occlusion.

To determine if this treatment interaction existed within 3 hours of symptom onset, we also revisited the NINDS rt-PA Stroke Study baseline CT scans using the ASPECTS. Readers were blinded to treatment assignment as well as to outcomes, with only information regarding symptom laterality and the suspicion for acute ischemic stroke. When the ASPECTS was applied, a significant improvement in the detection of EIC (57%) was noted. Higher ASPECTS values (ASPECTS > 7) were associated with a greater magnitude of benefit from rt-PA (NNT = 5) and a trend toward reduced mortality.

The surprise in the study was that significantly abnormal CT scans (ASPECTS = 3 – 7) still benefited from rt-PA (NNT = 8). Overall, the ASPECTS did not distinguish patients who should or should not receive thrombolytic agents. The only group in which rt-PA did not demonstrate a benefit or survival advantage was the ASPECTS less than 3 group, with extensive EIC in the MCA territory. This, however, represented a small proportion of the patients in the trial (<3%), which limited statistical interpretation [23].

The main difference between the PROACT-II and NINDS rt-PA Stroke Study was the preselection of MCA occlusions in PROACT-II, which ensures the presence of perfusion abnormalities and tissue penumbra in most patients [24].

We have previously shown that an ASPECTS of 10 is only associated with anterior circulation occlusion in 15% of cases; hence, patients with normal CT scans may not be ideal targets for thrombolysis in the absence of intracranial occlusion (no penumbra). In contrast, an ASPECTS of 5 or less was associated with intracranial occlusion 100% of the time [25].

We suspect that the robust effect of rt-PA in the "good" CT scan group would be amplified if a target thrombus was seen, and brain at risk was thus identified (expected with MCA occlusion). In the PROACT-II, all high ASPECTS patients (small regions of baseline infarction) had such MCA occlusions (large penumbras), thus explaining the robust effect of intra-arterial pro-urokinase at a high ASPECTS.

In addition, the importance of EIC may increase over time, with such changes more likely to represent irreversible injury. PROACT-II patients were treated much later than NINDS rt-PA Stroke Study patients, and, in fact, half of the NINDS rt-PA Stroke Study patients were treated "ultraearly," within 90 minutes of symptom onset [24]. It is likely that CT ischemic change may be more relevant for thrombolytic decision making in the 3- to 6-hour time window, as demonstrated by the PROACT-II and ECASS-1 results. EIC may be a less critical factor, which is overwhelmed by the importance of time after ictus in the early and ultra-early patient groups [3,26].

The relative importance of the individual characteristics of EIC (sulcal effacement, parenchymal hypoattenuation, and distortion of gray-white differentiation) has also been cast in doubt. The frequently seen subtle signs of ischemia on CT scans may not always represent irreversible injury [27]. Regions of ischemic brain showing severe hypoattenuation (attenuation lower than normal white matter) as a manifestation of tissue edema are likely irreversibly damaged; however, the reversibility—or even the physiologic significance—of subtle hypoattenuation is not unequivocally proven [12].

Alternatively, EIC manifesting as cortical sulcal effacement because of hypoperfusion on baseline CT may frequently be reversible. Recent work has suggested that sulcal effacement without hypodensity is attributable to increased cerebral blood volume (CBV) and reperfused areas of the brain. These areas have not consistently resulted in infarction on follow-up imaging [28,29]. Modification of ASPECTS methodology may be required to disregard the potentially reversible EIC finding of sulcal effacement.

Although a low admission ASPECTS is strongly correlated with a poor outcome, poor outcomes also occur in many patients despite a high admission ASPECTS. In some cases, this may be because the ASPECTS does not address ischemic change in other vascular territories in which a strategically placed infarct can leave a major disability, such as the anterior cerebral artery, posterior cerebral artery, or vertebrobasilar territories. Alternatively, the CT ASPECTS does not fully reflect potential progression of an ischemic penumbra. Newer contrast-enhanced CT techniques, such as blood-pool analysis from CT angiography (CTA) source images (SIs) [30,31] or CT perfusion studies [32–34], are now available using multislice CT scanners. These more accurately detect the "core" and "penumbra" than does conventional CT, and hence provide better delineation of infarcted and salvageable brain tissue, respectively.

Advanced imaging and the Alberta Stroke Program Early CT Score

Perfused blood volume measurements (blood pool) [35], which can be obtained from the source data of the CT angiogram, correlate significantly with final infarct volume and clinical outcome. This technique identifies areas of brain with reduced amounts of contrast enhancement, which is equivalent to low CBV within a collapsed vascular bed, thereby delineating areas of brain tissue destined to infarct.

Schramm and colleagues [36] found that the combination of CT, CTA, and CTA-SI was comparable to that of MR-DWI in identifying ischemic regions likely to infarct. CTA-SI is useful in predicting final infarct volume [37,38]. Brain tissue with a low CBV appears as a region without enhancement on CTA-SI, effectively delineating regions of severe ischemia. Using a follow-up ASPECTS as a surrogate for final infarct size, the CTA-SI ASPECTS provided a more accurate estimate of tissue destined for infarction than did the NCCT ASPECTS alone [39].

The value of combined CT, CTA, and CTA-SI over NCCT in predicting clinical outcome has also been demonstrated using a scale that differs from the ASPECTS [40]. It is important to recognize that low attenuation on NCCT and low blood pool on CTA-SI likely imply different pathophysiologic processes, which might in part be complementary, as discussed in the article by Kucinski elsewhere in this issue. Specifically, a CTA-SI region showing lack of enhancement provides an estimate of reduced blood volume, whereas NCCT measures shift in brain tissue water. It is the net uptake of water into brain regions with a CBF less than 12 mL per 100 g/min [41,42] that causes hypoattenuation.

Large shifts of water are needed for the human eye to visualize hypoattenuation. Animal studies have shown that a 1% increase in brain water content results in a radiographic attenuation decrease of 2 to 3 Hounsfield units (HU) [43,44]. We have found this concept to be especially useful in patients who present early into their events and may not yet have readily detectable changes on their admission CT scans. The clinical implications of early hypodensity, however, are not yet established [45,46].

Additional information available from CT may have an impact on the clinical utility of the ASPECTS with NCCT and CTA-SI. The hyperdense MCA sign reflects an M1 MCA occlusion [47] and predicts poor outcome with systemic thrombolysis [48]. This sign may suggest a large clot burden in the MCA, with poor or no residual flow, rendering systemic (intravenous) thrombolysis therapies largely ineffective. An intra-arterial lysis approach in these patients may lead to a better outcome [49].

Similarly, the MCA dot sign [50], hyperdensity of multiple small arteries in the Sylvian fissure (seen as dots), reflects occlusion of distal M2 or M3 MCA branches [51]. The dot sign, present in 16% of thrombolysis-treated patients, has not been demonstrated to have a treatment-modifying effect to date.

Dense artery signs in other major cerebral arteries, including the internal carotid, vertebral, and basilar arteries, have been documented [52] and shown to predict poor clinical outcome [53], although this is likely to be a considerably weaker effect than is present with the MCA hyperdense sign (Michael H. Lev, MD, unpublished data from the "STOPStroke" Trial, 2005). Calcification and high hematocrit can lead to overinterpretation [54] of hyperdense artery signs; however, when detected accurately, they are highly specific (but relatively insensitive) surrogates of vascular occlusion, which is the optimal target for thrombolytic intervention, as discussed below.

CTA can be used to characterize the presence and level of vascular thrombosis more accurately [55]. The sensitivity and specificity of CTA are excellent for diagnosing large vessel occlusion [56]. Identification of a major vascular occlusion in the setting of a CT scan with minimal EIC represents a likely target for reperfusion strategies, as demonstrated in the PROACT-II ASPECTS analysis (and as noted repeatedly in the article by Xavier and Farkas in this issue). CTA may also help to decide whether a combined intravenous rt-PA and intra-arterial intervention is warranted, by confirming a proximal or persistent arterial occlusion after rt-PA treatment. CTA might also be useful in coma evaluation by quickly ruling out basilar occlusion [57] as well as for rapid eval-

A

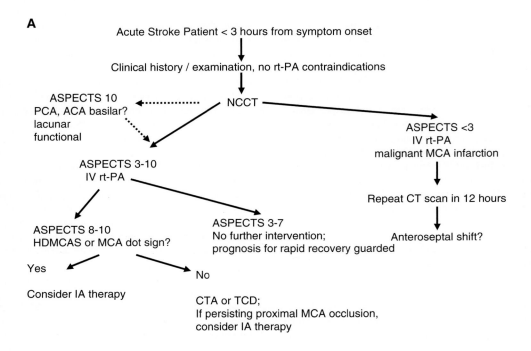

B

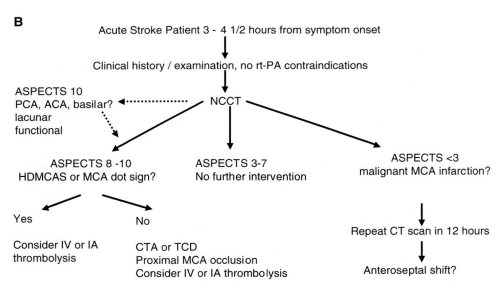

Fig. 3. (*A*) Algorithm for CT imaging less than 3 hours from symptom onset in acute stroke treatment. (*B*) Algorithm for CT imaging 3 to 4.5 hours from symptom onset in acute stroke treatment. (*C*) Algorithm for CT imaging 4.5 to 6 hours from symptom onset in acute stroke treatment. (*D*) Algorithm for CT imaging more than 6 hours from symptom onset in acute stroke treatment. ACA, anterior cerebral artery; ASPECTS, Alberta Stroke Program Early CT Score; CTA, CT angiography; HDMCAS, hyperdense middle cerebral artery sign; IA, intra-arterial; IV, intravenous; MCA, middle cerebral artery; NCCT, noncontrast CT; PCA, posterior cerebral artery; rt-PA, recombinant tissue plasminogen activator; TCD, transcranial Doppler.

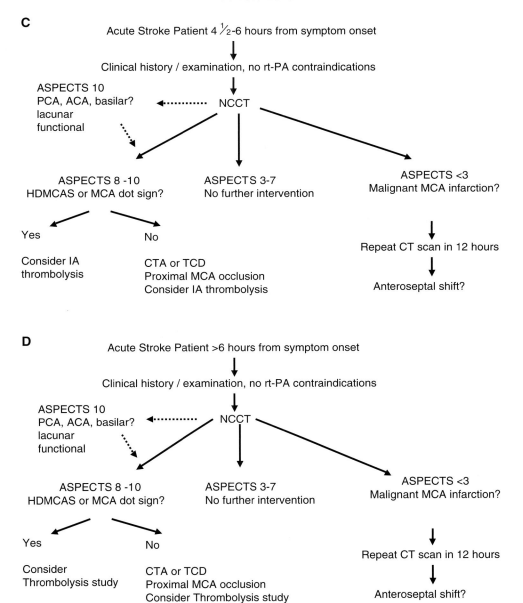

Fig. 3 (*continued*).

uation of extracranial carotid disease [58] when it is deemed necessary to obtain this information in the acute setting, especially given the added benefits of early revascularization [59].

The future is quite bright for NCCT and CT bolus techniques. MR imaging may be technologically superior but, for now, is limited by scanner availability and patient contraindications (eg, agitation,

metal, claustrophobia, weight >280 lb, extensive monitoring devices). Rapid evaluation of the hyperacute stroke patient seems adequate for most triage decisions with CT-based techniques alone, particularly when time is of the essence. The role of CT and CT bolus techniques at later time windows is debatable and must be compared with MR imaging techniques.

Practical clinical utility of the Alberta Stroke Program Early CT Score

The less-than-3-hour patient

We use the ASPECTS as a prognostic tool less than 3 hours from stroke onset (Fig. 3A). If ASPECTS values are low, we anticipate a lack of major clinical recovery or response from thrombolysis, even with successful recanalization, and council families accordingly. The ASPECTS is an independent predictor of clinical outcome [19].

We do not, however, exclude patients from intravenous rt-PA therapy based on the extent of EIC, unless it involves the entire MCA territory (ASPECTS < 3). A low ASPECTS may portend subsequent clinical deterioration in the form of malignant MCA infarction. Indeed, we have previously published that extensive EIC in the MCA territory predicts malignant MCA infarction [60] and that a repeat CT scan within 12 hours is warranted. A moderate to low ASPECTS can still factor in other decision making, especially when considering novel therapies beyond intravenous rt-PA.

We currently do not advocate an additional intra-arterial rescue approach if EIC is extensive (ASPECTS < 5). Patients with a good admission CT scan (high ASPECTS), however, are typically excellent candidates for aggressive measures to achieve recanalization, which might include a combined intravenous and intra-arterial approach (see the discussion on the "bridging trial" in the article by Xavier and Farkas in this issue).

We do, however, advocate additional vascular imaging with transcranial Doppler (TCD) [61] or CTA in such patients, especially if of a young age, to confirm a proximal vascular occlusion (M1, M2, or internal carotid artery), unless a clear hyperdense MCA sign or MCA dot sign is present. Either technique can also be used during intravenous rt-PA infusion to determine if proximal intracranial occlusion persists.

The 3- to 6-hour patient

The ASPECTS is likely a more valuable semi-quantitative score beyond the first 3 hours after symptom onset (Fig. 3B and C). Treatment with intravenous rt-PA normally has a limited but statistically significant benefit in the 180- to 270-minute time window. The NNT that results in 1 additional patient achieving clinical recovery to independence with intravenous rt-PA is as high as 20 in this group [26]. The challenge is to identify which patient represents that 1 in 20.

Based on our PROACT-II ASPECTS evaluation, we hypothesize that patients with a high ASPECTS in the setting of an MCA occlusion seem to be the ideal candidates for intervention. Specifically, for this highly selected target population, we advocate intravenous rt-PA in the 180- to 270-minute time window, based on pooled analysis of the available data, and an intra-arterial lysis strategy in the 270- to 360-minute time window, based on the PROACT-II data. We require emergency CTA to confirm MCA occlusion in all such patients with a high ASPECTS, unless an unequivocal hyperdense MCA sign is present on unenhanced CT. Clinical trials in development are targeting this group to confirm that it represents an appropriate target population.

The more-than-6-hour patient

The ASPECTS might also be useful in the more-than-6-hour time window Fig. 3D) as well as in patients with so-called "wake-up" strokes [62,63]. A subgroup of such patients is likely to have a salvageable penumbra, which can be spared infarction if recanalization can be achieved, as demonstrated in the Desmoteplase in Acute Ischemic Stroke (DIAS) Trial, a phase II MR imaging–based 9-hour window acute stroke thrombolysis trial (discussed at length in the article by Rowley in the next issue of *Neuroimaging Clinics of North America*). Despite this 9-hour delay in treatment, successful recanalization was associated with a good outcome in a highly selected population with MR diffusion- perfusion mismatch [64].

We hypothesize that those patients with a high admission ASPECTS and MCA occlusions represent a similar subgroup likely to benefit from delayed thrombolysis. Indeed, a pilot clinical trial is currently underway to evaluate the safety of intravenous rt-PA in wake-up stroke patients with (1) good admission CT scans (high ASPECTS), (2) poor admission clinical examination findings (ie, large "imaging/clinical mismatch"), and (3) CTA-proven MCA occlusion (Michael Hill, MD, personal communication, 2005). Comparison studies are needed to assess if this "clinical" penumbra prediction correlates with other penumbral predictors, such as MR-DWI/perfusion-weighted imaging mismatch [65,66] or CT CBV/cerebral blood flow mismatch [67,68].

Summary

In the setting of acute stroke evaluation, CT is a workhorse—it is accessible, versatile, available, inexpensive, and, most importantly, fast. Its use extends beyond that of identifying ICH. We have emphasized the importance of clinical assessment, supported by a systematic approach to unenhanced CT interpretation using the ASPECTS for determining the extent of EIC. The use of CT bolus techniques (providing vascular CTA, CTA-SIs, and quantitative CT perfusion maps) can augment the clinical information obtained from unenhanced CT. CT is likely to remain the workhorse of acute stroke imaging for some time to come.

References

[1] Handschu R, Garling A, Heuschmann PU, et al. Acute stroke management in the local general hospital. Stroke 2001;32:866–70.

[2] National Institute of Neurological Disorders and Stroke rt-PA Stroke Study Group. Tissue plasminogen activator for acute ischemic stroke. N Engl J Med 1995;333: 1581–7.

[3] Marler JR, Tilley BC, Lu M, et al. Early stroke treatment associated with better outcome: the NINDS rt-PA Stroke Study. Neurology 2000;55:1649–55.

[4] NINDS tPA Stroke Study Group. Generalized efficacy of tPA for acute stroke: subgroup analysis of the NINDS tPA Stroke Trial. Stroke 1997;28:2119–25.

[5] Hacke W, Kaste M, Fieschi C, et al for the ECASS Study Group. Intravenous thrombolysis with recombinant tissue plasminogen activator for acute hemispheric stroke: the European Cooperative Acute Stroke Study (ECASS). JAMA 1995;274:1017–25.

[6] Barber PA, Demchuk AM, Zhang J, et al for the ASPECTS study group. Validity and reliability of a quantitative computed tomography score in predicting outcome in hyperacute stroke before thrombolytic therapy. Lancet 2000;355:1670–4.

[7] Silver B, Demaerschalk B, Merino JG, et al. Improved outcomes in stroke thrombolysis with prespecified imaging criteria. Can J Neurol Sci 2001;28:113–9.

[8] Hacke W, Kaste M, Fieschi C, et al for the ECASS Study Group. Intravenous thrombolysis with recombinant tissue plasminogen activator for acute hemispheric stroke: the European Cooperative Acute Stroke Study (ECASS). JAMA 1995;274:1017–25.

[9] von Kummer R, Allen KL, Holle R, et al. Acute stroke: usefulness of early CT findings before thrombolytic therapy. Radiology 1997;205:327–33.

[10] Hacke W, Kaste M, Fieschi C, et al. Randomised double blind placebo-controlled trial of thrombolytic therapy with intravenous alteplase in acute ischaemic stroke (ECASS II). Lancet 1998;352:1245–51.

[11] Adams Jr HP, Brott TG, Furlan AJ, et al. Guidelines for thrombolytic therapy for acute stroke: a supplement to the guidelines for the management of patients with acute ischemic stroke. A statement for healthcare professionals from a Special Writing Group of the Stroke Council, American Heart Association. Circulation 1996;94:1167–74.

[12] Lyden P. Early major ischemic changes on computed tomography should not preclude use of tissue plasminogen activator. Stroke 2003;34:821–2.

[13] National Institute of Neurological Disorders and Stroke rt-PA Stroke Study Group. Tissue plasminogen activator for acute ischemic stroke. N Engl J Med 1995;333: 1581–7.

[14] Schriger D, Kalafut M, Starkman S, et al. Cranial computed tomography interpretation in acute stroke. Physicians' accuracy in determining eligibility for thrombolytic therapy. JAMA 1998;279:1293–7.

[15] Grotta JC, Chiu D, Lu M, et al. Agreement and variability in the interpretation of early CT changes in stroke patients qualifying for intravenous rtPA therapy. Stroke 1999;30:1528–33.

[16] Wardlaw JM, Dorman PJ, Lewis SC, et al. Can stroke physicians and neurologists identify signs of early cerebral infarction on CT? J Neurol Neurosurg Psychiatry 1999;67:651–3.

[17] Barber PA, Demchuk AM, Zhang J, et al for the ASPECTS Study Group. Hyperacute stroke: the validity and reliability of a novel quantitative CT score in predicting outcome prior to thrombolytic therapy. Lancet 2000;355:1670–4.

[18] Hill MD, Buchan AM for the Canadian Alteplase for Stroke Effectiveness Study (CASES) Investigators. Thrombolysis for acute ischemic stroke: results of the Canadian Alteplase for Stroke Effectiveness Study. Can Med Assoc J 2005;172:1307–12.

[19] Pexman JHW, Barber PA, Hill MD, et al. Use of the Alberta Stroke Program Early CT Score (ASPECTS) for assessing CT scans in patients with acute stroke. AJNR Am J Neuroradiol 2001;22:1534–42.

[20] Coutts SB, Demchuk AM, Barber PA, et al for the VISION Study Group. Interobserver variation of ASPECTS in real time. Stroke 2004;35(Suppl):e103–5.

[21] Barber PA, Hill MD, Eliasziw M, et al. A comparative analysis of CT with magnetic resonance diffusion weighted imaging in hyperacute stroke. J Neurol Neurosurg Psychiatry, in press.

[22] Hill MD, Rowley HA, Adler F, et al for the PROACT-II Investigators. Selection of acute ischemic stroke patients for intra-arterial thrombolysis with pro-urokinase by using ASPECTS. Stroke 2003;34:1925–31.

[23] Demchuk AM, Hill MD, Barber PA, et al. Importance of early ischemic computed tomography changes using ASPECTS in NINDS rtPA stroke study. Stroke 2005, in press.

[24] Furlan A, Higashida R, Wechsler L, et al. Intra-arterial prourokinase for acute ischemic stroke. The PROACT II study: a randomized controlled trial. Prolyse in Acute Cerebral Thromboembolism. JAMA 1999;282: 2003–11.

[25] Barber PA, Demchuk AM, Hill MD, et al. The probability of middle cerebral artery MRA flow signal abnormality with quantified CT ischaemic change:

targets for future therapeutic studies. J Neurol Neurosurg Psychiatry 2004;75:1426–30.

[26] Hacke W, Donnan G, Fieschi C, et al for the ATLANTIS Trials Investigators, ECASS Trials Investigators, and NINDS rt-PA Study Group Investigators. Association of outcome with early stroke treatment: pooled analysis of ATLANTIS, ECASS, and NINDS rt-PA stroke trials. Lancet 2004;363:768–74.

[27] Jaillard A, Hommel M, Baird AE, et al. Significance of early CT signs in acute stroke: a CT scan-diffusion MRI study. Cerebrovasc Dis 2002;13:47–56.

[28] Butcher KS, Lee SB, Parsons M, et al for the EPITHET Investigators. Increased blood volume maintains viability in tissue with isolated focal swelling on CT in acute stroke [abstract]. Stroke 2005;36:418.

[29] Na DG, Kim EY, Ryoo JW, et al. CT sign of brain swelling without concomitant parenchymal hypoattenuation: comparison with diffusion and perfusion-weighted MR imaging. Radiology 2005;235:992–8.

[30] Ezzeddine MA, Lev MH, McDonald CT, et al. CT angiography with whole brain perfused blood volume imaging: added clinical value in the assessment of acute stroke. Stroke 2002;33:959–66.

[31] Coutts SB, Lev MH, Eliasziw M, et al. ASPECTS on CTA source images versus unenhanced CT: added value in predicting final infarct extent and clinical outcome. Stroke 2004;35:2472–6.

[32] Wintermark M, Reichhart M, Thiran JP, et al. Prognostic accuracy of cerebral blood flow measurement by perfusion computed tomography, at the time of emergency room admission, in acute stroke patients. Ann Neurol 2002;51:417–32.

[33] Koenig M, Kraus M, Theek C, et al. Quantitative assessment of the ischemic brain by means of perfusion-related parameters derived from perfusion CT. Stroke 2001;32:431–7.

[34] Wintermark M, Fischbein NJ, Smith WS, et al. Accuracy of dynamic perfusion CT with deconvolution in detecting acute hemispheric stroke. AJNR Am J Neuroradiol 2005;26:104–12.

[35] Lev MH, Segal AZ, Farkas J, et al. Utility of perfusion-weighted CT imaging in acute middle cerebral artery stroke treated with intra-arterial thrombolysis. Prediction of final infarct volume and clinical outcome. Stroke 2001;32:2021–8.

[36] Schramm P, Schellinger PD, Fiebach JB, et al. Comparison of CT and CT angiography source images with diffusion-weighted imaging in patients with acute stroke within 6 hours after onset. Stroke 2002;33:2426–32.

[37] Lev MH, Segal AZ, Farkas J, et al. Utility of perfusion-weighted CT imaging in acute middle cerebral artery stroke treated with intra-arterial thrombolysis: prediction of final infarct volume and clinical outcome. Stroke 2001;32:2021–8.

[38] Ezzeddine MA, Lev MH, McDonald CT, et al. CT angiography with whole brain perfused blood volume imaging: added clinical value in the assessment of acute stroke. Stroke 2002;33:959–66.

[39] Coutts SB, Lev MH, Eliasziw M, et al. ASPECTS on CTA source images versus unenhanced CT: added value in predicting final infarct extent and clinical outcome. Stroke 2004;35(11):2472–6.

[40] Nabavi DG, Kloska SP, Nam EM, et al. MOSAIC: Multimodal Stroke Assessment Using Computed Tomography: novel diagnostic approach for the prediction of infarction size and clinical outcome. Stroke 2002;33:2819–26.

[41] Schuier FJ, Hossmann KA. Experimental brain infarcts in cats. II. Ischemic brain edema. Stroke 1980;11:593–601.

[42] Dzialowski I, Weber J, Doerfler A, et al. Brain tissue water uptake after middle cerebral artery occlusion assessed with CT. J Neuroimaging 2004;14:42–8.

[43] Unger E, Littlefield J, Gado M. Water content and water structure in CT and MR signal changes: possible influence in detection of early stroke. AJNR Am J Neuroradiol 1988;9:687–91.

[44] Dzialowski I, Weber J, Doerfler A, et al. Brain tissue water uptake after middle cerebral artery occlusion assessed with CT. J Neuroimaging 2004;14(1):42–8.

[45] Warach S. Stroke neuroimaging. Stroke 2003;34:345–7.

[46] Hill MD, Coutts SB, Pexman JH, et al. CTA source images in acute stroke. Stroke 2003;34:835–7.

[47] Bastianello S, Pierallini A, Collonnese C, et al. Hyperdense middle cerebral artery CT sign: comparison with angiography in the acute phase of ischemic supratentorial infarction. Neuroradiology 1991;33:207–11.

[48] Demchuk AM, Tanne D, Hill MD, et al. Predictors of good outcome after intravenous alteplase for acute ischemic stroke: the Multicenter tPA Acute Stroke Survey. Neurology 2001;57:474–80.

[49] Bendszuz M, Urbach H, Ries F, et al. Outcome after local intra-arterial fibrinolysis compared with the natural course of patients with a dense middle cerebral artery on early CT. Neuroradiology 1998;40:54–8.

[50] Barber PA, Demchuk AM, Hudon ME, et al. The hyperdense sylvian fissure MCA "dot" sign. A CT marker of acute ischemia. Stroke 2001;32:84–8.

[51] Leary MC, Kidwell CS, Villablanca JP, et al. Validation of computed tomographic middle cerebral artery "dot" sign: an angiographic correlation study. Stroke 2003;34:2636–40.

[52] Schuknecht B, Ratzka M, Hofmann E. The "dense artery sign"—major cerebral artery thromboembolism demonstrated by computed tomography. Neuroradiology 1990;32:98–103.

[53] Wardlaw JM, Mielke O. Early signs of brain infarction at CT: observer reliability and outcome after thrombolytic treatment—systematic review. Radiology 2005;235:444–53.

[54] Rauch RA, Bazan III C, Larsson EM, et al. Hyperdense middle cerebral arteries identified on CT as a false sign of vascular occlusion. AJNR Am J Neuroradiol 1993;14:669–73.

[55] Verro P, Tanenbaum LN, Borden NM, et al. The role

of CT angiography in acute ischemic stroke: a prospective study. Stroke 2002;33:276–8.

[56] Lev MH, Farkas J, Rodriguez VR. CT angiography in the rapid triage of patients with hyperacute stroke to intraarterial thrombolysis: accuracy in the detection of large vessel thrombus. J Comput Assist Tomogr 2001; 25:520–8.

[57] Brandt T, Knauth M, Wildermuth S, et al. CT angiography and Doppler sonography for emergency assessment in acute basilar artery ischemia. Stroke 1999; 30:606–12.

[58] Josephson SA, Bryant SO, Mak HK, et al. Evaluation of carotid stenosis using CT angiography in the initial evaluation of stroke and TIA. Neurology 2004; 63:457–60.

[59] Rothwell PM, Eliasziw M, Gutnikov SA, et al. Sex difference in the effect of time from symptoms to surgery on benefit from carotid endarterectomy for transient ischemic attack and nondisabling stroke. Stroke 2004;35:2855–61.

[60] Krieger DW, Demchuk AM, Kasner SE, et al. Early clinical and radiological predictors of fatal brain swelling in ischemic stroke. Stroke 1999;30:287–92.

[61] Saqqur M, Alexandrov AV, Hill MD, et al. Deriving transcranial Doppler criteria for rescue intra-arterial thrombolysis: multicenter experience from the Interventional Management of Stroke (IMS-1) study. Stroke 2005;36(4):865–8.

[62] Fink JN, Kumar S, Horkan C, et al. The stroke patient who woke up: clinical and radiological features, including diffusion and perfusion MRI. Stroke 2002; 33:988–93.

[63] Nadeau J, Fang J, Kapral MK, et al on behalf of the Investigators for the Registry of the Canadian Stroke Network. Outcome after stroke upon awakening. Can J Neurol Sci 2005;32:232–6.

[64] Hacke W, Albers G, Al-Rawi Y, et al. The Desmoteplase in Acute Ischemic Stroke Trial (DIAS): a phase II MRI-based 9-hour window acute stroke thrombolysis trial with intravenous desmoteplase. Stroke 2005;36: 66–73.

[65] Schellinger PD, Fiebach JB, Hacke W. Imaging-based decision making in thrombolytic therapy for ischemic stroke: present status. Stroke 2003;34:575–83.

[66] Chalela JA, Kang DW, Luby M, et al. Early magnetic resonance imaging findings in patients receiving tissue plasminogen activator predict outcome: insights into the pathophysiology of acute stroke in the thrombolysis era. Ann Neurol 2004;55:105–12.

[67] Wintermark M, Reichhart M, Cuisenaire O, et al. Comparison of admission perfusion computed tomography and qualitative diffusion- and perfusion-weighted magnetic resonance imaging in acute stroke patients. Stroke 2002;33:2025–31.

[68] Koroshetz WJ, Lev MH. Contrast computed tomography scan in acute stroke: "you can't always get what you want but…you get what you need." Ann Neurol 2002;51:415–6.

ELSEVIER
SAUNDERS

Neuroimag Clin N Am 15 (2005) 421 – 440

NEUROIMAGING
CLINICS OF
NORTH AMERICA

The Evolving Role of Acute Stroke Imaging in Intravenous Thrombolytic Therapy: Patient Selection and Outcomes Assessment

John Sims, MD[a,b,c], Lee H. Schwamm, MD[b,c,d],*

[a]*Stroke and Neurovascular Regulation Laboratory, Charlestown, MA, USA*
[b]*Harvard Medical School, Boston, MA, USA*
[c]*TeleStroke and Acute Stroke Services, Department of Neurology, Massachusetts General Hospital, Boston, MA, USA*
[d]*Clinical Research Center, Massachusetts Institute of Technology, Boston, MA, USA*

Imaging has played an indispensable role in the treatment of ischemic stroke with intravenous (IV) tissue plasminogen activator (tPA). Previously, the role of brain imaging was limited to the exclusion of intracerebral hemorrhage or massive early infarction. This limitation reflected the available technology and the absence of rapidly attainable vascular imaging. Currently, brain imaging has been proposed as a method for identifying patients likely to respond favorably or unfavorably to IV thrombolysis. In the future, imaging may allow us to expand the time window of the treatment for IV thrombolysis, test new thrombolytic strategies more rapidly, and better assign patients to available treatments. It also may help to reduce the complications of brain hemorrhage or edema, enhance lytic activity, and assist with prognosis before and after thrombolysis. This article reviews past applications of imaging for IV lysis triage to understand how the stage was set for current developments. Ongoing trials that use a broader array of imaging modalities are evaluated, and potential future applications of imaging for thrombolytic therapy are identified.

Shortened therapeutic time forces a transition from vascular to parenchymal imaging for patient selection in clinical trials of thrombolysis

Thrombolysis in stroke was first described in the 1950s [1], and the first randomized trial of intravenous thrombolysis was performed in 1964 [2], 8 years before the development of computer-assisted tomography. Previously, stroke trials had used contrast angiography to diagnose vascular occlusion and assess the efficacy of recanalization in eight pilot studies of intravenous thrombolysis [3–9]. These proof-of-principle studies demonstrated recanalization rates of 33% in treated arteries versus 5% in controls [10], but patients were treated relatively late in the course of stroke evolution. These trials made great strides in enrolling patients in a new "acute stroke" time window of 24 hours but discovered that radiographic success at recanalization was not always associated with tissue salvage and clinical improvement.

These studies (Table 1) [4,7,11–21] provided the foundation for the first large multicenter, placebo-controlled, randomized trial of intravenous thrombolysis, the European Cooperative Acute Stroke Study (ECASS) [11]. In ECASS, treatment with IV

This work was supported by a grant from the Craig H. Neilsen Foundation.

* Corresponding author. Department of Neurology, Massachusetts General Hospital, 55 Fruit Street, VBK915, Boston, MA 02114.

  E-mail address: Lschwamm@partners.org (L.H. Schwamm).

Table 1
Comparison of the brain imaging criteria used in the major randomized trials of intravenous thrombolytics conducted prior to the US Food and Drug Administration approval of recombinant tissue plasminogen

First author, year [Ref.]	N	Intravenous drug	Window of enrollment from onset	Imaging modality/exclusions	Required imaging follow-up	Outcome
Abe, 1981 [17]	107	Urokinase	14 d	CT/ICH	CT if indicated	No difference in mortality
Atarashi, 1985 [18]	286	Urokinase	5 d	CT/ICH	CT if indicated	No difference in mortality
Ohtomo, 1985 [19]	350	Urokinase	5 d	CT/ICH	CT if indicated	No difference in mortality
Mori, 1992 [4]	31	rtPA:duteplase	6 h	CT/ICH or visible infarct angiography/patent vessel	CT at 1, 2, 7 and 30 d	No difference in mortality or ICH
Yamcuchi, 1993 [7]; Wardlaw, 2005 [16]	98	rtPA:duteplase	6 h	CT/hemorrhage angiography/patent vessel	CT if indicated	No difference in mortality or ICH
Haley, 1993 [15]	27	rtPA:alteplase (activase)	3 h	CT/ICH	CT at 1 and 7 d and 30 mo	No difference in mortality or ICH
NINDS, 1995 [20]	624	rtPA:alteplase (activase)	3 h	CT/ICH	CT at 1 and 7–10 d and 3 mo	Less death and dependency in the treated group despite significant increase in fatal and symptomatic hemorrhage
Hacke, 1995 [11]	620	rtPA:alteplase (actilyse)	6 h	CT/ICH or visible infarct	CT if indicated	Trend toward less death and dependency in treated group, with significant increase in fatal and symptomatic hemorrhage
Morris, 1995 [21]	20	Streptokinase	6 h	CT/ICH	CT if indicated	No difference in mortality or ICH
MAST–I, 1995 [14]	313	Streptokinase	6 h	CT/ICH	CT if indicated	Trend toward less death and dependency in treated group, with significant increase in fatal and symptomatic hemorrhage
MAST–E, 1996 [12]	310	Streptokinase	6 h	CT/ICH	CT if indicated	No difference in death and dependency in treated group, with significant increase in fatal and symptomatic hemorrhage
Donan, 1996 [13]	340	Streptokinase	4 h	CT/ICH	CT at 7–10 d	No difference in death and dependency in treated group, with significant increase in fatal and symptomatic hemorrhage

tPA was initiated within 6 hours of symptom onset, which was much earlier than in previous trials. To shorten the door-to-needle time to an acceptable range, investigators were forced to sacrifice vascular imaging before patients were enrolled and to rely on the clinical diagnosis of stroke and the absence of hemorrhage on CT to identify candidates. This paradigm shift allowed for the rapid enrollment of patients at the price of a loss of specificity and increased heterogeneity in patient selection.

Occurring simultaneously with ECASS, three large randomized trials of intravenous thrombolysis with streptokinase were performed using a similar enrollment strategy without vascular imaging [12–14]. All three streptokinase trials showed excessive rates of intracranial hemorrhage without improved outcomes in survivors and with unacceptably high mortality in the first 10 days. To avoid brain hemorrhage and increase the patients' chances of recovery, the pilot dose-ranging clinical trial of IV tPA [4,15] explored the possibility of very early enrollment. The pivotal National Institutes of Neurological Disorders and Stroke (NINDS) IV tPA trial pushed early treatment to the limit by reducing the tPA dose to its minimum effective concentration. Given that a stratified enrollment required half the patients to be imaged as well as treated within 90 minutes of stroke onset, it is not surprising that there was no inclusion of vascular imaging and that many centers were pressed to complete simple unenhanced CT scans in the allotted time, albeit solely for the exclusion of hemorrhage and not for assessing patients for parenchymal hypodensity. This strategy finally unlocked the door to successful thrombolysis in acute ischemic stroke and defined the standards against which all future trials would be judged. Only the unsuccessful Japanese IV duteplase trials used vascular imaging findings (ie, angiographic occlusion) as a criterion for the diagnosis and patient eligibility for thrombolysis [4,7,16], but to do this the investigators had to use a window of up to 6 hours after stroke onset, similar to the later trials of catheter-based thrombolysis.

Unenhanced CT in acute stroke thrombolysis: how abnormal is too abnormal and how reliable is it?

With the shift from vascular to parenchymal imaging, rapid clinical diagnosis became more important. Many patients imaged within 24 hours of stroke symptoms had no "detectable" abnormality on review of printed films of unenhanced brain CT at the standard window width and center level settings. This meant that CT scanning could be relied on to exclude brain hemorrhage and other conditions mimicked by ischemic stroke (eg, brain tumor) and to identify more mature ischemic strokes that were associated with substantial hypodensity. Of the original thrombolytic trials, only the Japanese trials and ECASS sought to exclude patients with these large or advanced infarctions and used visible hypodensity on CT scanning as an exclusion criterion [4,11].

Despite the reliance on CT to exclude brain hemorrhage, the data suggest that emergency physicians, neurologists, and radiologists identify acute intracerebral hemorrhage based on CT scans with at best 80% sensitivity [22]. The accuracy for detecting hypodensity and early ischemic signs on standard CT scans is even worse, typically less than 65%, even by experienced stroke physicians and neuroradiologists [22,23]. Two early thrombolysis trials excluded patients with an abnormal CT scan [4,7,16], and the ECASS trial was designed to exclude patients with large strokes (ie, CT scanning with diffuse swelling or parenchymal hypodensity in more than one third of the middle cerebral artery [MCA] territory). In ECASS, 17% (109/620) of patients had protocol violations, with almost half (52/109) involving the inadequate reading of the CT scan as determined by a prespecified central review. Among the protocol violators for CT exclusions there was much higher mortality in the treated versus placebo patients (48% versus 28%, respectively) [24].

Past imaging metrics to predict and monitor outcomes and complications: could early changes on CT predict hemorrhage or poor outcome?

Unenhanced brain CT scanning in many of the trials was used to document hemorrhagic transformation of ischemic stroke after treatment. This imaging was acquired between 1 and 10 days after treatment. Many studies have performed post-hoc analyses with an attempt to identify characteristics on the pretreatment scans that would predict poor outcomes.

All of the streptokinase studies suffered from excessive morbidity because of intracranial hemorrhage; however, a meta-analysis of these trials showed no association between early CT changes and bleeding [25]. Most symptomatic hemorrhages, whether within the infarcted tissue or at an anatomically distinct site, occurred within the first few days after treatment. As a result, most trials restricted the classification of clinically symptomatic hemorrhages to the first 36 to

72 hours, although the Cochrane database includes the first 7 to 10 days [16]. Post-treatment CT scanning was used in ECASS to monitor for hemorrhage, but only radiological descriptors were used to assign classifications (eg, hemorrhagic transformation or parenchymal hematoma), rather than clinical interpretations (eg, symptomatic versus asymptomatic). Among those CT protocol violators who were treated with tPA despite early infarct signs, the rate of hemorrhage was 40% [24]. In the NINDS trial [26], a follow-up CT scan was required at 24 hours and at 7 to 10 days after the onset of stroke. Nine percent of patients with intracranial hemorrhage showed evidence of cerebral edema on CT scanning, compared with 4% of the study population. There was a significant increase in symptomatic hemorrhage in the tPA-treated patients versus controls (6.4% versus 0.6%, respectively; $P = .001$). This data initially suggested that early cerebral edema as defined by hypodensity on CT scanning might predict hemorrhage. However, a follow-up analysis demonstrated that, after adjusting for stroke severity (National Institutes of Health Stroke Scale), there was no association between early ischemic changes seen on CT scans and outcome [27]. By contrast, favorable outcome in the Standard Treatment with Alteplase to Reverse Stroke (STARS) tPA study [28] was associated with the absence of hypodensity involving more than 33% of the MCA territory or a dense MCA sign on CT scanning.

Imaging markers of vessel and tissue reperfusion

Transfemoral contrast angiography was used in early IV thrombolysis trials to define large-vessel recanalization endpoints and to enroll subjects. These studies have demonstrated that acute revascularization is associated with smaller infarcts [5] and that there is a greater likelihood of revascularization in more distal MCA occlusions [5,29]. The absence of CT hypodensity with good collateral blood supply on angiography performed within 5 hours of stroke onset predicted early improvement [30].

A more rapid alternative to positron emission tomography (PET) for measuring tissue reperfusion uses xenon gas administration concurrently with CT scanning to determine quantitative cerebral blood flow. Patients who were admitted with higher cerebral blood flow (CBF), as measured by xenon-CT, experienced a greater resolution of their neurologic deficit [31,32]. However, vessel recanalization without tissue reperfusion (the "no reflow" phenomenon)

does not salvage ischemic tissue, and other methods of tissue imaging need to be explored.

Single-photon emission CT (SPECT) scanning with a technetium-99m–labeled D,L-hexamethylpropylene amine oxime has been used to assess tissue reperfusion in thrombolysis-treated patients. One study [33] showed that streptokinase-treated patients had slightly better reperfusion rates at 24 hours compared with untreated patients (65% versus 52%, respectively). Regardless of treatment, patients with reperfusion at 24 hours had significantly less mortality and disability compared with those who had not undergone reperfusion [33,34].

One of the first studies [35] to use transcranial Doppler (TCD) ultrasonography to monitor vessel recanalization status was the Australian Streptokinase (ASK) trial, in which a subset of patients (N = 37) underwent assessment with SPECT or TCD ultrasonography to assess reperfusion status as a marker of efficacy. Treated patients had greater rates of reperfusion or recanalization (93% versus 50%, respectively; $P = .01$), but there were no differences in clinical outcomes assessed at 3 months.

TCD ultrasonography can demonstrate early recanalization, and the presence or absence of occlusion correlates well with both conventional angiography [36] and CT angiography (CTA) [37]. When TCD ultrasonography was used to detect residual flow around a clot, as described in the thrombolysis in brain ischemia (TIBI) scale [38], vessels with a flow of TIBI grade 1 through 3 were twice as likely to reestablish complete early recanalization than did clots that had no residual flow (TIBI grade 0). TCD monitoring has confirmed early angiographic studies, which have shown that recanalization depends on clot location [5,29]. Most patients with carotid occlusion do not demonstrate TCD ultrasonography evidence of recanalization after IV thrombolysis [39,40]. Indeed, the likelihood of recanalization appears greater for MCA (distal) versus internal carotid artery (proximal) occlusions [41]. However, early tPA-induced recanalization of a carotid or MCA occlusion typically results in a marked improvement of clinical outcomes compared with those without reperfusion. Recanalization of the middle cerebral artery within 2 hours of treatment is significantly associated with improved functional outcome and less mortality [42]. In contrast, patients who have an M1 occlusion and late recanalization by TCD ultrasonography (≥ 6 hours) may be at a higher risk for symptomatic hemorrhage [43]. Moreover, the TIBI grade correlates with initial severity, clinical outcome, and mortality [44].

Continuous TCD monitoring could identify patients who will benefit from bridging therapy with

Table 2
Comparison of the brain imaging criteria used in the major trials of intravenous thrombolytics conducted after the US Food and Drug Administration approval of recombinant tissue plasminogen

First author (study), year [Ref.]	N	Intravenous drug	Window of enrollment from onset	Imaging modality/exclusions	Required imaging follow-up	Outcome
Hacke (ECASS II), 1998 [48]	800	rtPA:alteplase (actilyse)	6 h	CT/ ICH or infarct > 1/3 MCA	CT if indicated	No overall benefit, less death and dependency in treated group was impacted by an increase in fatal and symptomatic hemorrhage
Clark (ATLANTIS A), 2000 [49]	142	rtPA:alteplase (activase)	3–6 h	CT/ hemorrhage	CT if indicated	Trend toward more death and dependency in treated group, with significant increase in fatal and symptomatic hemorrhage
Clark (ATLANTIS B), 1999 [50]	613	rtPA:alteplase (activase)	3–5 h	CT/ ICH or infarct > 1/3 MCA	CT if indicated	No difference in death or dependency, with significant increase in fatal and symptomatic hemorrhage
Wardlaw (Chinese UK), 2003 [16]	465	Urokinase	6 h	CT/ ICH or visible infarct	CT if indicated	No difference in death or dependency, with trend in increase in fatal and symptomatic hemorrhage

catheter-based techniques or other strategies. Early reocclusion after IV tPA, as documented by TCD ultrasonography, may occur in 34% of patients [45]. Early reocclusion documented by TCD ultrasonography is associated with increased mortality, although these patients do better than those who never had reperfusion [45]. In addition to monitoring patency, ultrasound energy also can enhance clot lysis. TCD ultrasonography has been shown to increase the rate of MCA recanalization [46] but also may increase the rate of intraparenchymal hemorrhage [47]. Although it is less sensitive and specific for occlusion or stenosis than other vascular imaging methods, TCD ultrasonography provides a superior method for continuous monitoring of vessel status.

Role of imaging after National Institutes of Neurological Disorders and Stroke: patient characterization and triage and expanding the role of acute CT

After the approval of alteplase for the treatment of acute ischemic stroke, many more patients began to receive the open-label drug, and the opportunities increased to explore imaging characteristics associated with better patient outcomes (Table 2) [16,48–50]. The creation of stroke teams increased the percentage of patients eligible for thrombolysis by decreasing both the door-to-CT and door-to-needle times [51]. With mounting pressure to make a rapid clinical diagnosis, the reliance on CT increased at a time

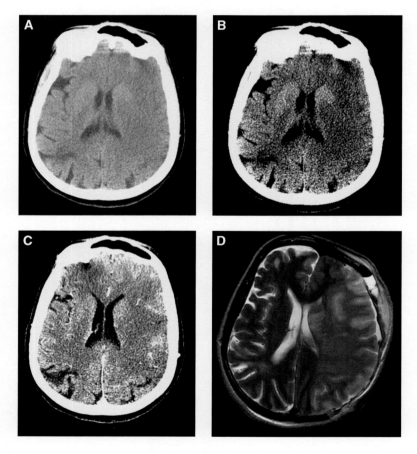

Fig. 1. Optimizing CT imaging. (*A*) Noncontrast CT (NCCT) scanning, routinely performed, shows a subtle hypodensity throughout the left hemisphere. (*B*) NCCT scan performed in the same slice (*A*) but windowed to optimize contrast. The optimized contrast shows a more obvious loss of gray-white differentiation and a large territory at risk. (*C*) CTA source image after bolus of dye has been given to image the vessels. This image also confirms the decrease in perfusion of dye into the left hemisphere seen in (*B*). (*D*) FLAIR MR image obtained 1 day after the patient underwent hemicraniectomy. This image confirms the regions identified in (*B*) and (*C*) with some posterior extension of the lesion.

when low-cost digital imaging workstations were becoming increasingly affordable.

Although it is rapid and available widely, a review of conventional CT images fails to identify ischemic changes in up to 10% of cases imaged within 6 hours of onset, although most of the false-negatives occur within the first 3 hours [52]. Early signs of ischemia on CT scans include subtle gray matter hypodensity, loss of cortical ribbon, sulcal effacement, or a hyperdense middle cerebral artery sign. Large and obvious hypodensities seen on CT scans are often a poor prognostic sign, even when obtained within 5 hours of onset. Hypodensity covering more than 50% of the MCA territory caused by a MCA trunk occlusion has been associated with a mortality rate of 85% [53].

One method to improve CT scan lesion conspicuity, and hence diagnostic accuracy, is by varying the center level and window width Hounsfield unit display ranges (Fig. 1). Such a method can improve the sensitivity of detecting ischemic injury by 20%

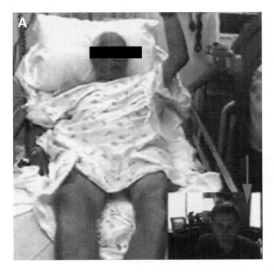

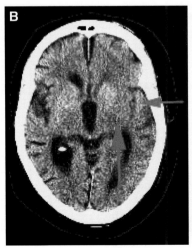
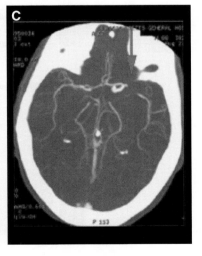

Fig. 2. (*A*) Still frame from the telemedicine-enabled stroke evaluation (Telestroke) examination by the neurologist at home (*arrow*), examining the patient through the camera located at the foot of the bed. Right arm weakness can be appreciated with the patient's arms held up, and the patient's left-gaze preference continued throughout the examination. (*B*) Unenhanced CT scan of the brain obtained 15 minutes after symptom onset viewed from the remote stroke physician's home through teleradiology. Subtle signs of early ischemia include loss of the normal outline of the posterior left putamen (*large arrow*) and loss of the insular stripe (*small arrow*). (*C*) Follow-up CT angiography performed 4 hours after symptom onset shows a continued left middle cerebral artery occlusion (*arrow*).

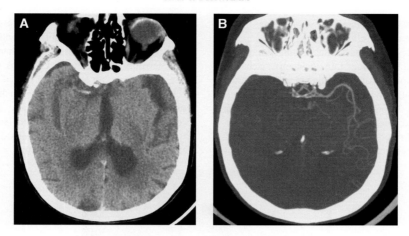

Fig. 3. CT angiography. (*A*) Dense right MCA sign is shown. (*B*) CTA maximum intensity map reconstruction demonstrating occlusion of the right MCA.

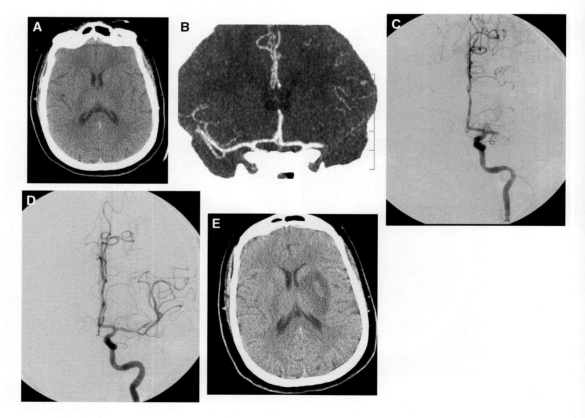

Fig. 4. CT angiography performed for acute triage treatment. (*A*) NCCT scan at symptom onset shows subtle hypodensity in putamen and internal capsule. (*B*) CTA maximum intensity map reconstruction demonstrating proximal M1 cutoff. (*C*) Conventional angiography confirms M1 occlusion. (*D*) After interventional procedure, M1 is opened and distal branches are shown. (*E*) NCCT scan obtained 2 days after the procedure showing limited infarct to deep structures with salvage of the rest of the MCA territory.

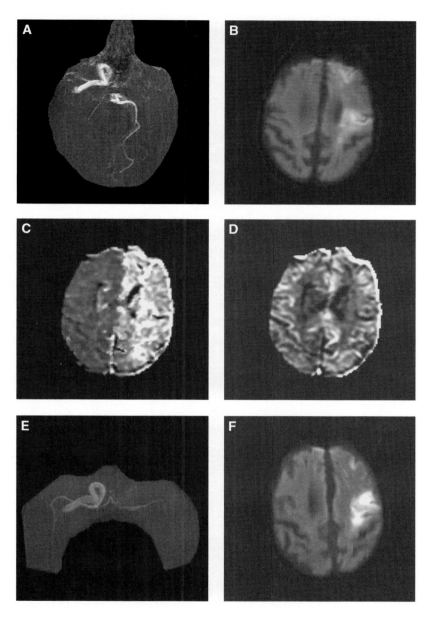

Fig. 5. MR diffusion-perfusion imaging study. (*A*) MR angiography obtained at onset of symptoms showing absence of flow in the distal left carotid, left anterior cerebral artery, and left MCA. (*B*) DWI shows a hazy involvement of the left anterior frontal pole and the supplementary motor cortex. (*C*) MTT shows an isolated hemisphere with delayed blood flow throughout. (*D*) CBV of the same region as MTT (*C*) shows well-preserved blood volume despite delayed flow. (*B*–*D*) Penumbral tissue with mismatch of DWI and CBV with MTT. (*E*) Repeat MR angiography obtained 1 day later after rheological therapy and induced hypertension. Improved blood flow is seen in the left MCA. (*F*) Repeat DWI obtained 1 day later (*E*). DWI reversal in the anterior pole is seen, indicating tissue salvage with development of the supplementary cortex infarct, but the remaining tissue is preserved.

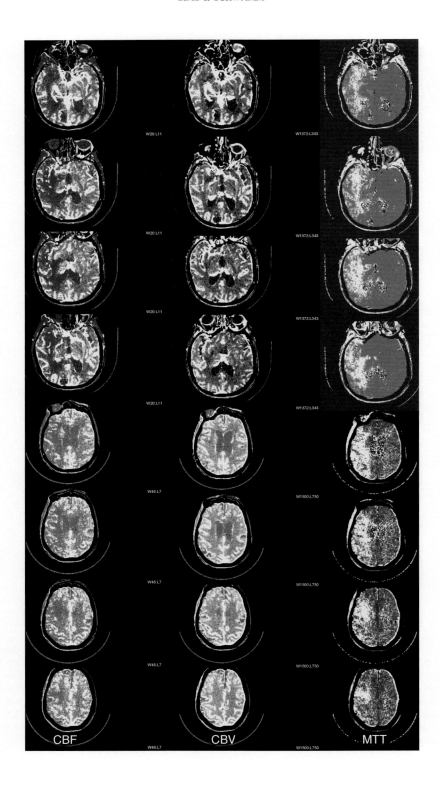

without sacrificing specificity [54]. Another approach involves the use of a simple technique for scoring CT images, which has been implemented in the Alberta Stroke Program Early CT Score (ASPECTS) methodology. This method, which divides the MCA territory into ten regions and then subtracts a point for each region involved, has proven to be useful in improving the reliability of CT assessment in acute stroke. It appears to correlate well with the initial NIHSS, the risk of symptomatic hemorrhage, and the clinical outcome, with ASPECTS scores less than 7 correlating with an increase in death and dependency [55].

Experience at community hospitals suggests a low rate of tPA use and a high rate of complications [56], which has been attributed to a lack of locally available acute stroke clinical and imaging expertise. To address these potential deficiencies, formal stroke center development and certification have been recommended and initiated [57,58]. For hospitals without available acute stroke expertise, telemedicine-enabled stroke care (TeleStroke) permits a remote review of digitally transferred CT data and a clinical evaluation of patients at smaller community hospitals to rapidly evaluate and treat eligible stroke patients with thrombolytic therapy, and then to admit or transfer them as needed [59–62]. These systems collapse the barriers of time and distance between patients and qualified providers, allowing for rapid interpretation of conventionally acquired neuroimaging (Fig. 2).

With the development and distribution of helical CT technology, scans can be acquired rapidly enough to permit angiographic imaging, as well as bolus-kinetic blood flow mapping based on functional methods pioneered in PET and MR imaging. During CTA image acquisition, the CT axial source images provide supplementary information on whole-brain collateral blood flow and tissue perfusion, which can increase the frequency of detecting regions of ischemia that correlate strongly with final infarct volume (see Fig. 1) [37,63–65]. The admission CTA and axial source images significantly improve accuracy over that of the initial clinical assessment and unenhanced CT imaging alone in the determination of infarct location, site of vascular occlusion, and syndrome classification in acute stroke patients (Fig. 3) [66]. In addition, the degree of hypodensity on the axial source images predicts subsequent hem-

orrhagic transformation after catheter-based thrombolysis [67] and may prove relevant to the patient selection for IV tPA in the future.

Now validated, CT angiography provides a method of vascular imaging rapid enough to be used during the acute evaluation of ischemic stroke patients [68–70]. For the first time, it is possible to obtain rapid and highly accurate vascular imaging in the hyperacute phase of ischemic stroke (Fig. 4). CTA is safe and well tolerated, compares favorably to other vascular imaging modalities [64,68], provides greater anatomic detail than TCD, and is more rapid than MR angiography or conventional angiography [63,71]. Several centers have adopted CTA as the method performed in all thrombolysis candidates, as a surrogate for conventional angiography. CTA can characterize the vascular anatomy of patients with acute stroke syndromes, identify those with persistent occlusion after IV tPA who might benefit from bridging to off-label catheter-based thrombolysis [70], or exclude those without large vessel vascular occlusion. This latter feature is important because the presence of a large vessel occlusion seen on CTA before IV thrombolysis may predict a worse outcome and a greater complication rate [71,72], and evidence of persistent occlusion by CTA and poor collateral perfusion on CTA source images may predict infarct growth and poorer outcomes [64,73].

Conventional and functional MR imaging in acute stroke: transforming the landscape

The development of MR diffusion-weighted imaging (DWI) dramatically improved the ability to detect ischemic tissue within minutes of a symptom onset [74], and challenged CT scanning as the preferred initial imaging study in acute stroke. The sensitivity for ischemic lesion detection in the early time window (≤6 hours), most notably for brainstem and lacunar infarctions, is superior to both unenhanced CT scanning and conventional MR imaging [75]. In one study [76], DWI detected 97% of lesions, conventional MR imaging detected 58% of lesions, and unenhanced CT detected 40% of lesions. This early diagnostic advantage provided by DWI largely evaporates 12 hours or later after symptom onset. DWI lesion volumes greater than 89 cm^3 may predict

Fig. 6. CT perfusion scan. CBF (*left*) demonstrates a large decrease in blood flow throughout the temporal lobe. CBV (*middle*) is more normal than the CBF, with a subtle decrease in the deep white matter on the right in the fourth image from the top. MTT (*right*) shows a significant delay in blood flow on all of the slices, indicating a large mismatch between the region of brain with slow flow and the loss of CBV, which correlates well with final infarct volume.

early neurologic deterioration [77]. DWI also can improve accuracy in determining ischemic stroke causes, timing, and subtype, which may play a critical role in the testing interventions for specific stroke subtypes [78–81]. Initially, it was believed that DWI represented an irreversible ischemic lesion. More recently, limited reversibility of DWI lesions after reperfusion with thrombolysis has been reported [82–84]. These reports are supported by findings that suggest regions of restricted diffusion may reflect both an infarct core as well as salvageable penumbral tissue [85].

In addition to providing unparalleled detection of severely ischemic tissue, MR imaging can provide concurrent whole-brain qualitative perfusion indices. Results of MR imaging first-pass bolus-kinetic techniques suggest that reduced cerebral blood volume (CBV) lesions may be superior to DWI lesions as the best predictors of final infarct volume [86]. Mean transit time (MTT) and CBF are sensitive but not specific and tend to overestimate final infarct volume [87]. A mismatch between DWI and CBV lesions predicts infarct growth [86]. A mismatch between DWI or CBV and CBF or MTT defines penumbral tissue (Fig. 5) [86,87]. The presence of MCA trunk occlusion increases the likelihood of such a mismatch and is associated with infarct volume expansion and poorer outcomes [77,88,89]. Contrary to previous conceptions about the pace of infarct evolution, the mismatch and salvageable tissue can be identified 12 hours or longer after symptom onset [90]. Although the volume of tissue comprising penumbra decreases with time [91,92], survival of the penumbra at later time points can result in improved neurologic recovery [92].

Because of the rigid time windows for acute stroke evaluation and lingering concerns about insensitivity to subarachnoid hemorrhage, most centers do not perform MR imaging soon enough to screen candidates for IV tPA. The role of MR imaging may be largely in defining candidates for catheter-based thrombolysis and in laying the foundation for extending the time window for the next generation of IV thrombolysis drugs, as described elsewhere.

Future role of imaging: paradigm shift from wall clock to tissue clock and extending the window for intravenous thrombolysis: the holy grail of imaging

The ECASS I, ECASS II, and Alteplase Thrombo-Lysis for Acute Noninterventional Therapy in Ischemic Stroke (ATLANTIS B) [50] studies have attempted to extend the window of thrombolytic eligibility and therefore have excluded patients if one third or more of the MCA territory showed ischemic change. This is based on evidence that suggests a lack of benefit in these patients and a higher risk of symptomatic hemorrhage [93]. The ECASS II [48] and ATLANTIS studies were unsuccessful (Table 2) [46,94,95]. A successful extension of the therapeutic time window for thrombolysis in a clinical trial was achieved only in the catheter-based trial of pro-urokinase (Prolyse in Acute Cerebral Thromboembolism: PROACT II) [96], in which patients with angiographic evidence of MCA occlusion benefited from clot lysis that was initiated up to 6 hours after symptom onset.

To extend the benefits of IV thrombolysis to a more substantial number of patients, the selection paradigms will need to shift away from a simple, temporal selection to a more sophisticated assessment of the "tissue clock," the biologic consequences of physiologic disruptions to blood flow at the tissue level. Patients who present swiftly to the hospital but with advanced tissue injury may be more likely to experience poor outcomes compared with those who present much later but with preserved tissue architecture and substantial regions of threatened yet viable brain. A recent meta-analysis [97] of over 3000 patients in six randomized placebo-controlled trials with IV recombinant (r)tPA that used risk-adjustment for factors predicting poor clinical outcome, confirms the benefit of IV tPA therapy within 3 hours of onset and suggests a gradually tapering benefit from 5 to 6 hours of onset.

MR imaging of the cerebral metabolic rate of oxygen ($CMRO_2$) use, based on tissue blood flow and oxygen extraction, may help define tissue heterogeneity within penumbral regions of the brain. It may distinguish tissue with reduced perfusion or high oxygen extraction from tissue with a well-compensated reduction in perfusion that is not truly at risk [98]. The early use of the DWI–perfusion-weighted imaging mismatch has suggested that the appropriate selection of patients can improve outcomes [99,100]. Strategies to determine "tissue at risk" could also involve bolus-kinetic perfusion models based on CT scanning (Fig. 6) [73,101,102], MR imaging, or other novel modalities. This approach is being applied already in a new generation of acute stroke thrombolytic trials seeking to increase therapeutic time and efficacy. It has been applied in two completed dose-escalation trials of IV desmetoplase (Desmetoplase In Acute ischemic Stroke [DIAS] study [94] and the Dose Escalation study of Desmetoplase in Acute ischemic Stroke [DEDAS] study [95]) (Table 3). In

Table 3
Clinical reperfusion trials using imaging characteristics to extend the window of thrombolytic eligibility or to enhance thrombolysis

First author (study), year [Ref.]	N	Intravenous drug	Window of enrollment from onset	Imaging modality/exclusions	Required imaging follow-up	Outcome
Alexandrov (activase CLOTBUST), 2004 [46]	126	rtPA:alteplase ± continuous TCD	3 h	CT/ICH; TCD/no occlusion	TCD to assess recanalizaton	Higher rates of recanalization in treated group, with trend toward better functional outcome
Hacke (DIAS II), 2005 [94]	102	rtPA:desmetoplase	9 h	MR imaging + MRA/DWI-perfusion mismatch <20%	MRA <8 h, MR imaging at 30 d	Higher rates of reperfusion and functional outcome in treated group, with no difference in fatal and symptomatic hemorrhage
Furlan (DEDAS II), 2005 [95]	38	rtPA:desmetoplase	9 h	MR imaging + MRA/diffusion/perfusion mismatch <20%	MRA <8 h, MR imaging at 30 d	Trend toward higher rates of reperfusion and functional outcome in treated group at highest dose, with no difference in fatal and symptomatic hemorrhage

Table 4
Ongoing clinical reperfusion trials using imaging characteristics to extend the window of thrombolytic eligibility

First author (study), year [Ref.]	N	Intravenous drug	Window of enrollment from onset	Imaging modality/exclusions	Required imaging follow-up	Outcome
Hacke (DIAS-2 III), 2005 [94]	182	rtPA:desmetoplase	9 h	MR imaging + MRA or CT + CTP + CTA/DWI-perfusion mismatch<20%	MR imaging at 30 d	Functional outcome and lesion size
Hacke (actilyse ECASS III), 2003 [105]	800	rtPA:alteplase	3–4 h	CT/ICH	CT various time points	Functional outcome
Butcher (actilyse EPITHET), 2005 [103]	100	rtPA:alteplase	3–6 h	MR imaging + MRA/no DWI-perfusion mismatch	MR imaging + MRA at 3–5 d and MR imaging at 90 d	Lesion growth by imaging
Kane (activase and actilyse IST3), 2005 [106]	6000	rtPA:alteplase	6 h	CT or MR imaging/ICH	CT at 1 d	Functional outcome
Ciccone (actilyse SYNTHESIS), 2005 [107]	350	rtPA:alteplase with intravenous vs. intra-arterial administration	3 h	CT/ICH; angiography for intra-arterial patients/patent vessel		Functional outcome
Stroke Trials (activase DEFUSE), 1998 [104]	80	rtPA:alteplase	3–6 h	CT and MR imaging/ICH or infarct>1/3 MCA		Functional outcome
Dunn (ROSIE), 1999 [108]	144	rtPA:reteplase + abciximab	3–24 h	CT/ICH; MR imaging/microbleeds or no DWI-perfusion mismatch	MR imaging at 1 d	Safety, perfusion lesion reduction, and functional outcome

an effort to extend the treatment window, both studies used MR imaging techniques to identify penumbral tissue and support the concept that recanalization of tissue at risk may be associated with improved outcomes [94,95]. This new paradigm is the basis for the next generation of clinical reperfusion trials currently enrolling stroke patients (the Echoplanar Imaging Thrombolysis Evaluation Trial [EPITHET] study [103], the Diffusion-weighted imaging Evaluation For Understanding Stroke Evolution [DEFUSE] [104] study, DIAS II [94], the MR and Recanalization of Stroke Clots Using Embolectomy [MR RESCUE] trial, and the ReoPro Retavase Reperfusion of Stroke Safety Study Imaging Evaluation [ROSIE] study) (Table 4) [102–108].

The newer imaging techniques, which combine vascular anatomic and functional with parenchymal imaging, may be critical for selecting patients with proximal carotid or MCA stem occlusions who may benefit from bridging to catheter-based therapies after the initiation of IV thrombolytics (Fig. 7) [109–113]. New targets for imaging assessment include the identification of microbleeds, which may be risk factors for intracranial hemorrhage after tPA, by T2-weighted gradient echo MR imaging [114–116] or leptomeningeal enhancement, which may predict early blood–brain barrier breakdown and subsequent malignant edema, on fluid-attenuated inversion-recovery (FLAIR) MR sequences [117].

Molecular imaging also may play a larger role in the future, identifying vulnerable plaque [118] in the proximal vascular tree or defining clot composition to aid in the selection of the optimal thrombolytic strategy. Fibrin labeling may improve the resolution of MR angiography in identifying small, distal clots [119,120], and MR spectroscopy may more accurately identify penumbral tissue and distinguish salvageable from nonsalvageable tissue [121].

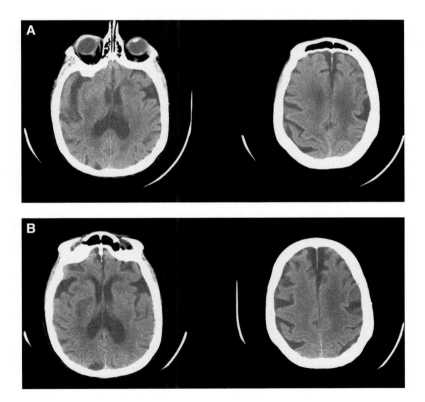

Fig. 7. CT perfusion scans correlate with tissue salvage (compare with Fig. 6). (*A*) NCCT scan at two slice levels demonstrating early hypodensity in the deep white matter (*right*). This region corresponds to the CBV decrease shown in Fig. 6. (*B*) NCCT scan at same two levels taken 2 days later after MCA occlusion was lysed. These images show progression of the early infarct identified in (*A*) and the CBV in Fig. 6 but demonstrate a limited extension of the infarct into the salvage penumbra represented in the MTT in Fig. 6.

Summary

Advances in brain imaging, from the first-generation CT scanning performed 30 years ago to the advent of transcranial Doppler and functional MR imaging, have revolutionized acute stroke care. These techniques have made it possible to finally identify a group of acute stroke patients who could benefit from thrombolytic therapy. These modalities hold the promise of further refining patient classification to permit a higher therapeutic index for current IV thrombolytic drugs and to extend the window of treatment so that many more patients can have the chance of the rapid recovery afforded by these agents. As these tools have grown more powerful, the paradigm has shifted toward more aggressive initial imaging and patient stratification before treatment.

References

[1] Sloan MA. Thrombolysis and stroke: past and future. Arch Neurol 1987;44(7):748–68.

[2] Meyer J, Gilroy J, Barnhart M. Anticoagulants plus streptokinase therapy in progressive stroke. JAMA 1964;189:373.

[3] Jansen O, von Kummer R, Forsting M, et al. Thrombolytic therapy in acute occlusion of the intracranial internal carotid artery bifurcation. AJNR Am J Neuroradiol 1995;16(10):1977–86.

[4] Mori E, Yoneda Y, Tabuchi M, et al. Intravenous recombinant tissue plasminogen activator in acute carotid artery territory stroke. Neurology 1992;42(5):976–82.

[5] Wolpert SM, Bruckmann H, Greenlee R, et al for the rt-PA Acute Stroke Study Group. Neuroradiologic evaluation of patients with acute stroke treated with recombinant tissue plasminogen activator. AJNR Am J Neuroradiol 1993;14(1):3–13.

[6] von Kummer R, Hacke W. Safety and efficacy of intravenous tissue plasminogen activator and heparin in acute middle cerebral artery stroke. Stroke 1992;23(5):646–52.

[7] Yamaguchi T, Kikuchi H, Hayakawa T, et al. Intravenous tissue plasminogen activator in acute thromboembolic stroke: a placebo-controlled double-blind trial. Berlin: Springer; 1993.

[8] Yamaguchi T, Kikuchi H, Hayakawa T, et al. Clinical efficacy and safety of intravenous tissue plasminogen activator in acute embolic stroke: a randomized double-blind, dose-comparison study of duteplase. Tokyo: Springer; 1995.

[9] von Kummer R, Forsting M, Sartor K, et al. Intravenous plasminogen activator in acute stroke. Boston: Springer; 1991.

[10] Caplan LR. Treatment. In: Caplan's stroke: a clinical

approach. 3rd edition. Boston: Butterworth Heinemann; 2000. p. 126.

[11] Hacke W, Kaste M, Fieschi C, et al for the European Cooperative Acute Stroke Study (ECASS). Intravenous thrombolysis with recombinant tissue plasminogen activator for acute hemispheric stroke. JAMA 1995;274(13):1017–25.

[12] The Multicenter Acute Stroke Trial–Europe Study Group. Thrombolytic therapy with streptokinase in acute ischemic stroke. N Engl J Med 1996;335(3):145–50.

[13] Donnan GA, Davis SM, Chambers BR, et al for the Australian Streptokinase (ASK) Trial Study Group. Streptokinase for acute ischemic stroke with relationship to time of administration. JAMA 1996;276(12):961–6.

[14] Multicentre Acute Stroke Trial–Italy (MAST-I) Group. Randomised controlled trial of streptokinase, aspirin, and combination of both in treatment of acute ischaemic stroke. Lancet 1995;346(8989):1509–14.

[15] Haley Jr EC, Brott TG, Sheppard GL, et al for the TPA Bridging Study Group. Pilot randomized trial of tissue plasminogen activator in acute ischemic stroke. Stroke 1993;24(7):1000–4.

[16] Wardlaw J, del Zoppo G, Yamaguchi T, et al. Thrombolysis for acute ischaemic stroke. Cochrane Database Syst Rev 2005;2:CD000213.

[17] Abe T, Kazama M, Naito I, et al. Clinical evaluation for efficacy of tissue cultured urokinase (TCUK) on cerebral thrombosis by means of multi-centre double blind study. Blood vessels 1981;12:321–41.

[18] Atarashi J, Ohtomo E, Araki G, et al. Clinical utility of urokinase in the treatment of acute stage cerebral thrombosis: multi-center double blind study in comparison with placebo. Clinical Evaluation 1985;13:659–709.

[19] Ohtomo E, Araki G, Itoh E, et al. Clinical efficacy of urokinase in the treatment of cerebral thrombosis: multi-center double-blind study in comparison with placebo. Clinical Evaluation 1985;15(3):711–31.

[20] The National Institute of Neurological Disorders and Stroke rt-PA Stroke Study Group. Tissue plasminogen activator for acute ischemic stroke. N Engl J Med 1995;333(24):1581–7.

[21] Morris AD, Ritchie C, Grosset DG, et al. A pilot study of streptokinase for acute cerebral infarction. QJM 1995;88(10):727–31.

[22] Schriger DL, Kalafut M, Starkman S, et al. Cranial computed tomography interpretation in acute stroke: physician accuracy in determining eligibility for thrombolytic therapy. JAMA 1998;279(16):1293–7.

[23] Wardlaw JM, Dorman PJ, Lewis SC, et al. Can stroke physicians and neuroradiologists identify signs of early cerebral infarction on CT? J Neurol Neurosurg Psychiatry 1999;67(5):651–3.

[24] Fisher M, Pessin MS, Furian AJ. ECASS: lessons for future thrombolytic stroke trials. European Cooperative Acute Stroke Study. JAMA 1995;274(13):1058–9.

[25] Cornu C, Boutitie F, Candelise L, et al for the Thrombolysis in Acute Stroke Pooling Project. Streptokinase in acute ischemic stroke: an individual patient data meta-analysis. Stroke 2000;31(7):1555–60.

[26] The NINDS t-PA Stroke Study Group. Intracerebral hemorrhage after intravenous t-PA therapy for ischemic stroke. Stroke 1997;28(11):2109–18.

[27] Patel SC, Levine SR, Tilley BC, et al. Lack of clinical significance of early ischemic changes on computed tomography in acute stroke. JAMA 2001;286(22):2830–8.

[28] Albers GW, Bates VE, Clark WM, et al for the Standard Treatment with Alteplase to Reverse Stroke (STARS) study. Intravenous tissue-type plasminogen activator for treatment of acute stroke. JAMA 2000;283(9):1145–50.

[29] del Zoppo GJ, Poeck K, Pessin MS, et al. Recombinant tissue plasminogen activator in acute thrombotic and embolic stroke. Ann Neurol 1992;32(1):78–86.

[30] Toni D, Fiorelli M, Bastianello S, et al. Acute ischemic strokes improving during the first 48 hours of onset: predictability, outcome, and possible mechanisms: a comparison with early deteriorating strokes. Stroke 1997;28(1):10–4.

[31] Firlik AD, Rubin G, Yonas H, et al. Relation between cerebral blood flow and neurologic deficit resolution in acute ischemic stroke. Neurology 1998;51(1):177–82.

[32] Kilpatrick MM, Yonas H, Goldstein S, et al. CT-based assessment of acute stroke: CT, CT angiography, and xenon-enhanced CT cerebral blood flow. Stroke 2001;32(11):2543–9.

[33] Baird AE, Donnan GA, Austin MC, et al. Reperfusion after thrombolytic therapy in ischemic stroke measured by single-photon emission computed tomography. Stroke 1994;25(1):79–85.

[34] Overgaard K, Sperling B, Boysen G, et al. Thrombolytic therapy in acute ischemic stroke: a Danish pilot study. Stroke 1993;24(10):1439–46.

[35] Yasaka M, O'Keefe GJ, Chambers BR, et al for the Australian Streptokinase Trial Study Group. Streptokinase in acute stroke: effect on reperfusion and recanalization. Neurology 1998;50(3):626–32.

[36] Burgin WS, Malkoff M, Felberg RA, et al. Transcranial doppler ultrasound criteria for recanalization after thrombolysis for middle cerebral artery stroke. Stroke 2000;31(5):1128–32.

[37] Wildermuth S, Knauth M, Brandt T, et al. Role of CT angiography in patient selection for thrombolytic therapy in acute hemispheric stroke. Stroke 1998;29(5):935–8.

[38] Labiche LA, Malkoff M, Alexandrov AV. Residual flow signals predict complete recanalization in stroke patients treated with TPA. J Neuroimaging 2003;13(1):28–33.

[39] Christou I, Felberg RA, Demchuk AM, et al. Intravenous tissue plasminogen activator and flow improvement in acute ischemic stroke patients with internal carotid artery occlusion. J Neuroimaging 2002;12(2):119–23.

[40] Christou I, Burgin WS, Alexandrov AV, et al. Arterial status after intravenous TPA therapy for ischaemic stroke: a need for further interventions. Int Angiol 2001;20(3):208–13.

[41] Linfante I, Llinas RH, Selim M, et al. Clinical and vascular outcome in internal carotid artery versus middle cerebral artery occlusions after intravenous tissue plasminogen activator. Stroke 2002;33(8):2066–71.

[42] Labiche LA, Al-Senani F, Wojner AW, et al. Is the benefit of early recanalization sustained at 3 months? a prospective cohort study. Stroke 2003;34(3):695–8.

[43] Molina CA, Montaner J, Abilleira S, et al. Timing of spontaneous recanalization and risk of hemorrhagic transformation in acute cardioembolic stroke. Stroke 2001;32(5):1079–84.

[44] Demchuk AM, Burgin WS, Christou I, et al. Thrombolysis in brain ischemia (TIBI) transcranial Doppler flow grades predict clinical severity, early recovery, and mortality in patients treated with intravenous tissue plasminogen activator. Stroke 2001;32(1):89–93.

[45] Alexandrov AV, Grotta JC. Arterial reocclusion in stroke patients treated with intravenous tissue plasminogen activator. Neurology 2002;59(6):862–7.

[46] Alexandrov AV, Molina CA, Grotta JC, et al. Ultrasound-enhanced systemic thrombolysis for acute ischemic stroke. N Engl J Med 2004;351(21):2170–8.

[47] Eggers J, Koch B, Meyer K, et al. Effect of ultrasound on thrombolysis of middle cerebral artery occlusion. Ann Neurol 2003;53(6):797–800.

[48] Hacke W, Kaste M, Fieschi C, et al for the Second European-Australasian Acute Stroke Study Investigators. Randomised double-blind placebo-controlled trial of thrombolytic therapy with intravenous alteplase in acute ischaemic stroke (ECASS II). Lancet 1998;352(9136):1245–51.

[49] Clark WM, Albers GW, Madden KP, et al. The rtPA (alteplase) 0- to 6-hour acute stroke trial, part A (A0276g): results of a double-blind, placebo-controlled, multicenter study: thromblytic therapy in acute ischemic stroke study investigators. Stroke 2000;31(4):811–6.

[50] Clark WM, Wissman S, Albers GW, et al. Recombinant tissue-type plasminogen activator (Alteplase) for ischemic stroke 3 to 5 hours after symptom onset: the ATLANTIS Study: a randomized controlled trial. JAMA 1999;282(21):2019–26.

[51] Koennecke HC, Nohr R, Leistner S, et al. Intravenous tPA for ischemic stroke team performance over time, safety, and efficacy in a single-center, 2-year experience. Stroke 2001;32(5):1074–8.

[52] von Kummer R, Nolte PN, Schnittger H, et al. Detectability of cerebral hemisphere ischaemic infarcts by CT within 6 h of stroke. Neuroradiology 1996;38(1):31–3.

[53] von Kummer R, Meyding-Lamade U, Forsting M, et al. Sensitivity and prognostic value of early CT in occlusion of the middle cerebral artery trunk. AJNR Am J Neuroradiol 1994;15(1):9–18 [discussion: 16–8].

[54] Lev MH, Farkas J, Gemmete JJ, et al. Acute stroke: improved nonenhanced CT detection–benefits of soft-copy interpretation by using variable window width and center level settings. Radiology 1999;213(1):150–5.

[55] Barber PA, Demchuk AM, Zhang J, et al for the ASPECTS Study Group. Validity and reliability of a quantitative computed tomography score in predicting outcome of hyperacute stroke before thrombolytic therapy: Alberta Stroke Programme early CT score. Lancet 2000;355(9216):1670–4.

[56] Katzan IL, Furlan AJ, Lloyd LE, et al. Use of tissue-type plasminogen activator for acute ischemic stroke: the Cleveland area experience. JAMA 2000; 283(9): 1151–8.

[57] Alberts MJ, Hademenos G, Latchaw RE, et al for the Brain Attack Coalition. Recommendations for the establishment of primary stroke centers. JAMA 2000;283(23):3102–9.

[58] Schwamm LH, Pancioli A, Acker III JE, Goldstein LB, et al. Recommendations for the establishment of stroke systems of care: recommendations from the American Stroke Association's Task Force on the Development of Stroke Systems. Stroke 2005;36(3): 690–703.

[59] Shafqat S, Kvedar JC, Guanci MM, et al. Role for telemedicine in acute stroke. Feasibility and reliability of remote administration of the NIH stroke scale. Stroke 1999;30(10):2141–5.

[60] Schwamm LH, Rosenthal ES, Hirshberg A, et al. Virtual TeleStroke support for the emergency department evaluation of acute stroke. Acad Emerg Med 2004;11(11):1193–7.

[61] Wang S, Gross H, Lee SB, et al. Remote evaluation of acute ischemic stroke in rural community hospitals in Georgia. Stroke 2004;35(7):1763–8.

[62] Audebert HJ, Kukla C, Clarmann von Claranau S, et al. Telemedicine for safe and extended use of thrombolysis in stroke: the Telemedic Pilot Project for Integrative Stroke Care (TEMPiS) in Bavaria. Stroke 2005;36(2):287–91.

[63] Lev MH, Nichols SJ. Computed tomographic angiography and computed tomographic perfusion imaging of hyperacute stroke. Top Magn Reson Imaging 2000;11(5):273–87.

[64] Schramm P, Schellinger PD, Fiebach JB, et al. Comparison of CT and CT angiography source images with diffusion-weighted imaging in patients with acute stroke within 6 hours after onset. Stroke 2002;33(10):2426–32.

[65] Coutts SB, Lev MH, Eliasziw M, et al. ASPECTS on CTA source images versus unenhanced CT: added value in predicting final infarct extent and clinical outcome. Stroke 2004;35(11):2472–6.

[66] Ezzeddine MA, Lev MH, McDonald CT, et al. CT angiography with whole brain perfused blood volume imaging: added clinical value in the assessment of acute stroke. Stroke 2002;33(4):959–66.

[67] Schwamm LH, Rosenthal ES, Swap CJ, et al. Hypoattenuation on CTA source images predicts risk of intracerebral hemorrhage and outcome after intra-arterial reperfusion therapy. AJNR Am J Neuroradiol 2005;26(7):1798–803.

[68] Knauth M, von Kummer R, Jansen O, et al. Potential of CT angiography in acute ischemic stroke. AJNR Am J Neuroradiol 1997;18(6):1001–10.

[69] Shrier DA, Tanaka H, Numaguchi Y, et al. CT angiography in the evaluation of acute stroke. AJNR Am J Neuroradiol 1997;18(6):1011–20.

[70] Lev MH, Farkas J, Rodriguez VR, et al. CT angiography in the rapid triage of patients with hyperacute stroke to intraarterial thrombolysis: accuracy in the detection of large vessel thrombus. J Comput Assist Tomogr 2001;25(4):520–8.

[71] Sims JR, Rordorf G, Smith EE, et al. Arterial occlusion revealed by CT angiography predicts NIH stroke score and acute outcomes after IV tPA treatment. AJNR Am J Neuroradiol 2005;26(2): 246–51.

[72] Verro P, Tanenbaum LN, Borden NM, et al. CT angiography in acute ischemic stroke: preliminary results. Stroke 2002;33(1):276–8.

[73] Lev MH, Segal AZ, Farkas J, et al. Utility of perfusion-weighted CT imaging in acute middle cerebral artery stroke treated with intra-arterial thrombolysis: prediction of final infarct volume and clinical outcome. Stroke 2001;32(9):2021–8.

[74] Sorensen AG, Buonanno FS, Gonzalez RG, et al. Hyperacute stroke: evaluation with combined multi-section diffusion-weighted and hemodynamically weighted echo-planar MR imaging. Radiology 1996; 199(2):391–401.

[75] Fiebach JB, Schellinger PD, Jansen O, et al. CT and diffusion-weighted MR imaging in randomized order: diffusion-weighted imaging results in higher accuracy and lower interrater variability in the diagnosis of hyperacute ischemic stroke. Stroke 2002;33(9): 2206–10.

[76] Mullins ME, Schaefer PW, Sorensen AG, et al. CT and conventional and diffusion-weighted MR imaging in acute stroke: study in 691 patients at presentation to the emergency department. Radiology 2002; 224(2):353–60.

[77] Arenillas JF, Rovira A, Molina CA, et al. Prediction of early neurological deterioration using diffusion- and perfusion-weighted imaging in hyperacute middle cerebral artery ischemic stroke. Stroke 2002; 33(9):2197–203.

[78] Takahashi K, Kobayashi S, Matui R, et al. The differences of clinical parameters between small multiple ischemic lesions and single lesion detected by diffusion-weighted MRI. Acta Neurol Scand 2002; 106(1):24–9.

[79] Gass A, Ay H, Szabo K, et al. Diffusion-weighted MRI for the "small stuff": the details of acute cerebral ischaemia. Lancet Neurol 2004;3(1):39–45.

[80] Lee LJ, Kidwell CS, Alger J, et al. Impact on stroke subtype diagnosis of early diffusion-weighted magnetic resonance imaging and magnetic resonance angiography. Stroke 2000;31(5):1081–9.

[81] Ay H, Oliveira-Filho J, Buonanno FS, et al. Diffusion-weighted imaging identifies a subset of lacunar infarction associated with embolic source. Stroke 1999;30(12):2644–50.

[82] Grant PE, He J, Halpern EF, Wu O, et al. Frequency and clinical context of decreased apparent diffusion coefficient reversal in the human brain. Radiology 2001;221(1):43–50.

[83] Schaefer PW, Hassankhani A, Putman C, et al. Characterization and evolution of diffusion MR imaging abnormalities in stroke patients undergoing intra-arterial thrombolysis. AJNR Am J Neuroradiol 2004;25(6):951–7.

[84] Kidwell CS, Saver JL, Mattiello J, et al. Thrombolytic reversal of acute human cerebral ischemic injury shown by diffusion/perfusion magnetic resonance imaging. Ann Neurol 2000;47(4):462–9.

[85] Guadagno JV, Warburton EA, Aigbirhio FI, et al. Does the acute diffusion-weighted imaging lesion represent penumbra as well as core? a combined quantitative PET/MRI voxel-based study. J Cereb Blood Flow Metab 2004;24(11):1249–54.

[86] Schaefer PW, Hunter GJ, He J, et al. Predicting cerebral ischemic infarct volume with diffusion and perfusion MR imaging. AJNR Am J Neuroradiol 2002;23(10):1785–94.

[87] Schlaug G, Benfield A, Baird AE, et al. The ischemic penumbra: operationally defined by diffusion and perfusion MRI. Neurology 1999;53(7):1528–37.

[88] Barber PA, Davis SM, Darby DG, et al. Absent middle cerebral artery flow predicts the presence and evolution of the ischemic penumbra. Neurology 1999;52(6):1125–32.

[89] Rordorf G, Koroshetz WJ, Copen WA, et al. Regional ischemia and ischemic injury in patients with acute middle cerebral artery stroke as defined by early diffusion-weighted and perfusion-weighted MRI. Stroke 1998;29(5):939–43.

[90] Marchal G, Beaudouin V, Rioux P, et al. Prolonged persistence of substantial volumes of potentially viable brain tissue after stroke: a correlative PET-CT study with voxel-based data analysis. Stroke 1996;27(4):599–606.

[91] Darby DG, Barber PA, Gerraty RP, et al. Pathophysiological topography of acute ischemia by combined diffusion-weighted and perfusion MRI. Stroke 1999;30(10):2043–52.

[92] Markus R, Reutens DC, Kazui S, et al. Hypoxic tissue in ischaemic stroke: persistence and clinical consequences of spontaneous survival. Brain 2004; 127(Pt 6):1427–36.

[93] von Kummer R, Allen KL, Holle R, et al. Acute stroke: usefulness of early CT findings before thrombolytic therapy. Radiology 1997;205(2):327–33.

[94] Hacke W, Albers G, Al-Rawi Y, et al. The Desmoteplase in Acute Ischemic Stroke Trial (DIAS): a phase II MRI-based 9-hour window acute stroke thrombolysis trial with intravenous desmoteplase. Stroke 2005;36(1):66–73.

[95] Furlan A. Dose escalation study of desmetoplase in acute ischemic stroke. Presented at the International Stroke Conference. New Orleans, Louisiana, February 2–4, 2005.

[96] Furlan A, Higashida R, Wechsler L, et al. Intra-arterial prourokinase for acute ischemic stroke: the PROACT II study: a randomized controlled trial: prolyse in acute cerebral thromboembolism. JAMA 1999;282(21):2003–11.

[97] Hacke W, Donnan G, Fieschi C, et al. Association of outcome with early stroke treatment: pooled analysis of ATLANTIS, ECASS, and NINDS rt-PA stroke trials. Lancet 2004;363(9411):768–74.

[98] Lee JM, Vo KD, An H, Celik A, et al. Magnetic resonance cerebral metabolic rate of oxygen utilization in hyperacute stroke patients. Ann Neurol 2003; 53(2):227–32.

[99] Rother J, Schellinger PD, Gass A, et al. Effect of intravenous thrombolysis on MRI parameters and functional outcome in acute stroke less than 6 hours. Stroke 2002;33(10):2438–45.

[100] Parsons MW, Barber PA, Chalk J, et al. Diffusion- and perfusion-weighted MRI response to thrombolysis in stroke. Ann Neurol 2002;51(1):28–37.

[101] Wintermark M, Reichhart M, Cuisenaire O, et al. Comparison of admission perfusion computed tomography and qualitative diffusion- and perfusion-weighted magnetic resonance imaging in acute stroke patients. Stroke 2002;33(8):2025–31.

[102] Wintermark M, Reichhart M, Thiran JP, et al. Prognostic accuracy of cerebral blood flow measurement by perfusion computed tomography, at the time of emergency room admission, in acute stroke patients. Ann Neurol 2002;51(4):417–32.

[103] Butcher KS. Echoplanar imaging thrombolysis evaluation trial: EPITHET. Presented at the 30th International Stroke Conference. New Orleans, Louisiana, February 2–4, 2005.

[104] Stroke Trials Directory Website. Diffusion-weighted imaging evaluation for understanding stroke evolution. Available at: http://www.strokecenter.org/trials/TrialDetail.asp?ref=588&browse=D. Accessed March 8, 2005.

[105] Hacke W, Kaste M, Fieschi C, et al. A placebo controlled trial of alteplase (rt-PA) in acute ischemic hemispheric stroke where trhombolysis is initiated between 3 and 4 hours after stroke onset. ECASS III. Presented at the International Stroke Conference. Phoenix, Arizona, 2003.

[106] Kane I, Sandercock P, Lindley R for Group I-C. Third international stroke trial. Presented at the

30th International Stroke Conference. New Orleans, Louisiana, February 2–4, 2005.

[107] Ciccone A, Boccardi E, Cantisani TA, et al. A randomized comparison of intra-arterial with intra-venous thrombolysis for acute ischemic stroke: the SYNTHESIS Trial. Presented at the 30th International Stroke Conference. New Orleans, Louisiana, February 2–4, 2005.

[108] Dunn B, Warach S. ReoPro retavase reperfusion of stroke safety study: imaging evaluation. Presented at the 30th International Stroke Conference. New Orleans, LouisianaA, February 2–4, 2005.

[109] Lee KY, Kim DI, Kim SH, et al. Sequential combination of intravenous recombinant tissue plasminogen activator and intra-arterial urokinase in acute ischemic stroke. AJNR Am J Neuroradiol 2004;25(9):1470–5.

[110] Zaidat OO, Suarez JI, Santillan C, et al. Response to intra-arterial and combined intravenous and intra-arterial thrombolytic therapy in patients with distal internal carotid artery occlusion. Stroke 2002;33(7): 1821–6.

[111] Keris V, Rudnicka S, Vorona V, et al. Combined intraarterial/intravenous thrombolysis for acute ischemic stroke. AJNR Am J Neuroradiol 2001;22(2): 352–8.

[112] Lewandowski CA, Frankel M, Tomsick TA, et al, for the Emergency Management of Stroke (EMS) Bridging Trial. Combined intravenous and intra-arterial r-TPA versus intra-arterial therapy of acute ischemic stroke. Stroke 1999;30(12):2598–605.

[113] Broderick JP, Tomsick TA. Interventional management of stroke study: part II (IMS II). Presented at the 30th International Stroke Conference. New Orleans, Louisiana, February 2–4, 2005.

[114] Tsushima Y, Aoki J, Endo K. Brain microhemorrhages detected on T2*-weighted gradient-echo MR images. AJNR Am J Neuroradiol 2003;24(1):88–96.

[115] Nighoghossian N, Hermier M, Adeleine P, et al. Old microbleeds are a potential risk factor for cerebral bleeding after ischemic stroke: a gradient-echo T2*-weighted brain MRI study. Stroke 2002;33(3): 735–42.

[116] Derex L, Nighoghossian N, Hermier M, et al. Thrombolysis for ischemic stroke in patients with old microbleeds on pretreatment MRI. Cerebrovasc Dis 2004;17(2–3):238–41.

[117] Latour LL, Kang DW, Ezzeddine MA, et al. Early blood-brain barrier disruption in human focal brain ischemia. Ann Neurol 2004;56(4):468–77.

[118] Barber PA, Foniok T, Kirk D, Buchan AM, et al. MR molecular imaging of early endothelial activation in focal ischemia. Ann Neurol 2004;56(1):116–20.

[119] Botnar RM, Perez AS, Witte S, et al. In vivo molecular imaging of acute and subacute thrombosis using a fibrin-binding magnetic resonance imaging contrast agent. Circulation 2004;109(16):2023–9.

[120] Winter PM, Caruthers SD, Yu X, et al. Improved molecular imaging contrast agent for detection of human thrombus. Magn Reson Med 2003;50(2):411–6.

[121] Zhou J, Payen JF, Wilson DA, et al. Using the amide proton signals of intracellular proteins and peptides to detect pH effects in MRI. Nat Med 2003;9(8): 1085–90.

ELSEVIER
SAUNDERS

Neuroimag Clin N Am 15 (2005) 441 – 453

Catheter-Based Recanalization Techniques for Acute Ischemic Stroke

Andrew R. Xavier, MD[a], Jeffrey Farkas, MD[b],*

[a]*Department of Neurosciences, University of Medicine and Dentistry–New Jersey Medical School, Newark, NJ, USA*
[b]*Interventional Neuroradiology, Maimonides Medical Center, Brooklyn, NY, USA*

Most patients with acute ischemic stroke have thromboembolic material occluding large cerebral vessels, and hence disruption of cerebral blood flow [1–3]. If the arterial occlusion is relieved in a timely manner, a substantial reduction in the size and severity of the cerebral infarction can be achieved [4–7], with significant improvement in the level of disability among survivors [8].

For nearly a decade, the only recanalization strategy for acute ischemic stroke approved by the US Food and Drug Administration (FDA) was intravenous thrombolysis using tissue-type plasminogen activator (t-PA), alteplase (Genentech, San Francisco, California). Since its approval in 1995, t-PA has become a widely implemented strategy in the management of acute ischemic stroke, propelling the development of numerous primary stroke centers. The widespread clinical application of this strategy has confirmed its usefulness in a narrowly selected group of patients; the narrow selection criteria have, however, excluded most patients from receiving this therapy [9,10].

Widespread clinical use has also highlighted some of the serious limitations of intravenous t-PA that were originally observed in the clinical trials. Intravenous t-PA has only a limited role to play in the setting of a large thromboembolic burden, as seen in patients with acute occlusions of the internal carotid artery (ICA), proximal middle cerebral artery (MCA) [11], and basilar artery (BA). It works best in the

setting of a smaller clot burden, with occlusions of distal intracerebral branches [12]. Clinically, this translates into a better response in mild to moderate stroke, as compared with only a modest benefit in severe ischemic stroke [13]. Hence, supplemental or alternate treatment strategies might be essential to manage patients with more proximal occlusions. In addition, a significant proportion of patients excluded from intravenous t-PA might benefit from alternative recanalization strategies, such as catheter-directed thrombolysis (Fig. 1).

The intra-arterial approach to thrombolysis has the following advantages: (1) higher concentrations of thrombolytic agents can be administered locally without inducing excessive systemic thrombolysis, (2) better dose titration with angiographic visualization of clot lysis, and (3) mechanical devices for clot retrieval and lysis. Recent FDA approval of the Mechanical Embolus Removal in Cerebral Ischemia (Merci) retrieval device (Concentric Medical, Mountain View, California; Fig. 2) has made one such technology available for routine clinical use; a number of other devices are in various stages of investigation.

With the availability of more than one therapeutic approach, the treatment of acute ischemic stroke has started to move away from a "one size fits all" mentality to the development of increasingly complex algorithms aimed at rapid evaluation of patients with acute neurologic syndromes as well as to triage to different treatment pathways. Diagnostic neuroimaging has kept pace with these rapid developments in stroke therapeutics. We now have the diagnostic imaging tools to evaluate suspected stroke patients in a timely manner and to obtain noninvasive real-

* Corresponding author.
E-mail address: jfarkas@maimonidesmed.org
(J. Farkas).

1052-5149/05/$ – see front matter © 2005 Elsevier Inc. All rights reserved.
doi:10.1016/j.nic.2005.06.007

neuroimaging.theclinics.com

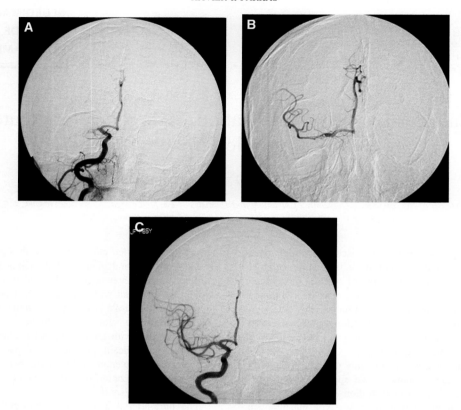

Fig. 1. (*A*) Digital subtraction angiogram (DSA), anteroposterior (AP) view, shows occlusion of the proximal right MCA. (*B*) Microcatheter injection after the 8-mg infusion of recombinant tissue-type plasminogen activator (rt-PA)), using catheter-directed thrombolysis. There has been restoration of antegrade flow in the MCA (degree of flow restoration must be judged on the basis of the guide catheter angiogram and not from the microcatheter injection). (*C*) After intra-arterial thrombolysis (rt-PA, 12.5 mg), there has been complete recanalization of the MCA.

time information about the integrity of the cerebral circulation and viability of brain parenchyma. More rational treatment decisions can be made when the clinical status and hemodynamic status of the patient are known. Therapeutic options based on incomplete evaluations cannot be subscribed to. If we limit the imaging evaluation, we are too often limiting the therapeutic options.

Imaging rationale

The goal of therapy is to restore perfusion to the ischemic but potentially salvageable brain parenchyma ("viable penumbra") rather than to the irreversibly damaged brain tissue ("infarct core"). In severely ischemic regions, the integrity of the blood-brain barrier may already be compromised and re-

establishing perfusion might actually do more harm in the form of reperfusion injury and hemorrhage. Depending on the degree of ischemia, this may occur within minutes (Fig. 3). Conversely, patients with borderline ischemic blood flow may benefit from reperfusion therapy much later than the traditional 3- to 6-hour time window (Fig. 4).

The endovascular treatment strategy varies depending on the identification and location of a large vessel occlusion. Patients with small distal occlusions do not benefit from emergent diagnostic angiography. Valuable time would be wasted in pursuing angiography, not to mention the potential complications and expense. Diagnostic arteriography should be reserved for those patients for whom therapeutic maneuvers are also likely be performed.

Determining the cause and location of the occlusive lesion before angiography allows the interventionalist to save valuable time by planning the

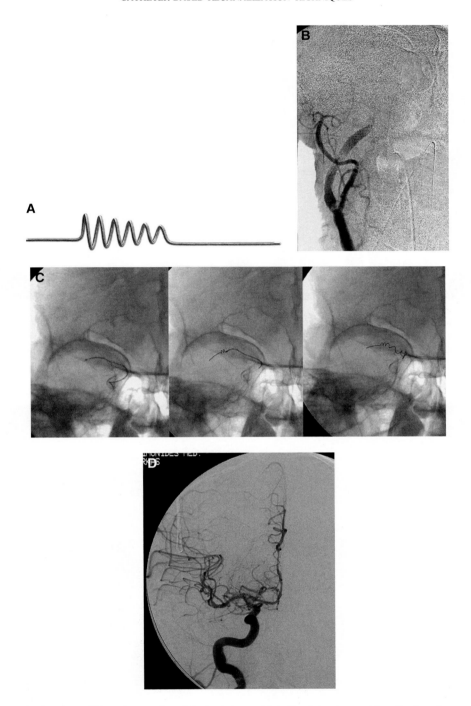

Fig. 2. (*A*) Merci retriever. This corkscrew-shaped device is inserted into the clot and can retrieve the thrombus, supplementing or obviating the need for thrombolytic medication. (*B*) Late-phase right internal carotid angiogram demonstrating an occlusion of the distal extracranial ICA. CTA (not shown) confirms that there is a thrombus in the distal right ICA extending to the MCA. (*C*) Images demonstrate progressive deployment of the Merci retriever into the right MCA. (*D*) After clot retrieval, excellent flow has been re-established in the right MCA and ICA.

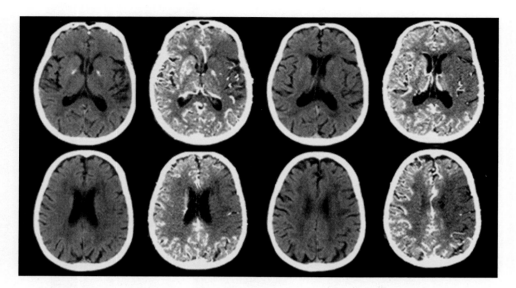

Fig. 3. Unenhanced CT (*odd columns*), with corresponding CTA source images (*even columns*) in a patient with an acute left MCA occlusion. Whereas the noncontrast study demonstrates subtle ischemic hypodensity of the gray matter compared with the white matter, the CTA source perfusion images clearly demonstrate a severe blood volume deficit in the left MCA distribution. Despite early and successful reperfusion, this patient's final infarct size was large, as predicted by the CTA source perfusion images.

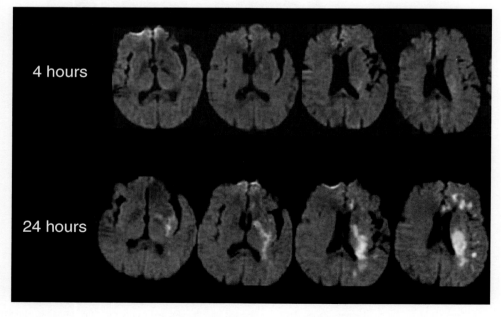

Fig. 4. Diffusion images obtained at 4 (*top row*) and 24 (*bottom row*) hours after the onset of stroke symptoms. Although this patient was symptomatic at 4 hours, there was minimal evidence for infarction. Delayed diffusion-weighted imaging at 24 hours confirmed restricted diffusion consistent with cytotoxic edema and infarction.

treatment approach as the patient is being prepared. Treatment varies depending on whether the lesion is proximal or distal, whether there is underlying atherosclerotic stenosis at the occlusion site, and whether the proximal extracranial vessel is open or closed. In the setting of proximal arterial occlusions, the primary approach may be to attempt clot retrieval, such as with the Merci device, supplemented by direct catheter-directed thrombolysis. If there is severe stenosis proximal to the occlusion, treatment of the stenosis may be necessary before or immediately after restoring intracranial flow. Larger sized sheaths or specialized balloon guide catheters are necessary for stent placement or clot retrieval, whereas smaller and more easily placed guide catheters are all that is necessary for intra-arterial thrombolysis. Significant time could be saved by choosing the appropriate device up front.

Outcomes depend not only on appropriate therapy but on patient selection. Physicians who routinely treat acute stroke know that "time is brain"; however, time from symptom onset is only one crude marker for cerebrovascular status. Patient-specific factors can be more predictive and should be accounted for if possible. Radiologic assessment of cerebral perfusion is just beginning to be incorporated into therapeutic stroke trials. In the acute stroke setting, the least time-consuming study that can obtain all information necessary to triage patients adequately based on cerebral viability and perfusion status should ideally be performed. Ultimately, the type and complexity of the chosen imaging protocol depend on the specific therapeutic options that are available.

Noncontrast head CT

Noncontrast head CT is currently the standard examination that is universally obtained for all patients with new-onset neurologic symptoms. Although unenhanced CT can reliably differentiate between hemorrhagic and nonhemorrhagic causes of cerebral dysfunction, it cannot currently reliably detect ischemic stroke in the hyperacute state.

Definitive hypodensity on unenhanced CT typically reflects parenchyma destined for irreversible infarction. Patients with a normal CT scan and symptoms suggesting ischemia are considered to be ideal treatment candidates. The early ischemic signs (EISs) of stroke are often subtle; these earliest changes, such as effacement of sulci or subtle hypodensity, may not be easy to recognize. Early CT changes can be accentuated by manipulation of the window width

and center level review settings [14]. During the European Cooperative Study of Acute Stroke [15], there was a significant false-negative CT scan interpretation rate. It was this subgroup of treated patients who were thought by some to undermine the benefits of the study. Hence, even a noncontrast CT scan can provide much more information than ruling out hemorrhage in the acute setting, as discussed at length in other articles in this issue.

Advanced CT techniques for endovascular therapy triage

The addition of CT angiography (CTA) to routine unenhanced head CT provides critical information without lengthy imaging times or the necessity of moving the patient to another scanner. The data that CTA provides help to define the degree and severity of the ischemic insult. In an examination that takes only a few minutes, several additional pieces of information can be gleaned. CTA source images (CTA-SIs), which are blood volume weighted, help to determine the presence, location, and size of the territory likely to be irreversibly infarcted. Visualization of a large vessel occlusion on CTA is crucial in identifying patients who could benefit from aggressive treatments, such local intra-arterial thrombolysis. Even for patients with major clinical deficits, if a large vessel occlusion is not detected, attempts at intra-arterial thrombolysis might not only potentially waste valuable time but be futile. In such cases, alternative treatment options would be considered.

In a Canadian study [16], the perception of improving clinical deficits was cited as the most important reason not to treat otherwise eligible stroke patients aggressively. Follow-up revealed that a full one third of these patients died or remained dependent as a consequence of their admission ischemic insult. Clearly, initial clinical impressions can be misleading. A more complete understanding of the precise pathophysiology and hemodynamics of the ischemic insult, including knowledge of the collateral flow distribution, has the potential to improve physician decision making. If these patients had undergone CTA and a vascular occlusion had been identified, prompt treatment might have prevented delayed progressive neurologic deterioration. Conversely, had CTA been negative for a large vessel occlusion, withholding aggressive endovascular therapy is far more rational.

Some interventionists advocate immediate diagnostic arteriography based on clinical evaluation and time from onset. The reasoning is to prevent delays in therapy. Proceeding directly to angiography, however, without specific confirmation of vascular occlusion, could result in a significant number of patients who undergo the risks of angiography but do not qualify for intra-arterial therapy. Given the nontrivial angiographic complication rate, rapid noninvasive imaging to determine who best qualifies for intra-arterial therapy could be of value. Specifically, CTA could be used to identify patients with large vessel occlusions [17]. Multiple studies have confirmed the accuracy of CTA in identifying such occlusions.

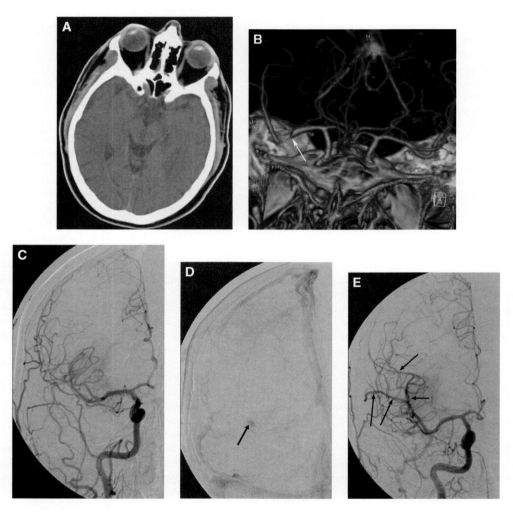

Fig. 5. (*A*) Unenhanced CT scan of a 48-year-old left-handed man 1 hour status post onset of left hemiplegia and aphasia (National Institute of Health Stroke Scale [NIHSS] score of 22). No definite hyperdense vessel is present. (*B*) Volume-rendered CTA image demonstrates complete occlusion of the right distal M1 segment of the MCA. The CT angiogram was obtained 45 minutes after the infusion of intravenous recombinant tissue-type plasminogen activator (rt-PA) at a dose of 0.6 mg/kg ("bridging therapy" in anticipation of further intra-arterial treatment to be performed). At the time of the CTA, there was no clinical improvement. (*C*) Same patient 30 minutes later; digital subtraction angiography of the right internal carotid artery demonstrates that the MCA has reopened. (*D*) Careful evaluation demonstrates a persistent occlusion of the inferior division of the right MCA; the delayed-phase angiogram demonstrates enhancing embolic occlusion (*arrow*). Clinically, the patient has started to move his right leg, yet he remains aphasic and hemiplegic in the upper extremity. (*E*) Intra-arterial rt-PA (4 mg) has been administered to the inferior division of the right MCA, which has now recanalized. At this time, his right arm moves against gravity and his speech has improved. The 24-hour NIHSS score is 3. Arrows point to the recanalized inferior division MCA branch. Large vessel occlusions can sometimes be subtle on angiography, as in *C*.

Intra-arterial thrombolysis

Interventionalists have applied a large variety of agents in the treatment of acute cerebrovascular occlusions. t-PA is currently the most frequently used agent for intra-arterial thrombolysis in acute ischemic stroke. It is a naturally occurring enzyme that activates plasminogen into active plasmin, which dissolves fibrin, causing thrombolysis.

We treated 40 acute ischemic stroke patients who were not candidates for intravenous thrombolysis with intra-arterial t-PA over a 40-month period.

The patients were aged 65 ± 17 years (range: 21–94 years), and 22 were men. Twenty-three (58%) had arterial occlusions in the MCA; 11 (28%) had occlusions in the ICA, 4 (10%) had occlusions in the BA, and 1 (2%) had an occlusion in the anterior cerebral artery (ACA). One patient had spontaneous recanalization during the initial diagnostic angiogram. The mean National Institutes of Health Stroke Scale (NIHSS) score on admission was 19. The mean t-PA dose was 9 mg (range: 3–24 mg). Recanalization to thrombolysis in myocardial infarction (TIMI) grade II or III was seen in 92% of

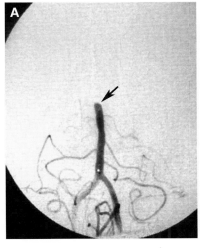
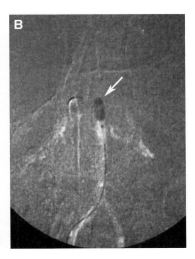
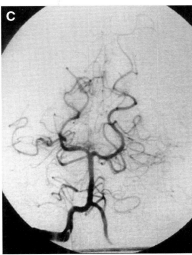

Fig. 6. (*A*) Anteroposterior digital subtraction angiography image demonstrating an acute top of a BA occlusion; the black arrow points to the distal BA. The patient has received urokinase at a total dose of 600,000 U without significant recanalization. (*B*) Roadmap image demonstrating balloon angioplasty with a 4-mm × 10-mm Endeavor device (*arrow*), which was inflated twice. (*C*) After angioplasty, there is complete recanalization of the basilar tip, without visualized distal embolic occlusions.

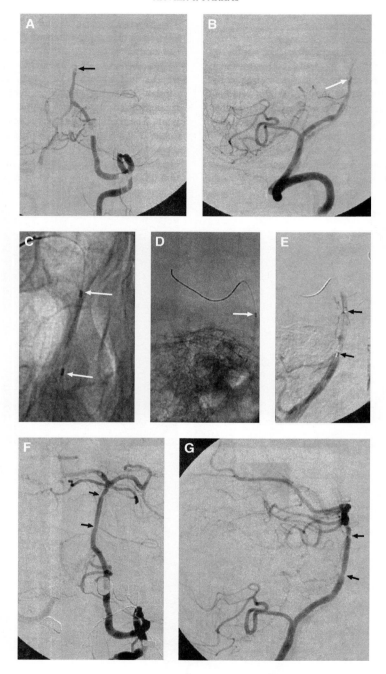

Fig. 7. A 33-year-old man with new-onset headache, followed by 30 minutes of being "locked in." He was awake but unable to move. AP (*A*) and lateral (*B*) digital subtraction angiography (DSA) images show narrowing of the middle BA. The BA beyond the anterior inferior cerebral arteries is intermittently occluded (*arrow*). The findings are consistent with BA dissection. (*C* and *D*) AP and lateral DSA images show a stent being brought into position in the middle BA (*arrows*). (*E*) Lateral DSA view of the BA with the stent, just before deployment, confirms good stent positioning (*arrows*). (*F* and *G*) AP and lateral DSA images show that the deployed stent is in a good position, with excellent restoration of flow throughout the BA. Immediately after stent placement, there is proximal and distal arterial spasm (*arrows*). (*H*) CT angiogram volume reconstruction image of the BA demonstrating the basilar stent and the recanalized artery.

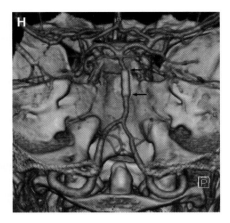

Fig. 7 (*continued*).

the patients. The neurologic outcome was good in 17 (43%) patients, but 5 (12%) patients died. Symptomatic cerebral hemorrhage occurred in 3 patients (7%). The outcome was good in 14 (60%) patients with MCA occlusions and in 3 (27%) patients with ICA occlusions. The outcome was poor in 4 patients with BA occlusions and in the 1 patient with an ACA occlusion.

Until its recent withdrawal and reintroduction into the US market, urokinase was the most widely used intra-arterial thrombolytic agent for acute ischemic stroke. Urokinase is a naturally occurring enzyme that activates plasminogen in a nonspecific manner. It has been the subject of numerous nonrandomized trials and series [18–25]. Pro-urokinase is a proenzyme precursor of urokinase; this second-generation thrombolytic agent is activated to urokinase by fibrin-bound plasmin, resulting in superior fibrin specificity [26]. Its role in acute ischemic stroke has been evaluated by the Prolyse in Acute Cerebral Thromboembolism (PROACT) I and II trials.

PROACT II [27] was the first randomized multicenter clinical trial to demonstrate the efficacy of intra-arterial thrombolysis in patients with acute MCA stroke of less than 6 hours' duration. The study, conducted in 54 centers across the United States and Canada, randomized 180 patients at a ratio of 2:1 to receive intra-arterial pro-urokinase and heparin at a dose of 9 mg (n = 121) or heparin alone (n = 59). The recanalization rate was 66% in the pro-urokinase group and 18% in the control group. The frequency of symptomatic intracranial hemorrhage was 10% in the treatment group and 2% in the control group. A significantly larger number of patients (P = .047) treated with pro-urokinase showed good clinical recovery compared with control patients, as demonstrated by a modified Rankin Scale score of 2 or less at 3 months (40% versus 25%). Higher rates of recanalization were seen in patients who received high-dose versus low-dose heparin, although these same patients had more intracranial hemorrhage as well. Clinically, we prefer a low-dose heparinization scheme when treating patients with intra-arterial t-PA. On average, during a typical intra-arterial lysis case, the patient receives a one-time bolus (2000 U) of intravenous heparin.

Other thrombolytic agents that have been used for intracranial thrombolysis include streptokinase and reteplase. Because of its adverse effects, streptokinase is no longer used. There is limited information about the newer second- and third-generation thrombolytic agents.

Glycoprotein IIb-IIIa inhibitors are also used in conjunction with thrombolytic medications. These agents block the final common pathway for platelet aggregation and, theoretically, should not function as thrombolytic agents. Thrombolytic agents often promote platelet activation, however, causing rapid rethrombosis and partial occlusion. These agents have traditionally been administered intravenously but are being used increasingly with catheter-directed intra-arterial thrombolysis. The appropriate dose for each IIb-IIIa agent varies significantly from center to center. In some centers, cardiac dosages are being used, whereas a modified escalating dose is used during intra-arterial therapy in others.

Combination intra-arterial and lytic ("bridging") therapy

A major limitation of intra-arterial thrombolysis is the inevitable delay associated with angiography and microcatheter navigation to the site of arterial occlusion. Hence, a promising strategy has been to combine the early benefit of intravenous thrombolytic therapy with the more definitive response of an endovascular approach (Fig. 5) [11,28–31]. A theoretic disadvantage would be the potential for increased vascular access difficulties, including puncture site hematoma and bleeding. Our own clinical experience as well as data from coronary trials has found that this is not a significant cause of mortality or morbidity, however.

This strategy has been studied in the Emergency Management of Stroke (EMS) Bridging Trial, a phase II, multicenter, double-blind, randomized trial. That study evaluated the use of combined intravenous and intra-arterial t-PA in patients with acute ischemic stroke presenting within 3 hours of symptom onset

[11]. A total of 35 patients with an NIHSS score greater than 5 were randomized at a ratio of 1:1 to receive intravenous t-PA or placebo (0.6 mg/kg), followed directly by arterial catheterization. After a microcatheter was placed in the proximity of the thrombus, t-PA (2 mg) was infused, followed by an infusion at a rate of 10 mg/h with a maximum intra-arterial dose of 20 mg to achieve definitive recanalization. The median baseline NIHSS score was 16 in the combined intravenous/intra-arterial arm, which dropped to 11 and 7 at 24 hours and 7 days, respectively. Recanalization rates were better (81% versus 50%; $P = .03$) in the combined group, suggesting that this strategy might have better results than a purely intra-arterial approach. A further extension of this study is underway, where the intra-arterial t-PA is administered by a special microcatheter that is capable of generating ultrasound pulses, adding a component of mechanical clot disruption.

Another combination approach takes advantage of the synergic roles played by traditional thrombolytic medications and glycoprotein IIb-IIIa inhibitors. Initial reports suggest improved recanalization rates without excessive complications.

Mechanical thrombolysis

Although the recanalization rates and safety associated with intra-arterial lysis have steadily improved over the last decade, there are still a number of patients who are resistant to pharmacologic thrombolysis. These patients could benefit from a strategy combining pharmacologic thrombolysis with mechanical clot disruption. In addition to treating resistant clots, mechanical methods could help to accelerate the process of thrombolysis, thereby reducing time to recanalization. These mechanical maneuvers include wire and microcatheter manipulation through the clot and balloon angioplasty of stenotic vessels and resistant thrombus (Fig. 6) [32–34].

Most intracerebral occlusions are emboli from proximal donor sites, with the actual site of occlusion being normal in most cases. In addition, proximal cerebral and basilar arteries are rich with perforating branches; hence, treating acute embolic occlusions with stent deployment in those locations has generally not resulted in good outcomes. Only in selected cases do we use intracranial stents to treat acutely ischemic patients. Examples may be patients with ischemia secondary to hypoperfusion or those with known or suspected atherosclerotic occlusions or occlusions secondary to vessel dissections (Figs. 7 and 8).

Some have compared acute ischemic stroke treatment with acute myocardial infarction. Although the treatment for acute myocardial ischemia is increasingly angioplasty and stenting, this approach cannot be applied routinely to stroke. The pathophysiology of acute myocardial infarction is that of acute plaque rupture with occlusion. There is almost always disease of the underlying vessel, such that therapy is aimed at restoring blood flow and repairing the underlying lesion to prevent recurrence. The most common cause of ischemic stroke is acute embolic occlusion; hence, mechanical removal of the offending thrombus should be the goal of therapy. Angioplasty and stenting may recanalize a vessel locally, but multiple distal emboli can have severe clinical consequences as well. Potentially, a better approach to large embolic debris in accessible locations would be the use of thrombus-retrieval devices, and a better approach to that in nonaccessible locations would currently be lytic therapy.

The FDA has recently approved the Concentric clot retrieval device for routine clinical use in acute ischemic stroke within 9 hours of onset. The concentric retriever is a flexible and tapered nickel titanium wire with a helically shaped distal tip that can be deployed intra-arterially to entrap and retrieve large vessel intracerebral clots. The safety and efficacy of the Concentric clot retrieval device for up to 8 hours after symptom onset in patients with an angiographic-

Fig. 8. (A) A 58-year-old man with repeated episodes of expressive aphasia over the prior 3 hours, despite treatment with antiplatelet agents and full anticoagulation. A volume-rendered reconstruction of the left cervical ICA shows a flow gap in the distal vessel. The fact that there is visualization of the ICA distal to the occlusion typically implies slow antegrade flow (vessels usually back-thrombose to the nearest nonoccluded branch). (B) Anteroposterior digital subtraction angiography late-phase view demonstrates critical stenosis of the left ICA, with hairline antegrade flow (*arrows*). (C) After crossing the lesion with a microcatheter and placement of a balloon-expandable stent, there has been excellent restoration of antegrade flow (*arrows*). (D) Volume-rendered CT angiogram at 3 days after therapy shows the ICA to be patent status post stent placement. Once the flow had been re-established, the patient had no further symptoms. (E) Mean transit time of CT perfusion image from admission (before treatment) demonstrates a significant delay in the left temporal lobe transit time (*normal gray matter flow is blue, reduced gray matter flow is green*). Once the left ICA flow had been re-established, the patient had no further neurologic events.

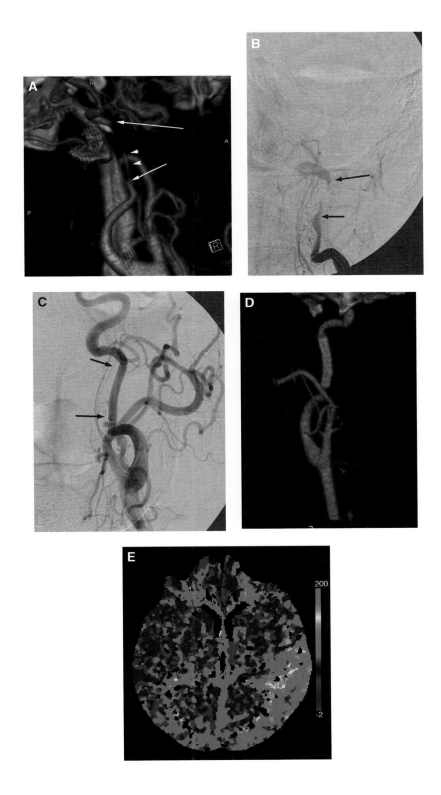

ally proven large vessel occlusion was evaluated in the Merci I and II trials.

Patients were eligible for enrollment if they were 18 years of age or older, had an NIHSS score of 10 or greater (phase I) or 8 or greater (phase II), and had less than one-third MCA territory hypodensity on baseline CT scanning. Three retriever models were used during the study. The results from 114 treated patients have been presented. Primary end point measures were recanalization (TIMI grade II or III) and occurrence of major complications. Secondary end points included target vessel status using CT angiography at 24 hours and neurologic and functional outcome (NIHSS, modified Rankin Scale) at 24 hours, 5 days or day of discharge, 30 days after treatment (phase I), and 90 days after treatment (phase II). The recanalization rate was 54%, and the serious adverse event rate was 14%.

The key to successful treatment using the Merci device is careful preoperative evaluation. The currently available Merci guide sheaths are quite large (7 and 9 French). Introduction of this catheter usually requires an exchange. Preselecting those patients for whom the retriever can be used can save considerable time. This can be done if CTA or MR angiography (MRA) is obtained before thrombolysis. Patients with distal MCA occlusion may benefit more from standard thrombolytic therapy than from the Merci retrieval device. Again, planning is essential to select patients for therapy.

A number of other clot retrieval devices as well as devices for endovascular thrombectomy are in various stages of development. Animal and in vitro models have shown that mechanical clot disruption improves drug delivery and efficacy during thrombolysis. This effect may be attributable to the increased surface area of the clot that is exposed to the thrombolytic agent [35,36]. Mechanical energy transmitted through ultrasound waves is also now being used as an adjuvant to thrombolysis [37,38]. This can be applied externally using transcranial Doppler (TCD) or internally via a microcatheter. A microcatheter called "E.K.O.S." is currently in the evaluation process; it releases ultrasound energy from its tip to enhance thrombolysis.

Summary: endovascular treatment pearls

Decision making in acute stroke endovascular therapy can be difficult. Ischemic stroke is an unforgiving disease; there is little time for planning. Time is of the essence, and there is a minimal margin of error. Even when procedures are technically suc-

cessful, patient outcome is variable. Triage decisions need to be based on the patient's prognosis with versus without treatment, and all parties involved must understand this clearly. Advanced preoperative imaging that includes assessment of vascular and tissue status, in conjunction with clinical status, offers the best prospect of optimizing outcome prediction.

Improved patients outcomes should increase with experience. Treating the most symptomatic vascular lesion early is important. In patients with intracranial and extracranial occlusions, the intracranial lesion should be treated first if possible. In most cases, symptoms are caused by the intracranial occlusion. Finally, the stroke interventionalist should have modest but firm goals. There are many possible techniques to recanalize an occluded vessel, and with persistence and the proper tools, almost any acute occlusion can be successfully treated. Knowing when to be aggressive and when not to be is crucial for success.

References

[1] Solis OJ, Roberson GR, Taveras JM, et al. Cerebral angiography in acute cerebral infarction. Rev Interam Radiol 1977;2(1):19–25.

[2] Fieschi C, Argentino C, Lenzi GL, et al. Clinical and instrumental evaluation of patients with ischemic stroke within the first six hours. J Neurol Sci 1989; 91(3):311–21.

[3] Wolpert SM, Bruckmann H, Greenlee R, et al. Neuroradiologic evaluation of patients with acute stroke treated with recombinant tissue plasminogen activator. The rt-PA Acute Stroke Study Group. AJNR Am J Neuroradiol 1993;14(1):3–13.

[4] Jones TH, Morawetz RB, Crowell RM, et al. Thresholds of focal cerebral ischemia in awake monkeys. J Neurosurg 1981;54(6):773–82.

[5] Zivin JA, Lyden PD, DeGirolami U, et al. Tissue plasminogen activator. Reduction of neurologic damage after experimental embolic stroke. Arch Neurol 1988;45(4):387–91.

[6] Young AR, Touzani O, Derlon JM, et al. Early reperfusion in the anesthetized baboon reduces brain damage following middle cerebral artery occlusion: a quantitative analysis of infarction volume. Stroke 1997;28(3):632–7 [discussion: 7–8].

[7] National Institute of Neurological Disorders and Stroke (NINDS) rt-PA Stroke Study Group, NINDS. Effect of intravenous recombinant tissue plasminogen activator on ischemic stroke lesion size measured by computed tomography. Stroke 2000;31(12):2912–9.

[8] National Institute of Neurological Disorders and Stroke rt-PA Stroke Study Group. Tissue plasminogen activator for acute ischemic stroke. N Engl J Med 1995;333(24):1581–7.

[9] Katzan IL, Furlan AJ, Lloyd LE, et al. Use of tissue-

type plasminogen activator for acute ischemic stroke: the Cleveland area experience. JAMA 2000;283(9): 1151–8.

[10] del Zoppo GJ, Poeck K, Pessin MS, et al. Recombinant tissue plasminogen activator in acute thrombotic and embolic stroke. Ann Neurol 1992;32(1):78–86.

[11] Lewandowski CA, Frankel M, Tomsick TA, et al. Combined intravenous and intra-arterial r-TPA versus intra-arterial therapy of acute ischemic stroke: Emergency Management of Stroke (EMS). Bridging Trial. Stroke 1999;30(12):2598–605.

[12] Generalized efficacy of t-PA for acute stroke. Subgroup analysis of the NINDS t-PA Stroke Trial. Stroke 1997;28(11):2119–25.

[13] Chiu D, Krieger D, Vollar-Cordova C, et al. Intravenous tissue plasminogen activator for acute ischemic stroke—feasibility, safety, and efficacy in the first year of clinical practice. Stroke 1998;29:2119–25.

[14] Lev MH, Farkas J, Gemmete JJ, et al. Acute stroke: improved nonenhanced CT detection—benefits of softcopy interpretation by using variable window width and center level settings. Radiology 1999;213(1):150–5.

[15] Hacke W, Kaste M, Fieschi C, et al. Intravenous thrombolysis with recombinant tissue plasminogen activator for acute hemispheric stroke. The European Cooperative Acute Stroke Study (ECASS). JAMA 1995;274(13):1017–25.

[16] Barber PA, Zhang J, Demchuk AM, et al. Why are stroke patients excluded from TPA therapy? An analysis of patient eligibility. Neurology 2001;56(8):1015–20.

[17] Lev MH, Farkas J, Rodriguez VR, et al. CT angiography in the rapid triage of patients with hyperacute stroke to intraarterial thrombolysis: accuracy in the detection of large vessel thrombus. J Comput Assist Tomogr 2001;25(4):520–8.

[18] Ezura M, Kagawa S. Selective and superselective infusion of urokinase for embolic stroke. Surg Neurol 1992;38(5):353–8.

[19] Barnwell SL, Clark WM, Nguyen TT, et al. Safety and efficacy of delayed intraarterial urokinase therapy with mechanical clot disruption for thromboembolic stroke. AJNR Am J Neuroradiol 1994;15(10):1817–22.

[20] Higashida RT, Halbach VV, Barnwell SL, et al. Thrombolytic therapy in acute stroke. J Endovasc Surg 1994;1:4–15.

[21] Casto L, Caverni L, Camerlingo M, et al. Intra-arterial thrombolysis in acute ischaemic stroke: experience with a superselective catheter embedded in the clot. J Neurol Neurosurg Psychiatry 1996;60(6):667–70.

[22] Gonner F, Remonda L, Mattle H, et al. Local intra-arterial thrombolysis in acute ischemic stroke. Stroke 1998;29(9):1894–900.

[23] Jahan R, Duckwiler GR, Kidwell CS, et al. Intra-arterial thrombolysis for treatment of acute stroke: experience in 26 patients with long-term follow-up. AJNR Am J Neuroradiol 1999;20(7):1291–9.

[24] Suarez JI, Sunshine JL, Tarr R, et al. Predictors of clinical improvement, angiographic recanalization, and intracranial hemorrhage after intra-arterial thrombolysis for acute ischemic stroke. Stroke 1999;30(10): 2094–100.

[25] Ueda T, Sakaki S, Kumon Y, et al. Multivariable analysis of predictive factors related to outcome at 6 months after intra-arterial thrombolysis for acute ischemic stroke. Stroke 1999;30(11):2360–5.

[26] Pannell R, Gurewich V. Pro-urokinase: a study of its stability in plasma and of a mechanism for its selective fibrinolytic effect. Blood 1986;67(5):1215–23.

[27] Furlan A, Higashida R, Wechsler L, et al. Intra-arterial prourokinase for acute ischemic stroke. The PROACT II study: a randomized controlled trial. Prolyse in Acute Cerebral Thromboembolism. JAMA 1999;282(21):2003–11.

[28] Ernst R, Pancioli A, Tomsick T, et al. Combined intravenous and intra-arterial recombinant tissue plasminogen activator in acute ischemic stroke. Stroke 2000;31(11):2552–7.

[29] Keris V, Rudnicka S, Vorona V, et al. Combined intraarterial/intravenous thrombolysis for acute ischemic stroke. AJNR Am J Neuroradiol 2001;22(2):352–8.

[30] Hill MD, Barber PA, Demchuk AM, et al. Acute intravenous–intra-arterial revascularization therapy for severe ischemic stroke. Stroke 2002;33(1):279–82.

[31] Suarez JI, Zaidat OO, Sunshine JL, et al. Endovascular administration after intravenous infusion of thrombolytic agents for the treatment of patients with acute ischemic strokes. Neurosurgery 2002;50(2):251–60.

[32] Nesbit GM, Clark WM, O'Neill OR, et al. Intracranial intraarterial thrombolysis facilitated by microcatheter navigation through an occluded cervical internal carotid artery. J Neurosurg 1996;84(3):387–92.

[33] Barnwell SL, Clark WM, Nguyen TT, et al. Safety and efficacy of delayed intraarterial urokinase therapy with mechanical clot disruption for thromboembolic stroke. AJNR Am J Neuroradiol 1994; 15(10):1817–22.

[34] Ueda T, Sakaki S, Nochide I, et al. Angioplasty after intra-arterial thrombolysis for acute occlusion of intracranial arteries. Stroke 1998;29(12):2568–74.

[35] Mitchel JF, Shwedick M, Alberghini TA, et al. Catheter-based local thrombolysis with urokinase: comparative efficacy of intraluminal clot lysis with conventional urokinase infusion techniques in an in vivo porcine thrombus model. Cathet Cardiovasc Diagn 1997;41(3):293–302.

[36] Shangguan HQ, Gregory KW, Casperson LW, et al. Enhanced laser thrombolysis with photomechanical drug delivery: an in vitro study. Lasers Surg Med 1998;23(3):151–60.

[37] Alexandrov AV, Demchuk AM, Felberg RA, et al. High rate of complete recanalization and dramatic clinical recovery during tPA infusion when continuously monitored with 2-MHz transcranial Doppler monitoring. Stroke 2000;31(3):610–4.

[38] Akiyama M, Ishibashi T, Yamada T, et al. Low-frequency ultrasound penetrates the cranium and enhances thrombolysis in vitro. Neurosurgery 1998;43: 828–32.

ELSEVIER
SAUNDERS

Neuroimag Clin N Am 15 (2005) 455 – 466

NEUROIMAGING
CLINICS OF
NORTH AMERICA

Advanced MR Imaging of Acute Stroke: The University of California at Los Angeles Endovascular Therapy Experience

David S. Liebeskind, MD[a,*], Chelsea S. Kidwell, MD[a,b,c], on behalf of UCLA Thrombolysis Investigators[a,1]

[a]University of California at Los Angeles Stroke Center, UCLA Medical Center, Los Angeles, CA, USA
[b]Washington Hospital Center, Washington, DC, USA
[c]Georgetown University, Washington, DC, USA

Historical perspective

Endovascular therapy including intra-arterial thrombolysis has been performed at the University of California at Los Angeles (UCLA) for select cases of acute ischemic stroke since 1992 [1]. Endovascular therapy initially included pure intra-arterial thrombolysis or bridging intravenous (IV)–intra-arterial thrombolysis. Selective catheterization and local delivery of the thrombolytic agent at the site of the occlusive thrombus could be achieved with confirmation of vascular patency. In 2001, mechanical thromboectomy became the preferred procedure of

choice with the theoretical advantages of more rapid recanalization and lower rates of hemorrhage [2]. Intra-arterial thrombolysis was typically offered up to 6 hours from symptom onset in the anterior circulation and up to 24 hours in the posterior circulation, with mechanical thromboectomy being offered up to 8 hours from onset.

During the early years of endovascular thrombolysis, CT was used as the initial diagnostic imaging modality. In 1996, technological advances in MR imaging, including echo planar imaging capability, allowed for clinical implementation of diffusion- and perfusion-weighted imaging in the acute stroke setting. Emergent acquisition of MR imaging is feasible but requires a coordinated, multidisciplinary effort [3]. Standard noncontrast CT imaging or multimodal CT, including noncontrast CT, CT angiography, and CT perfusion, is now increasingly reserved for acute stroke cases with contraindications to MR imaging. Early application of advanced MR imaging techniques led to unusual observations in acute stroke [3,4]. Successive studies using comprehensive MR imaging protocols confirmed the complexity in the pathophysiology of this disorder. These investigations led to increased understanding of various imaging patterns and subtle correlates.

Endovascular techniques for recanalization were offered on a compassionate basis for cases beyond traditional time windows. UCLA investigators tested the hypothesis that imaging could be used to evaluate

This work was supported in part by grants from the American Heart Association (0170033N, CSK) and National Institute of Neurological Disorders and Stroke (K23 NS 02088, CSK; NS 39498/EB 002087, JRA; K24 NS 02092, JLS).

* Corresponding author. University of California at Los Angeles Stroke Center, UCLA Medical Center, 710 Westwood Plaza, Los Angeles, CA 90095.
E-mail address: davidliebeskind@yahoo.com (D.S. Liebeskind).

[1] *Additional UCLA Thrombolysis Investigators:* Jeffry R. Alger, PhD, Gary R. Duckwiler, MD, Y. Pierre Gobin, MD, Reza Jahan, MD, Bruce Ovbiagele, MD, Jeffrey L. Saver, MD, Sidney Starkman, MD, Paul M. Vespa, MD, J. Pablo Villablanca, MD, and Fernando Viñuela, MD.

1052-5149/05/$ – see front matter. Published by Elsevier Inc.
doi:10.1016/j.nic.2005.06.002

neuroimaging.theclinics.com

and select cases for intervention (Fig. 1), potentially optimizing acute stroke care. Although some individuals may benefit from revascularization at these later time points, it became clear that imaging would be required to identify other cases in which these therapeutic interventions may be futile or harmful. For cases beyond 3 hours from symptom onset, multimodal MR imaging screening is performed and endovascular treatment with mechanical thrombectomy or intra-arterial thrombolysis is considered. MR imaging studies have enriched clinical estimates of risk and benefit to select cases for further intervention. Simple paradigms, such as diffusion-perfusion mismatch, have been transformed into refined models that estimate the extent of ischemic core and penum-

bra [5]. Although certain MR imaging findings, such as extensive volumes of tissue with severe reductions in the apparent diffusion coefficient (ADC) may dissuade the treating physician from pursuing revascularization, calculations in the degree of mismatch are not routinely used for case selection. Preliminary imaging models incorporating ADC values and perfusion thresholds have been constructed from the large series of intra-arterial thrombolysis cases at UCLA, yet such models await prospective validation in clinical trials [6]. Prior reports on the MR imaging correlates of endovascular thrombolysis have examined recanalization, lesion patterns, the evolution of dynamic changes in diffusion and perfusion, and hemorrhage [3,5–11].

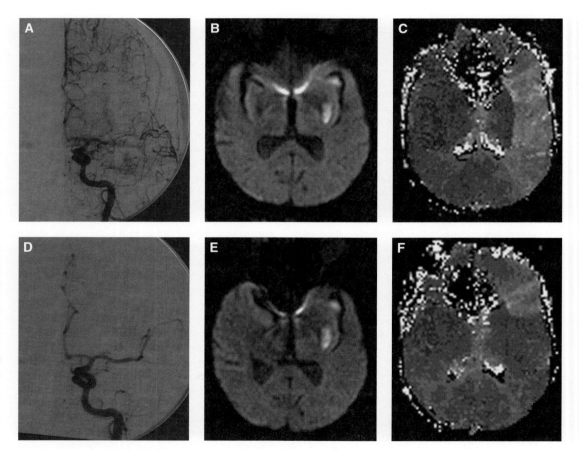

Fig. 1. Diffusion-perfusion MR imaging before and after mechanical thrombectomy in acute ischemic stroke. Proximal occlusion of left middle cerebral artery (*A*) associated with extensive mismatch between diffusion-weighted imaging (DWI) (*B*), and PWI time-to-peak contrast enhancement (TTP) (*C*) abnormalities. After thrombectomy, angiography reveals proximal recanalization with residual branch occlusion (*D*) and reduction in mismatch between DWI (*E*) and PWI TTP (*F*). (Courtesy of the UCLA Stroke Center, Los Angeles, CA; with permission.)

MR imaging sequences and protocols

The MR imaging protocols used for evaluation of acute stroke cases have evolved with the introduction of novel sequences. Maintaining stringent limits on overall acquisition time has been a priority. Maximizing the amount of imaging data available for therapeutic decision-making within the shortest amount of time is critical in the acute setting. Current stroke protocols take 5 to 20 minutes for acquisition. Typically the treating physicians accompany the patient from the emergency room to the MR imaging suite, concurrently evaluating clinical aspects of the case. Ascertainment of the clinical history and examination often continues in the MR imaging suite.

The standard interventional stroke protocol (Table 1) is performed on a 1.5 Tesla echo planar MR imaging scanner. Diffusion-weighted imaging (DWI) provides information regarding the diagnosis of ischemic stroke, including location, extent, and the potential etiology or cause. These sequences rapidly reflect ischemic sequelae associated with restriction in the diffusion of water molecules. Restricted diffusion has been principally ascribed to cytotoxic edema caused by the influx of water molecules associated with altered ion flux at the cellular membrane, although this swelling may also limit the diffusion of water molecules within the adjacent extracellular space [12]. ADC maps are automatically generated following acquisition of the diffusion sequence. These maps reveal diminished ADC values that precipitously decline following the onset of ischemia. ADC values persist at diminished levels for 72 to 96 hours before gradually increasing caused by concomitant development of vasogenic edema [13].

A gradient recalled echo (GRE) sequence is used for the detection of acute and chronic intracranial hemorrhage, including cerebral microbleeds. GRE sequences are susceptibility-weighted and detect the paramagnetic effects of blood break-down products

[14]. This sequence often detects signal loss associated with susceptibility effects of intraluminal thrombus in the proximal cerebral arteries [14]. In 2003, following completion of the Hemorrhage and Early MR Imaging Evaluation (HEME) study [10], MR imaging was adopted as the sole screening modality for acute stroke, eliminating the CT to rule out hemorrhage.

A fluid attenuated inversion recovery (FLAIR) sequence is acquired as time permits or if the treating team believes that the study will provide important information for therapeutic decisions. FLAIR sequences reveal early parenchymal changes associated with ischemia and prior cerebral lesions that may be indicative of disease burden. FLAIR may also demonstrate vascular hyperintensity caused by slow, retrograde collateral flow distal to the occlusive lesion [15].

Perfusion-weighted imaging (PWI) is performed using dynamic contrast enhancement with gadolinium (0.1 mmol/kg dose by way of power injector) and gradient-echo imaging. Perfusion maps of time-to-peak contrast enhancement (TTP) are automatically generated following acquisition of the perfusion sequence. Additional postprocessing techniques for the perfusion sequence are generally performed at a later time-point. These perfusion parameter maps typically include cerebral blood flow, cerebral blood volume, mean transit time (MTT), and time-to-peak of the residue function (Tmax), following deconvolution of an arterial input function identified from the contralateral middle cerebral artery and tissue concentration curves [16]. The TTP maps automatically generated at the time of scan acquisition are used for prompt evaluation of diffusion-perfusion mismatch, revealing perfusion delays caused by elongated collateral routes [17]. Tmax and MTT permit evaluation of transit phenomena following deconvolution.

Three-dimensional time-of-flight (TOF) MR angiography (MRA) of the intracranial circulation and occasionally two-dimensional TOF MRA of the

Table 1
University of California at Los Angeles interventional stroke MR imaging protocol

Sequence	TR (ms)	TE (ms)	TI (ms)	Flip angle (°)	Slice thickness (mm)	Gap (mm)	FOV	Matrix size
DWI/ADC[a]	6000	105	NA	90	5–7	0	220–240	128 × 128
GRE	800	15	NA	30	5–7	0	220–240	256 × 144
FLAIR	10,000	105	2400	120	5–7	0	220–240	256 × 132
PWI[b]	2000	46	NA	60	5–7	0	220–240	128 × 96
Intracranial MRA (3D-TOF)	44	6	NA	25	1	0	220–240	512 × 208
Extracranial MRA (2D-TOF)	27	6	NA	50	3	0	220–240	256 × 163

Abbreviations: FOV, field of view; NA, not applicable; TE, echo time; TI, inversion time; TR, repetition time.
  [a] b = 0 and 1000 s/m^2.
  [b] 0.1 mg/kg by way of antecubital vein at 5 cc/s.

extracranial circulation are acquired to identify large vessel occlusions that are the target of the endovascular therapies.

As part of a research protocol, follow-up MR imaging studies have been performed at 3 hours following treatment, day 5 through 7, and day 90. Serial acquisition of detailed MR imaging data allow for characterization of dynamic changes in diffusion and perfusion lesions and hemorrhagic sequelae during the acute and early subacute phases.

The imaging protocol is occasionally modified based on particular features of the clinical presentation. For instance, if cervicocephalic arterial dissection is suspect, axial fat-saturated T1-weighted images may be acquired. Alternatively, extracranial MRA may be added to the protocol if there is concern regarding the feasibility of catheter navigation during endovascular therapy if prominent carotid atherosclerosis is present. For patients eligible for IV tissue-type plasminogen activator (tPA), the preliminary sequences of the protocol may be acquired with interruption of the scan sequence to initiate thrombolysis. Following administration of the IV tPA bolus and initiation of the continuous infusion, the remainder of the MR imaging protocol is obtained. Because of varying time constraints, the standard protocol may also be abbreviated to expedite transfer of the patient to the angiography suite for endovascular therapies.

Defining ischemic core and penumbra

Numerous approaches have been used to define the ischemic penumbra in acute stroke [18]. The most clinically relevant approach is to define the penumbra as tissue that is at risk for infarction but still salvageable. The potential for salvage of these regions forms the basis for emergent thrombolytic interventions, including intra-arterial thrombolysis. Penumbral zones typically surround an area of irreversible ischemic injury or core infarction. Similarly, a region of hypoperfusion surrounding the peripheral extent of the penumbra may be described as benign oligemia or mild reductions in perfusion that do not impart significant risk for infarction [5]. Conceptual subdivisions have been used to describe ischemic lesions and may be defined with diffusion-perfusion MR imaging. Idealized schematics of circumferential zones may be helpful in describing ischemic pathology across large subsets of cases, yet the topography may vary considerably from case to case. Heterogeneity in the topography of core, penumbra, and adjacent regions of oligemia is determined by individual factors potentially reflecting tissue fea-

tures, such as ischemic tolerance caused by prior ischemic conditioning and vascular aspects, including the extent of collateral circulation [19].

The introduction of diffusion-perfusion MR imaging provided the ability to grossly depict the extent of core and penumbra in individual cases of acute stroke. Diffusion lesions were initially considered to represent the extent of ischemic core with perfusion lesions demonstrating more extensive regions of hypoperfusion incorporating ischemic penumbra. Mismatch or incongruous volumes of perfusion and diffusion on MR imaging provided a simple and practical means of defining penumbra (Fig. 2) [5,20]. Assessment of the extent of core and penumbra seemed critical to gauge the potential for tissue salvage with emergent thrombolysis. Although most diffusion lesions visualized at later time points seemed to reliably denote irreversible infarction, early studies performed at UCLA demonstrated that portions of the diffusion abnormality might reverse or resolve following reperfusion. Thrombolytic reversal of diffusion abnormalities in acute stroke was first demonstrated in a pilot study of intra-arterial thrombolysis cases at UCLA (Fig. 3) [3]. Serial MR imaging evaluation, including diffusion and perfusion sequences, was conducted in seven cases. This cohort included various supratentorial vascular lesions from proximal middle cerebral artery (MCA) to branch occlusions. Partial (Thrombolysis in Myocardial Ischemia [TIMI] grade 2) or complete (TIMI 3) recanalization was achieved in five and two cases, respectively. Post-treatment clinical improvement was invariable. Early follow-up MR imaging was acquired at a mean of 5.5 hours after recanalization (range 2.5–9.5 hours). Day-7 MR imaging was used

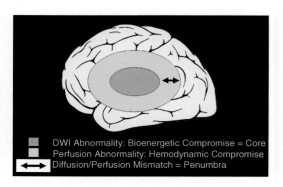

DWI Abnormality: Bioenergetic Compromise = Core
Perfusion Abnormality: Hemodynamic Compromise
Diffusion/Perfusion Mismatch = Penumbra

Fig. 2. MR imaging–defined penumbra employing the diffusion perfusion mismatch model where the perfusion deficit appears in purple, the diffusion deficit in yellow with penumbra equaling area of mismatch between two. (Courtesy of UCLA Stroke Center, Los Angeles, CA; with permission.)

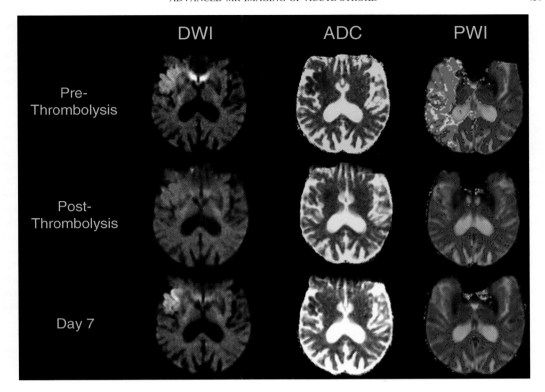

Fig. 3. Example of early reversal of diffusion and perfusion abnormalities followed by late secondary injury after vessel recanalization with intra-arterial thrombolysis. Top row shows pretreatment DWI, ADC maps, and PWI sequences from representative slice. Middle row shows same sequences 3 hours after treatment. Bottom row shows day-7 studies. Perfusion image shows color-coded map of time-to-peak of the residue function (Tmax) where red represents delay of greater than 8 seconds, yellow a delay greater than 6 seconds, green a delay greater than 4 seconds, and blue a delay greater than 2 seconds. (Courtesy of UCLA Stroke Center, Los Angeles, CA; with permission.)

to estimate final infarct volume. Overall, six out of seven cases demonstrated a reduction in the volumes of the DWI abnormalities and ADC lesion volumes. More dramatic changes in DWI and ADC lesion volumes were evident on review of individual cases.

Parallel changes in perfusion abnormalities were also evident (see Fig. 3) [3]. Baseline perfusion MR imaging performed in five cases revealed average mismatch of 79% (range 57%–94%). In four of these cases with serial perfusion imaging, there was complete resolution in the initial perfusion abnormalities. This study demonstrated the potential reversibility of diffusion and perfusion lesions. This finding changed the previously maintained perspective that diffusion abnormalities were synonymous with regions of core infarction. Instead, the diffusion abnormality was shown to contain regions of core and penumbra. The therapeutic implications of this novel finding suggest that DWI lesion growth might be amenable to early interventions.

A subsequent analysis of 13 patients treated with intra-arterial therapy demonstrated partial or complete reversal of diffusion abnormalities in 44% of patients [8]. Recently, Chalela and colleagues [21] reported partial or complete reversal in 33% of patients treated with IV thrombolysis. These findings of reversal of diffusion abnormalities have led to revision of the mismatch model, whereby the border between core and penumbra may lie deeper within a subset of the diffusion abnormality (Fig. 4) [5].

Perfusion studies have also revealed that the outer limit of the visually identified perfusion abnormality may overestimate the extent of tissue at risk or penumbra in acute stroke [6]. The evolution and regression of diffusion and perfusion lesions with intra-arterial thrombolysis suggested that baseline imaging data might be used to predict tissue fate. Diffusion abnormalities and the severity in reductions of ADC values may theoretically reflect the duration and severity of the initial ischemic insult. Similarly,

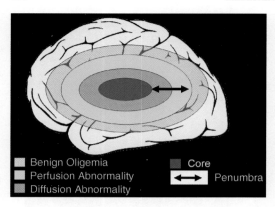

Benign Oligemia

Perfusion Abnormality

Diffusion Abnormality

Core

◄──► Penumbra

Fig. 4. Modified view of MR imaging defined penumbra where penumbra includes only portion of diffusion and perfusion deficits. (Courtesy of UCLA Stroke Center, Los Angeles, CA; with permission.)

the severity and extent of perfusion abnormalities may be predictive of tissue response to revascularization. An analysis of the perfusion MR imaging data in a series of MCA occlusions treated with IV tPA or combined IV and intra-arterial thrombolysis at UCLA surveyed baseline perfusion thresholds for tissue fate at day 7 following successful recanalization without hemorrhagic transformation [6]. The imaging data in this ideal subset of 14 stroke cases were analyzed on a voxel-by-voxel and patient-by-patient basis. Baseline DWI lesions ranged from 2.1 to 52.1 cm^3 (median 16.3 cm^3). Baseline perfusion abnormalities were defined by voxels with Tmax greater than 2 seconds. Baseline perfusion lesions ranged from 6.7 to 181.7 cm^3 (median 69.7 cm^3). A matched deficit was noted in one case, with 13 out of 14 cases demonstrating diffusion-perfusion mismatch at baseline.

Voxel-by-voxel analysis of tissue fate in 254,429 voxels across all cases demonstrated that approximately 20% evolved toward infarction [6]. The sensitivity, specificity, and positive and negative predictive values for infarction were determined for perfusion abnormalities based on various perfusion thresholds defined by the initial Tmax. Sensitivity and specificity for ultimate infarction were optimized for Tmax values between 6 and 8 seconds. Sensitivity values using these thresholds ranged from 53% to 71%, with sensitivity improving as Tmax increased. Although these numbers are modest in predictive power, this study further strengthened the concept of predictive models based on perfusion thresholds.

Concordant results for voxel-by-voxel and patient-by-patient analyses supported the predictive value of perfusion thresholds between Tmax 6 and 8 seconds [6]. These measures derived from post-

processed image data are not typically used in the acute setting, yet gross visual inspection of a perfusion lesion may overestimate final infarct volume. This study suggests that multivariate models incorporating specific perfusion thresholds might more reliably predict tissue fate. Although the perfusion thresholds used in this series were based on cases of successful recanalization, the perfusion parameters corresponded to critical values determined from other published series [22]. Only modest sensitivity and specificity values (50%–80%) for prediction of final infarction, however, were obtained in this study [6].

Despite these limitations, the diffusion-perfusion mismatch model provides a simple and practical means of estimating the penumbra in the acute stroke setting. Several trials are currently underway to validate the mismatch model for identifying the ischemic penumbra and whether diffusion-perfusion MR imaging can be used to select patients with recanalization therapies. In addition, several phase II clinical trials are underway employing the mismatch model to select patients for late recanalization therapies [23,24].

Alternative approaches to the mismatch model for identifying penumbra have been under investigation. A multivariate voxel-by-voxel model for predicting tissue fate has been developed incorporating quantitative information from the diffusion and perfusion sequences. Initial studies demonstrate an accuracy rate of 81% compared with 53% for mismatch estimates [5]. Following this study, the application of multivariate models incorporating ADC and perfusion values was used to predict clinical outcome with mechanical thrombectomy. Kidwell and colleagues [25] demonstrated that recanalization with a penumbral pattern resulted in a good clinical outcome (modified Rankin score 0–2) in 89% of cases at day 90 compared with only 14% for those devoid of penumbra. Prospective validation of predictive MR imaging models awaits further evaluation. As gross visualization of mismatch evident on comparison of diffusion and perfusion images may neglect penumbral regions within the diffusion abnormality, cases without mismatch are not currently excluded from endovascular therapy at UCLA. Novel MR imaging techniques, including measures of flow heterogeneity and oxygen status will further expand these evolving definitions of ischemia on MR imaging.

Diffusion-perfusion MR imaging of basilar occlusion

The studies reported in earlier discussion include only patients with anterior circulation occlusions. In an effort to compare and contrast the MR imaging changes and the underlying pathophysiology of the posterior circulation with the anterior circulation, a subsequent analysis was performed on patients with basilar artery occlusion treated with intra-arterial thrombolysis and imaging with diffusion-perfusion MR imaging [11]. Thrombolysis in the posterior circulation differs in numerous respects with regard to anterior circulation ischemia. In basilar occlusion, the conventional time window for revascularization is considerably extended compared with anterior circulation lesions. Furthermore, endovascular therapy may be offered more frequently on a compassionate basis caused by the morbid outcome of this disorder. From an imaging standpoint, the posterior circulation is also radically dissimilar to anterior circulation strokes. The regions of interest or territories at risk may be considerably smaller and more difficult to depict because of the vascular anatomy and differences in the topography or perfusion patterns.

A UCLA study described the MR imaging correlates in 10 cases of basilar occlusion [11]. Median National Institutes of Health Stroke Scale (NIHSS) score of 14 (range 4–28). The median time from onset to MR imaging was 4 hours and 10 minutes (range 2:30–30:05). The extent of the DWI lesion did not correlate with baseline neurological deficit, although a modest correlation was noted between the PWI lesion volume and baseline NIHSS score. Combined diffusion-perfusion data at baseline were

available in five cases. In all five cases, mismatch was evident involving the brainstem, cerebellum, and posterior cerebral hemispheres (Fig. 5). Mismatch volumes ranged from 49% to 99% (mean 73%). Early post-thrombolysis MR imaging demonstrated that the mean DWI lesion volume was substantially less than the initial perfusion abnormality, suggesting penumbral salvage. For the six cases with follow-up MR imaging performed at day 7, the mean DWI lesion did not progressively enlarge, yet DWI reversal was not apparent. The absence of diffusion reversibility previously demonstrated in the anterior circulation was ascribed to potential differences associated with the time to recanalization, because these posterior circulation lesions were treated much later. A subsequent case of basilar occlusion treated with mechanical thromboectomy demonstrated reversal of a pontine diffusion lesion [26].

Postischemic hyperperfusion

The UCLA group performed the first study characterizing postischemic hyperperfusion employing serial MR imaging studies [7]. A study of 14 cases of serial diffusion-perfusion MR imaging revealed early and late hyperperfusion, unexplained by changes in blood pressure or hemodynamic parameters (Fig. 6). Although 13 out of 14 cases demonstrated clinical

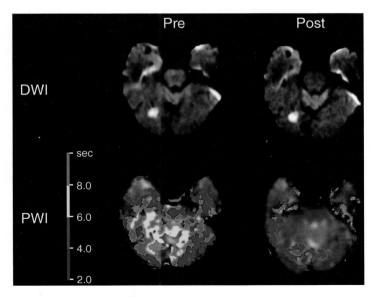

Fig. 5. Serial DWI-PWI (Tmax) images revealing marked reduction in mismatch accompanying basilar thrombolysis. (*From* Ostrem JL, Saver JL, Alger JR, et al. Acute basilar artery occlusion: diffusion-perfusion MRI characterization of tissue salvage in patients receiving intra-arterial stroke therapies. Stroke 2004;35(2):e33; with permission.)

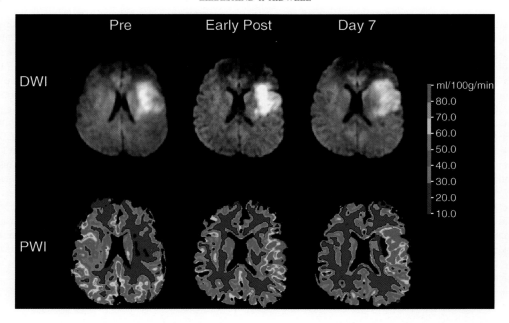

Fig. 6. Serial DWI-PWI (CBF) images demonstrating hyperperfusion in the left middle cerebral artery territory following intra-arterial thrombolysis (*From* Kidwell CS, Saver JL, Mattiello J, et al. Diffusion-perfusion MRI characterization of post-recanalization hyperperfusion in humans. Neurology 2001;57(11):2020; with permission).

improvement after the procedure, hyperperfusion was demonstrated in half of all cases and was associated with larger final infarct volumes (median 31.5 cm³ [range 5.2–73 cm³] versus 6.4 cm³ [range 0–40.6 cm³], $P < .05$). Relative cerebral blood flow measurements with respect to contralateral homologous regions were used to define hyperperfusion. Hyperperfusion was evident in 5 out of 12 (42%) cases with early postthrombolysis studies and 6 out of 11 (55%) day-7 studies. Cerebral blood volume measures in regions of hyperperfusion confirmed the presence of hyperemia, although hemorrhagic transformation was not associated with hyperperfusion. Most regions with early hyperperfusion following thrombolysis, and delayed hyperperfusion at day 7, ultimately infarcted. These hyperperfused voxels had lower baseline ADC values and more severe hypoperfusion at baseline.

The isolated time intervals for serial MR imaging evaluation performed in this study limited further evaluation of the time course in hyperperfusion. It seemed that the observed hyperperfusion in this series was non-nutritional because most of these regions progressed toward infarction. Impaired autoregulation and related aspects of vasodilatation following ischemia were implicated the cause of the observed hyperperfusion.

Late secondary ADC decline

An additional important observation emanating from the serial MR imaging studies was that of late secondary injury in patients with successful vessel recanalization [8]. Subacute or secondary reductions in ADC values were noticed in a subset of cases in which reversal of diffusion abnormalities was seen at the early timepoint (Fig. 7). Eighteen cases of anterior circulation ischemia treated with intra-arterial thrombolysis or combined IV and intra-arterial thrombolysis were studied. Reversal of diffusion abnormalities was apparent in 8 out of 18 (44%) cases shortly after recanalization, yet reappearance of diffusion lesions and secondary declines in the ADC values at day 7 were also apparent in 5 out of 8 (28%) cases. Sustained reversal was noted in 3 out of 8 (17%) cases. Patient age, time to recanalization, and the degree of recanalization were unrelated to the occurrence of secondary ADC decline. Voxel-by-voxel analyses revealed that baseline ADC values were predictive of secondary decline, because voxels with sustained reversal had a higher mean ADC value (663 μm²/sec) than those with secondary decline (617 μm²/sec). Hyperperfusion was unrelated to secondary ADC decline and there was no evidence of vascular re-occlusion in these cases. The cause of

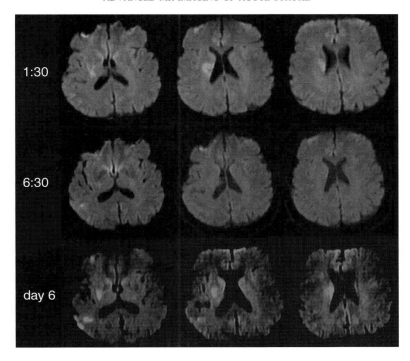

Fig. 7. Serial DWI depicting early reversal and subsequent reappearance of subcortical diffusion abnormality associated with right middle cerebral artery stroke at day 6. Cortical DWI abnormality associated with distal embolization evolves between the second and third study. (Courtesy of UCLA Stroke Center, Los Angeles, CA; with permission.)

secondary reductions in ADC following initial improvement remains unclear, although this phenomenon raises speculation regarding the need for therapeutic strategies that target secondary cellular injury. Reperfusion-related neuroprotective strategies may ultimately be used in combination with thrombolytic interventions [27].

Cerebral microbleeds

In the 1990s, several groups began characterizing the frequency, risk factors, and clinical correlates of cerebral microbleeds [14]. Microbleeds are clinically silent, punctate lesions caused by hemosiderin deposition and only demonstrated on MR imaging GRE sequences (Fig. 8). Early demonstration of scattered microbleeds posed a diagnostic dilemma because a prior history of intracranial hemorrhage is a contraindication thrombolysis [9]. These lesions have been reported in up to 6% of healthy elderly subjects and 26% of cases with prior ischemic stroke. Following a case of remote intracranial hemorrhage after thrombolysis at the site of a microbleed evident on baseline GRE, the UCLA group reported this unusual

complication and reviewed the prevalence of microbleeds before thrombolysis [9]. Susceptibility-weighted imaging or GRE sequences acquired before thrombolysis were reviewed in 41 cases. Microbleeds were evident in 5 out of 41 (12%) cases. Major

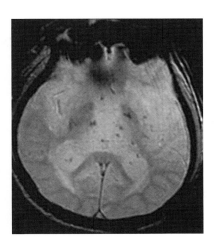

Fig. 8. Scattered microbleeds evident as hypointensity on GRE. (Courtesy of UCLA Stroke Center, Los Angeles, CA; with permission.)

symptomatic hemorrhage occurred in 1 of 5 patients with microbleeds compared with 4 of 36 patients without. Only 1 patient in the entire 41-patient cohort experienced any hemorrhagic transformation (HT) outside the acute ischemic field. In this patient, the symptomatic hemorrhage occurred directly at the site of a prior microbleed, contralateral to the acute ischemic event. This report provided the first suggestion that microbleeds may be a risk for hemorrhagic transformation following thrombolytic therapy. Subsequent case series have supported this hypothesis; however, further data are needed to determine the role of microbleeds in selecting patients for thrombolytic therapies.

MR imaging for the exclusion of intracranial hemorrhage

The extensive use of MR imaging in conjunction with CT before intra-arterial thrombolysis prompted questions regarding the use of MR imaging specifically for the exclusion of intracranial hemorrhage. CT was acquired in most cases solely to exclude the presence of hemorrhage that would obviate thrombolytic therapy, because most imaging data regarding ischemia were obtained from MR imaging. The arduous process of acquiring two diagnostic imaging studies before thrombolysis was labor and time intensive and later questionable once GRE sequences became available. The exquisite sensitivity of GRE sequences to static magnetic field inhomogeneity and the paramagnetic effects of deoxyhemoglobin and methemoglobin suggested that this sequence may

rival the traditional role of CT for detection of hyperacute intraparenchymal hemorrhage.

The HEME study was conducted at UCLA and the National Institutes of Health Stroke Center at Suburban Hospital [10]. For 200 acute stroke cases presenting within 6 hours of symptom onset, MR imaging was acquired and followed within 30 minutes by CT. All imaging was acquired within 90 minutes of emergency room presentation. Two neuroradiologists and two stroke neurologists conducted blind, independent review of CT and MR imaging for the presence of intracranial hemorrhage. All forms of intracranial hemorrhage were evaluated and intraparenchymal hemorrhages were subsequently classified as hematoma, petechial, or microbleeds. Although initially planned as a noninferiority study to demonstrate the role of MR imaging compared with the standards of CT, the study was later changed because an interim analysis revealed that MR imaging was detecting hemorrhages not illustrated with CT. Overall, 25 acute hemorrhages were noted on CT and MR imaging. In four additional cases, MR imaging revealed hemorrhagic transformation that was not apparent on CT (Fig. 9). In another four cases in which CT was positive, MR imaging was interpreted as negative for acute hemorrhage, yet chronic hemorrhage was suspect in three. This study corroborated the findings of a concurrent study evaluating the use of MR imaging for the detection of acute hemorrhage [28]. The HEME study included 34 cases treated with IV tPA, substantiating the role of MR imaging as a sole diagnostic imaging modality for comprehensive evaluation of acute stroke cases. The study also confirmed the su-

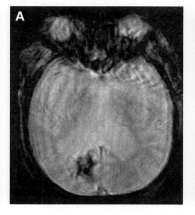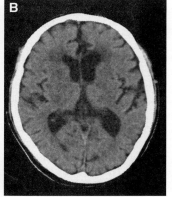

Fig. 9. GRE (*A*) demonstration of hemorrhagic transformation of an ischemic infarct not visualized on CT (*B*). (*From* Kidwell CS, Chalela JA, Saver JL, et al. Comparison of MRI and CT for detection of acute intracerebral hemorrhage. JAMA 2004;292(15):1827; with permission).

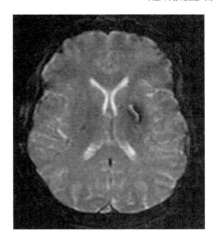

Fig. 10. Chronic, slit-like putaminal hemorrhage (hypointensity) illustrated on GRE. (Courtesy of UCLA Stroke Center, Los Angeles, CA; with permission.)

periority of GRE sequences compared with CT for detecting chronic hemosiderin deposition caused by prior intracranial hematomas (Fig. 10) and cerebral microbleeds.

Summary

An intensive early imaging approach using MR imaging before intra-arterial thrombolysis has provided considerable information regarding acute ischemic stroke, including the dynamic aspects of diffusion and perfusion abnormalities. Simple paradigms, such as diffusion-perfusion mismatch, have been transformed into refined models that estimate the extent of ischemic core and penumbra. MR imaging has also been advanced for the detection of intracranial hemorrhage, and may serve as the sole imaging modality before thrombolysis. Angiographic correlation at the time of thrombolysis has provided unique insight, delineating vascular correlates, including the degree of proximal arterial patency with recanalization and the extent of collateral flow. Although multivariate MR imaging models await prospective validation, these models may ultimately be used to optimize selection of ideal thrombolytic candidates.

References

[1] Jahan R, Duckwiler GR, Kidwell CS, et al. Intraarterial thrombolysis for treatment of acute stroke: experience in 26 patients with long-term follow-up. Am J Neuroradiol 1999;20(7):1291–9.

[2] Gobin YP, Starkman S, Duckwiler GR, et al. MERCI 1: a phase 1 study of mechanical embolus removal in cerebral ischemia. Stroke 2004;35(12):2848–54.

[3] Kidwell CS, Saver JL, Mattiello J, et al. Thrombolytic reversal of acute human cerebral ischemic injury shown by diffusion/perfusion magnetic resonance imaging. Ann Neurol 2000;47(4):462–9.

[4] Kidwell CS, Alger JR, Di Salle F, et al. Diffusion MRI in patients with transient ischemic attacks. Stroke 1999;30(6):1174–80.

[5] Kidwell CS, Alger JR, Saver JL. Beyond mismatch: evolving paradigms in imaging the ischemic penumbra with multimodal magnetic resonance imaging. Stroke 2003;34(11):2729–35.

[6] Shih LC, Saver JL, Alger JR, et al. Perfusion-weighted magnetic resonance imaging thresholds identifying core, irreversibly infarcted tissue. Stroke 2003;34(6): 1425–30.

[7] Kidwell CS, Saver JL, Mattiello J, et al. Diffusion-perfusion MRI characterization of post-recanalization hyperperfusion in humans. Neurology 2001;57(11): 2015–21.

[8] Kidwell CS, Saver JL, Starkman S, et al. Late secondary ischemic injury in patients receiving intraarterial thrombolysis. Ann Neurol 2002;52(6):698–703.

[9] Kidwell CS, Saver JL, Villablanca JP, et al. Magnetic resonance imaging detection of microbleeds before thrombolysis: an emerging application. Stroke 2002; 33(1):95–8.

[10] Kidwell CS, Chalela JA, Saver JL, et al. Comparison of MRI and CT for detection of acute intracerebral hemorrhage. JAMA 2004;292(15):1823–30.

[11] Ostrem JL, Saver JL, Alger JR, et al. Acute basilar artery occlusion: diffusion-perfusion MRI characterization of tissue salvage in patients receiving intraarterial stroke therapies. Stroke 2004;35(2):E30–4.

[12] van Gelderen P, de Vleeschouwer MH, DesPres D, et al. Water diffusion and acute stroke. Magn Reson Med 1994;31(2):154–63.

[13] Schlaug G, Siewert B, Benfield A, et al. Time course of the apparent diffusion coefficient (ADC) abnormality in human stroke. Neurology 1997;49(1): 113–9.

[14] Hermier M, Nighoghossian N. Contribution of susceptibility-weighted imaging to acute stroke assessment. Stroke 2004;35(8):1989–94.

[15] Maeda M, Yamamoto T, Daimon S, et al. Arterial hyperintensity on fast fluid-attenuated inversion recovery images: a subtle finding for hyperacute stroke undetected by diffusion-weighted MR imaging. Am J Neuroradiol 2001;22(4):632–6.

[16] Ostergaard L, Sorensen AG, Kwong KK, et al. High resolution measurement of cerebral blood flow using intravascular tracer bolus passages. Part II: experimental comparison and preliminary results. Magn Reson Med 1996;36(5):726–36.

[17] Calamante F, Gadian DG, Connelly A. Quantification of perfusion using bolus tracking magnetic resonance imaging in stroke: assumptions, limitations, and poten-

tial implications for clinical use. Stroke 2002;33(4): 1146–51.

[18] Fisher M. The ischemic penumbra: identification, evolution and treatment concepts. Cerebrovasc Dis 2004; 17(Suppl 1):1–6.

[19] Liebeskind DS. Collateral circulation. Stroke 2003; 34(9):2279–84.

[20] Baird AE, Warach S. Magnetic resonance imaging of acute stroke. J Cereb Blood Flow Metab 1998;18(6): 583–609.

[21] Chalela JA, Kang DW, Luby M, et al. Early magnetic resonance imaging findings in patients receiving tissue plasminogen activator predict outcome: Insights into the pathophysiology of acute stroke in the thrombolysis era. Ann Neurol 2004;55(1):105–12.

[22] Neumann-Haefelin T, Wittsack HJ, Wenserski F, et al. Diffusion- and perfusion-weighted MRI. The DWI/ PWI mismatch region in acute stroke. Stroke 1999; 30(8):1591–7.

[23] Hacke W, Albers G, Al-Rawi Y, et al. The Desmoteplase in Acute Ischemic Stroke Trial (DIAS): a phase II MRI-based 9-hour window acute stroke thrombolysis trial with intravenous desmoteplase. Stroke 2005; 36(1):66–73.

[24] Davis SM, Donnan GA, Butcher KS, et al. Selection of thrombolytic therapy beyond 3 h using magnetic resonance imaging. Curr Opin Neurol 2005;18(1): 47–52.

[25] Kidwell C, Starkman S, Jahan R, et al. Pretreatment MRI penumbral pattern predicts good clinical outcome following mechanical embolectomy [abstract]. Stroke 2004;35:294.

[26] Suzuki S, Kidwell CS, Starkman S, et al. Multimodal MRI and novel endovascular therapies in a patient ineligible for IV tPA. Stroke 2005, in press.

[27] Liebeskind DS. Neuroprotection from the collateral perspective. IDrugs 2005;8(3):222–8.

[28] Fiebach JB, Schellinger PD, Gass A, et al. Stroke magnetic resonance imaging is accurate in hyperacute intracerebral hemorrhage: a multicenter study on the validity of stroke imaging. Stroke 2004;35(2):502–6.

ELSEVIER
SAUNDERS

Neuroimag Clin N Am 15 (2005) 467–472

NEUROIMAGING
CLINICS OF
NORTH AMERICA

Index

Note: Page numbers of article titles are in **boldface** type.

A

Acetazolamide, as cerebral vasodilator, 373–374

Alberta Stroke Program, early CT score, 410
  advanced imaging and, 413–414
  and outcome prediction, 411–413
  in triage of acute stroke, **409–419**
  ischemic change on unenhanced CT and,
    410–411
  practical clinical utility of, 414–416

Amyloid angiopathy, cerebral, 266

Angiography, CT, 428
  in carotid artery stenosis, 354, 355, 356
  digital subtraction, in acute ischemic stroke,
    441, 442
  MR, to assess carotid artery stenosis, 353–357

Arterial occlusive disease, chronic, PET to study,
  344–347

Arterial-spin-labeling, to assess cerebrovascular
  reserve, 372

Arteriovenous malformations, intracerebral
  hemorrhage due to, 267

Asia, stroke in. See *Stroke, in Asia*.

Atheromatous disease, in Asia, 276, 277

Atherosclerosis, extracranial carotid artery, in Asia,
  276, 278

B

Balloon test occlusion, of carotid artery, 377

Benedikt's syndrome, 322

Blood flow, cerebral, assessment of, 343
  PET measurements of, 342

Blood volume, cerebral, PET measurements of,
  342–343

Brain infarction, hemorrhagic transformation of, 267

Brain tissue, ischemic, operational model of,
  249, 250

Brain tumors, intracerebral hemorrhage in, 267–268

Brainstem, hemorrhage of, 265
  key structures in, 299
  vascular stroke anatomy of, **297–324**
  vascularization of, 298–300
  venous structures of, 323

Brainstem stroke, clinical localization of,
  297–298, 299
  mechanisms of, 297

Bypass surgery, intracranial to extracranial, selection
  of patients for, 375–376

C

CADISIL, 278–279

Carbon dioxide, systemic partial pressure, to test
  cerebrovascular reactivity, 374

Carotid angiography, training, competency, and
  standards for, 392–393

Carotid angioplasty, and carotid endarterectomy, in
  high-risk patients, compared, 393
  training, competency, and standards for, 392–393

Carotid artery, balloon test occlusion of, 377
  dissection of, stenting of, 387
  extracranial, stenosis of, decision to treat,
    383–384
      endovascular trestment of, **383–395**
      hemodynamic factors in, 388–389
      heterogenous nature of, 385–388
  self-expanding stent device, 384

Carotid artery stenosis, and contralateral overstimu-
  lation, 358, 359
  assessment of, ultrasound, MR angiography, and
    CT for, 353–357

T

U

Changing Your Address?

Make sure your subscription changes too! When you notify us of your new address, you can help make our job easier by including an exact copy of your Clinics label number with your old address (see illustration below.) This number identifies you to our computer system and will speed the processing of your address change. Please be sure this label number accompanies your old address and your corrected address—you can send an old Clinics label with your number on it or just copy it exactly and send it to the address listed below.

We appreciate your help in our attempt to give you continuous coverage.
Thank you.

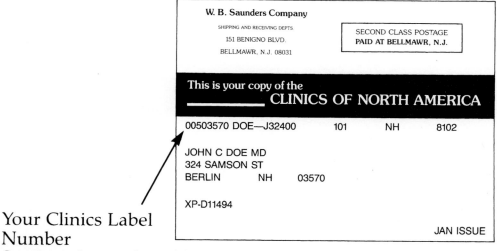

Your Clinics Label Number
Copy it exactly or send your label
along with your address to:
W.B. Saunders Company, Customer Service
Orlando, FL 32887-4800
Call Toll Free 1-800-654-2452

Please allow four to six weeks for delivery of new subscriptions and for processing address changes.